# Management of Patients with Pseudo-Endocrine Disorders

Michael T. McDermott
Editor

# Management of Patients with Pseudo-Endocrine Disorders

A Case-Based Pocket Guide

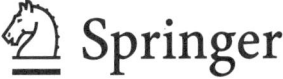

*Editor*
Michael T. McDermott
University of Colorado Hospital
Aurora, CO
USA

ISBN 978-3-030-22719-7    ISBN 978-3-030-22720-3 (eBook)
https://doi.org/10.1007/978-3-030-22720-3

© Springer Nature Switzerland AG 2019
This work is subject to copyright. All rights are reserved by the Publisher, whether the whole or part of the material is concerned, specifically the rights of translation, reprinting, reuse of illustrations, recitation, broadcasting, reproduction on microfilms or in any other physical way, and transmission or information storage and retrieval, electronic adaptation, computer software, or by similar or dissimilar methodology now known or hereafter developed.
The use of general descriptive names, registered names, trademarks, service marks, etc. in this publication does not imply, even in the absence of a specific statement, that such names are exempt from the relevant protective laws and regulations and therefore free for general use.
The publisher, the authors, and the editors are safe to assume that the advice and information in this book are believed to be true and accurate at the date of publication. Neither the publisher nor the authors or the editors give a warranty, expressed or implied, with respect to the material contained herein or for any errors or omissions that may have been made. The publisher remains neutral with regard to jurisdictional claims in published maps and institutional affiliations.

This Springer imprint is published by the registered company Springer Nature Switzerland AG
The registered company address is: Gewerbestrasse 11, 6330 Cham, Switzerland

*This book is dedicated to Libby, whose strength, courage, and love of life are a daily inspiration, and to Katie Cohen, Emily Cohen, Hayley McDermott, and Henry McDermott, for making life fun.*

# Preface

"Pseudo-endocrine patient" is a term that can be applied to many different types of patients that we see in our practices every day. They are those who believe they have an endocrine or metabolic disorder, despite previous normal testing, because of the misleading information they have gotten from a health-care provider, a personal trainer, a friend, a book, or the Internet. They may even have been given a diagnosis of a disorder that has not been scientifically proven to exist. They are those who may have true endocrine disorders but continue to have symptoms despite adequate treatment and normal on-treatment tests. They are patients who have been treated with excessive hormone doses or unproven and even dangerous treatments. They also include those whose conditions have been incorrectly diagnosed by lab testing interference or other assay issues.

We have all seen these types of patients. Many of us are trained in traditional medicine and practice evidence-based medicine, whenever there is evidence available. And we have very good tests and treatments for many of the maladies our patients suffer from. Yet we all see patients that have conditions or complaints, as described above, that challenge our ability to find evidence-based diagnostic tools and/or evidence-based treatments. We all deal with these patients and these situations in our own self-taught ways because there has been little or no organized effort to provide education during fellowship or thereafter regarding the best ways to evaluate and deliver good care to these patients. We would all like to do better.

The purpose of this book is to initiate an ongoing dialog about these issues and to begin to develop a framework for training, research, expert opinion, and eventually evidence-based guidelines to assist providers in dealing with this very important aspect of their practices. I have asked experienced colleagues from around the country, in academic institutions and in private practice, to contribute chapters describing, in case-based formats, their approaches and opinions regarding the optimal evaluation and management of patients with "pseudo-endocrine" disorders.

I did not attempt to suggest or encourage the authors to adopt any specific point of view. I asked them to write about the pseudo-endocrine disorders they most commonly see and that they think are the most important for us to recognize and discuss. Because some authors felt very strongly that they wanted to write about certain topics, you will see that there is some overlap among chapter titles and content. Rather than being repetitious, I found their various points of view on these topics to be interesting and enriching.

As you will see, these seasoned professionals vary significantly in their philosophies and opinions about the optimal evaluation and management strategies for these patients. Some believe in a straightforward scientific and evidence-based approach that emphasizes the robustness of our current testing paradigms and the safety and effectiveness of the currently available FDA-approved treatment modalities. Others prefer a modified approach that utilizes both evidence-based diagnostic and treatment recommendations and variable degrees of alternative medicine strategies in areas where no solid evidence base exists. All recommend honesty and compassion.

I greatly appreciate the time and effort these colleagues have devoted to their chapters and their dedication to forge ahead to develop guidance in this challenging area of endocrinology. I have learned a great deal by reading their chapters, and I hope that all our readers will similarly benefit.

Aurora, CO, USA　　　　　　　　　　Michael T. McDermott, MD

# Contents

1. **Pseudo-Endocrine Disorders: Definitions, Examples, and Considerations** .................... 1
   Michael T. McDermott

2. **Pseudo-Endocrine Disorders: My General Approach to Management of the Patient** .......... 15
   Michael T. McDermott

3. **Rogue Practitioners and Practices** ................ 23
   Michael T. McDermott

4. **Influence of the Internet in Endocrinology Practice** .................................. 31
   David R. Saxon

5. **Debunking Internet Myths: What Is the Best Approach?** .................................. 37
   Deirdre Cocks Eschler and Jonathan D. Leffert

6. **Bewildered by Biotin** ........................... 51
   Alicia Algeciras-Schimnich and Carol Greenlee

7. **Help, My Metabolism Is Low!** .................... 77
   Sean J. Iwamoto and Marc-Andre Cornier

8. **Idiopathic Postprandial Syndrome** ................ 91
   Helen M. Lawler

## Contents

9 **Pseudohypoglycemia** .......................... 99
Fadi Aboona, Sulmaz Zahedi,
and S. Sethu K. Reddy

10 **Chronic Fatigue**................................109
Margaret A Eagan

11 **Adrenal Fatigue** ...............................127
Michael T. McDermott

12 **Adrenal Insufficiency, "Relative Adrenal Insufficiency," or None of the Above?**.............139
Maria Vamvini and James V. Hennessey

13 **Pseudo-Cushing's Syndrome: A Diagnostic Dilemma** .....................................159
Teresa Brown, Regina Belokovskaya,
and Rachel Pessah-Pollack

14 **Pseudo-Cushing's Syndrome: Alcohol Abuse, Obesity, and Psychiatric Disorders**.................179
Janice M. Kerr

15 **Pseudopheochromocytoma**......................193
David R. Saxon and Lauren Fishbein

16 **Holistic Hypercalcemia** .........................203
Irene E. Schauer

17 **Low Testosterone: Determine and Treat the Underlying Disorder** .........................215
Kenneth Tompkins and Micol S. Rothman

18 **Inappropriate Use of Mifepristone to Treat Diabetes Mellitus** ..............................227
Eveline Waring and Beatrice Hull

19 **Insulin-like Growth Factor-1 Deficiency** ...........235
Thomas Ittoop and S. Sethu K. Reddy

| | | |
|---|---|---|
| **20** | **Non-thyroidal Hypothyroidism**................251 | |
| | James V. Hennessey | |

| | | |
|---|---|---|
| **21** | **Wilson's Syndrome (Low T3 Syndrome)**..........273 | |
| | Catherine J. Tang and Jeffrey R. Garber | |

| | | |
|---|---|---|
| **22** | **Reverse T3 Dilemma**..........................291 | |
| | Katarzyna Piotrowska and Mark Lupo | |

| | | |
|---|---|---|
| **23** | **Persistent Hypothyroid Symptoms Despite Adequate Thyroid Hormone Replacement**.........301 | |
| | Michael T. McDermott | |

| | | |
|---|---|---|
| **24** | **Low-Dose Naltrexone Treatment of Hashimoto's Thyroiditis**...................................317 | |
| | Michael T. McDermott | |

| | | |
|---|---|---|
| **25** | **Hashimoto Encephalopathy**.....................327 | |
| | Michael T. McDermott | |

| | | |
|---|---|---|
| **26** | **Non-thyroidal Illness Syndrome (Euthyroid Sick Syndrome)**................................331 | |
| | Michael T. McDermott | |

**Index**..........................................341

# Contributors

**Fadi Aboona, MD** Discipline of Medicine, Central Michigan University College of Medicine, Mt. Pleasant, MI, USA

**Alicia Algeciras-Schimnich, MD** Department of Laboratory Medicine and Pathology, Mayo Clinic, Rochester, MN, USA

Western Slope Endocrinology, Grand Junction, CO, USA

**Regina Belokovskaya, DO** Icahn School of Medicine at Mount Sinai Medical Center, Division of Endocrinology, Diabetes, & Bone Disease, New York, NY, USA

**Teresa Brown, DO** Icahn School of Medicine at Mount Sinai Medical Center, Division of Endocrinology, Diabetes, & Bone Disease, New York, NY, USA

**Marc-Andre Cornier, MD** Division of Endocrinology, Metabolism & Diabetes, University of Colorado School of Medicine, Anschutz Medical Campus, Aurora, CO, USA

CU Anschutz Health and Wellness Center, University of Colorado School of Medicine, Anschutz Medical Campus, Aurora, CO, USA

**Margaret A. Eagan, MD** Anschutz Health and Wellness Center, University of Colorado, Aurora, CO, USA

**Deirdre Cocks Eschler, MD** Renaissance School of Medicine at Stony Brook University, Stony Brook, NY, USA

Health Sciences Center, Level 16, Department of Medicine, Stony Brook, NY, USA

**Lauren Fishbein, MD** University of Colorado School of Medicine, Department of Medicine, Division of Endocrinology, Metabolism and Diabetes, Aurora, CO, USA

Rocky Mountain VA Medical Center, Division of Endocrinology, Aurora, CO, USA

**Jeffrey R. Garber, MD** Atrius Health, Boston, MA, USA

Division of Endocrinology, Diabetes, and Metabolism, Harvard Medical School, Beth Israel Deaconess Medical Center, Boston, MA, USA

**Carol Greenlee, MD** Department of Laboratory Medicine and Pathology, Mayo Clinic, Rochester, MN, USA

Western Slope Endocrinology, Grand Junction, CO, USA

**James V. Hennessey, MD** Division of Endocrinology, Diabetes and Metabolism, Beth Israel Deaconess Medical Center, Harvard Medical School, Boston, MA, USA

**Beatrice Hull, MD** Carolina Endocrine Associates, North Charleston, SC, USA

**Thomas Ittoop, MD** Central Michigan University College of Medicine, Mt. Pleasant, MI, USA

**Sean J. Iwamoto, MD** Division of Endocrinology, Metabolism & Diabetes, University of Colorado School of Medicine, Anschutz Medical Campus, Aurora, CO, USA

Division of Endocrinology, Rocky Mountain Regional VA Medical Center, VA Eastern Colorado Health Care System, Aurora, CO, USA

**Janice M. Kerr, MD** University of Colorado, Anschutz Medical Center, Aurora, CO, USA

**Helen M. Lawler, MD** University of Colorado School of Medicine, Division of Endocrinology, Metabolism, and Diabetes, Aurora, CO, USA

**Jonathan D. Leffert, MD** North Texas Endocrine Center, Dallas, TX, USA

**Mark Lupo, MD** Thyroid and Endocrine Center of Florida, Florida State University, College of Medicine, Sarasota, FL, USA

**Michael T. McDermott, MD** University of Colorado Hospital, Aurora, CO, USA

**Rachel Pessah-Pollack, MD** Icahn School of Medicine at Mount Sinai Medical Center, Division of Endocrinology, Diabetes, & Bone Disease, New York, NY, USA

**Katarzyna Piotrowska, MD** Thyroid and Endocrine Center of Florida, Sarasota, FL, USA

**S. Sethu K. Reddy, MD** Discipline of Medicine, Central Michigan University College of Medicine, Mt. Pleasant, MI, USA

**Micol S. Rothman, MD** University of Colorado, Department of Medicine, Division of Endocrinology, Aurora, CO, USA

**David R. Saxon, MD** Division of Endocrinology, Metabolism and Diabetes, Rocky Mountain Regional Veterans Affairs Medical Center, Aurora, CO, USA

University of Colorado School of Medicine, Department of Medicine, Division of Endocrinology, Metabolism and Diabetes, Aurora, CO, USA

Rocky Mountain VA Medical Center, Division of Endocrinology, Aurora, CO, USA

**Irene E. Schauer, MD** University of Colorado School of Medicine, Department of Medicine, Division of Endocrinology, Metabolism and Diabetes, Aurora, CO, USA

Rocky Mountain Regional VA Medical Center, Aurora, CO, USA

**Catherine J. Tang, MD** Division of Endocrinology, Diabetes, and Metabolism, Harvard Medical School, Beth Israel Deaconess Medical Center, Boston, MA, USA

**Kenneth Tompkins, MD** University of Colorado, Department of Medicine, Division of Endocrinology, Aurora, CO, USA

**Maria Vamvini, MD** Division of Endocrinology, Diabetes and Metabolism, Beth Israel Deaconess Medical Center, Harvard Medical School, Boston, MA, USA

**Eveline Waring, MD** Carolina Endocrine Associates, North Charleston, SC, USA

**Sulmaz Zahedi, MD** Discipline of Medicine, Central Michigan University College of Medicine, Mt. Pleasant, MI, USA

# Chapter 1
# Pseudo-Endocrine Disorders: Definitions, Examples, and Considerations

**Michael T. McDermott**

## What Is a Pseudo-Endocrine Disorder?

The term "pseudo-endocrine" disorder does not yet have a clear and distinct definition. The term could be used in reference to people who believe they have an endocrine or metabolic disorder because of information they received from another health care provider, a personal trainer, a family member or a friend and, despite previously appropriate normal testing, they request further unwarranted testing of their endocrine system or their hormones. It may apply to patients who have read about endocrine disorders (real and unproven) in books or on the Internet and may have even ordered hormone or metabolic testing online. It also refers to those who have been given "endocrine" diagnoses by providers based on symptoms alone without validated hormone testing. It can also be applied to patients who have true endocrine disorders for which they are being treated but continue to have

M. T. McDermott (✉)
University of Colorado Hospital, Aurora, CO, USA
e-mail: michael.mcdermott@cuanschutz.edu

© Springer Nature Switzerland AG 2019
M. T. McDermott (ed.), *Management of Patients with Pseudo-Endocrine Disorders*,
https://doi.org/10.1007/978-3-030-22720-3_1

symptoms despite appropriate therapy and normal on-treatment tests. And it also refers to patients with endocrine or metabolic conditions that were diagnosed correctly (or not) by other providers and who are treated for these conditions with excessive hormone doses or with unproven, inappropriate, and even dangerous medications. Alternatively, an endocrine diagnosis may have erroneously been made as a result of lab assay error due to supplements and other conditions that adversely affect the accuracy of various tests.

In this introductory chapter, I will show multiple case examples and patient emails that illustrate many of the issues regarding pseudo-endocrine disorders that I have regularly encountered throughout my many years in practice. Following these, I offer some thoughts about the complexity of the endocrine system and further considerations for the evaluation and care of these patients. I do believe that our current diagnostic tests provide a very good evaluation of the endocrine and metabolic milieu. However, I pose some honest questions about whether our current diagnostic armamentarium is sufficient to evaluate all aspects of our various multi-layered systems of hormone synthesis, secretion, transport, action, and feedback homeostasis.

My personal approach to the management of these issues in individual patients will be the subject of the next chapter. In the following chapter, I will address the more general issue of rogue practitioners and practices, reproduce two letters I have received from colleagues, and offer suggestions about what we might do as a community of professionals to curb these unethical practices. The subsequent chapters by my esteemed colleagues will then describe and discuss multiple specific topics and the authors' individualized approaches to evaluation and management of patients with these conditions.

# Case Examples

## *Case 1*

A 32-year-old woman has been experiencing fatigue, depression, and difficulty losing weight for 2 years. Thyroid tests that she ordered online have been normal except for a moderately low reverse T3.

---

PMH: Negative     Meds: Multiple supplements

PE: BP 122/84   P 80   Ht 5′6″   Wt 172 lb.

        Complete exam normal

Lab Report:     TSH 1.2 mU/l (nl: 0.45–4.5)

                Free T4 1.3 ng/dl (nl: 0.8–1.8)

                Free T3 3.1 pg/ml (nl: 2.3–4.2)

                Reverse T3 9 ng/dl (nl: 10–24)

---

She has read that thyroid tests don't accurately evaluate thyroid function. She requests more thorough thyroid testing and treatment to raise her reverse T3.

## *Case 2*

A 47-year-old woman has been experiencing fatigue for about 15 years but complains of "total exhaustion" progressively over the past year. She does not sleep well but does not snore. Her appetite is poor. Mild weight gain (5 lb.) has occurred in the past year. She cannot exercise due to severe fatigue.

---

PMH: Mononucleosis at age 18    Meds: Occasional prescription pain medication

PE: BP 128/70   P 80   Ht 5′8″   Wt 157 lb. (Orthostatic vitals negative)

        Complete exam normal

Lab:    Full-day salivary cortisol profile – diagnostic of "Adrenal Fatigue"

---

She requests to be treated for Adrenal Fatigue for which she says she has tested positive.

## Case 3

A 53-year-old man complains of muscle weakness, exercise intolerance, fatigue, lack of motivation, increased need for sleep, and difficulty concentrating for about 5 years, all following a motor vehicle accident with "whiplash injury." He read about post-traumatic hypopituitarism and has had online tests done. Thyroid and adrenal tests were normal but his growth hormone (GH) level was low and his Insulin-like Growth Factor 1 (IGF-1) level was low normal.

PMH: GERD, Colon Polyps   Meds: None

PE: BP 140/85   P 76   Ht 5'11"   Wt 208 lb.

Complete exam normal

Lab:   Growth Hormone 0.05 ng/ml (nl: 0.05–3.0)

IGF-1 82 ng/ml (nl: 60–220)

He requests treatment for Growth Hormone Deficiency.

## Case 4

A 38-year-old woman is self-referred for hormone evaluation because of chronic progressive fatigue. She began feeling fatigued at age 28, about 1 year after the birth of her second child. She also endorses hair loss, inability to lose weight, and persistent "brain fog." She has read extensively on the Internet and is convinced that this is a hormone disorder and is adamant that this is not due to depression. She has ordered some tests online (cycle day 4) and several are abnormal.

PMH: Negative   Meds: Vitamins

PE:   BP 129/74   P 74   Ht 5'7"   Wt 158 lb.   BMI 24.8 kg/m$^2$

General: Normal   Thyroid: Normal   Skin: Normal

*Tests from Online Orders (Cycle day 4; 10:00 AM)*:

| | |
|---|---|
| TSH 2.1 mU/l (nl: 0.45–4.5) | Free T4 1.0 ng/dl (nl: 0.78–1.81) |
| Free T3 2.4 pg/ml (nl: 2.3–4.2) | Reverse T3 23 ng/dl (nl: 10–24) |
| TPO Antibodies: Negative | Tg Antibodies: Negative |
| Cortisol 12 μg/dl (nl: 10–20) | ACTH 19 pg/ml (nl: 10–50) |
| Testosterone 27 ng/ml (nl: 30–95) | Estradiol 101 pg/ml (nl: 27–123) |
| Progesterone <1.5 ng/ml (nl < 1.5) | DHEA 188 μg/dl (nl: 145–395) |
| GH 0.04 ng/ml (nl: 0.05–3.0) | IGF-1 57 ng/ml (nl: 60–220) |

She is concerned that she has Wilson's Low T3 syndrome, Reverse T3 syndrome, and Growth Hormone Deficiency and requests advice and treatment for all of these conditions.

## *Case 5*

A 51-year-old man is referred by his PCP for exercise intolerance, muscle weakness, excess sweating, and difficulty concentrating for the past 4–5 years. He is a former college athlete. He eats a well-balanced diet, exercises regularly, and sleeps fairly well. Libido and sexual function are normal. He has five alcohol drinks/week and doesn't smoke. A general evaluation, including serum TSH and Testosterone, was normal. A naturopath advised thyroid support and adrenal support supplements, but he has not yet started these.

PMH: Colon polyps   Meds: Vitamins, minerals

PE:   BP 140/85   P 76   Ht 5'11"   Wt 208 lb.   BMI 29 kg/m$^2$

General: Normal   Thyroid: Normal   Skin: Normal

Labs: TSH 2.3 mU/l, Free T4 1.4 ng/dl (nl: 0.8–1.8)

Testosterone 390 ng/dl (nl: 275–1075)

IGF-1 132 ng/ml (nl: 60–220)

He would like a more complete hormone evaluation and consideration for testosterone therapy because he is a former athlete and believes that this testosterone level, while in the normal range, is low for him.

## Case 6

A 42-year-old man is referred for persistent hypothyroid symptoms despite LT4 therapy. Hypothyroidism was diagnosed 6 months ago. He still experiences fatigue, mild depression, and difficulty losing weight. He requests further thyroid testing and medication adjustment.

---

PMH: Hypothyroidism   Meds: Levothyroxine 150 μg/day

PE: BP 122/84   P 76   Ht 6′1″   Wt 203 lb.

      General Exam: Normal   Thyroid: Enlarged, granular

Lab:   TSH 1.6 mU/l (nl: 0.45–4.5)

      Free T4 1.4 ng/dl (nl: 0.8–1.8)

---

You say: "It's not your thyroid."

He says: "I was told you'd say that. But I believe it is. What else could it be? My previous doctor said that my TSH does not reflect my actual thyroid status but that my symptoms do. I want to take a natural thyroid hormone."

## Case 7

A 46-year-old woman is self-referred for hormone evaluation because of obesity and an inability to lose weight. She weighed 118 lb. at high school graduation. She gained 30 lb. with each of two pregnancies and retained ~15 lb. after each. She has gradually gained weight since then despite intermittent dieting and exercise programs. She also endorses fatigue, dry skin, and constipation.

Chapter 1. Pseudo-Endocrine Disorders: Definitions… 7

---

PMH: Negative    Meds: Vitamins, supplements

PE: BP 138/76    P 82    Ht 5′5″    Wt 194 lb.

General: Generalized obesity, mild buffalo hump, rosy cheeks

Thyroid: Normal size/consistency  Skin: Non-violaceous abdomen striae

Lab: TSH 1.9 mU/l (nl: 0.45–4.5), Free T4 1.1 ng/dl (nl: 0.8–1.8)

24 h Urine cortisol 29 µg (nl < 55 µg/24 h)

Serum cortisol <1.8 µg/dl after 1 mg Dexamethasone at bedtime

---

She is convinced that her weight gain and inability to lose weight must be a hormone problem.

## *Case 8*

A 33-year-old man complains of progressive fatigue and lack of motivation. His sleep habits are poor because he brings his work home with him and works until late at night. His interest in sex has waned but is still present. Erectile function is normal. His primary care provider evaluated him for these complaints but all lab tests, done in the afternoon on the day of his visit, were normal. However, because his testosterone level was in the lower one-third of the normal range, he visited a local "Low T" clinic. Additional testing was not done but he was given an injection of testosterone pellets. He noted some subjective improvement after this. The testosterone pellets were not covered by insurance. He presents to his local endocrinologist to verify that he has an ongoing need for these pellets so that insurance will cover them. He also asks if his low testosterone levels will cause him to be infertile. His serum testosterone level is 1173 ng/dl (nl: 300–1000).

## Case 9

A 55-year-old woman complains of hot flashes, insomnia, fatigue, and depression. Her naturopath recently prescribed a compounded hormone replacement product containing estrogens, progesterone, and testosterone. She has recently noted dark hair growing on her chin, which has never happened before since she is red-haired and fair-skinned. Her serum testosterone is 2129 ng/dl (nl: 20–80).

## Case 10

A 60-year-old woman was diagnosed with chronic fatigue syndrome 26 years ago. She was told that her thyroid and adrenal glands were underactive, but she is not sure exactly what tests were done. At that time, she was started on dexamethasone, levothyroxine, and liothyronine. Because of worsening symptoms, dextroamphetamine, modafinil, and midodrine were later sequentially added and various antidepressant medications were tried over the years. Despite these interventions, her symptoms worsened: she developed severe insomnia and she intermittently began considering suicide. She is referred to endocrinology for management of her hormone issues. Current medications: dexamethasone 0.5 mg every morning, levothyroxine 100 μg daily, liothyronine 15 μg in the morning and 10 μg in the afternoon, modafinil 200 mg BID, dextroamphetamine 5 mg BID, midodrine 5 mg TID, Zolpidem 10 mg HS, Bupropion XL 300 mg daily, cyclobenzaprine 10 mg TID, Lamotrigine 150 mg daily, linaclotide 145 mg daily, estradiol patch 0.1 mg/24 hours, and micronized progesterone cream 50 mg BID. Her fatigue continues to worsen, and her insomnia persists. She says: "Something has to be done about this. I can't go on feeling this way."

Chapter 1. Pseudo-Endocrine Disorders: Definitions... 9

## Email/Phone Questions (Unedited)

- Phone call from a 47-year-old woman with active severe Graves' disease for whom Methimazole treatment was recommended. "I don't want to take that medication because it might make me gain weight. A friend recommended that I try Naturethroid. Please send a prescription for Naturethroid to my pharmacy."
- For about a month, I have been having this sensation of bugs crawling on the right side of my head in my hair. Last night when I Googled, I was surprised to find that this is more common than I knew and can be caused by hypothyroid. Since it has been a long time since I have had my thyroid checked, it seems that it is time. So, might you be able to order the test and then prescribe as needed?
- Dr. McDermott ... I have just been diagnosed with conjunctival chalasis (the film that covers the eyeball) becomes very loose and wrinkles up causing discomfort and irritation as if there is something continually in your eye? One prospective study found that the prevalence of conjunctival chalasis in patients with autoimmune thyroid eye diseases was as high as 88%. I may have to have surgery. Would it help me to change to Armour? A shortage of T3 is supposed to contribute. Thanks,
- Dr. McDermott, I continue to struggle with exhaustion constantly and maybe that is just parenthood and need to improve my sleep habits. It is frustrating. I feel my best when pregnant honestly. What are your feelings on celiac connection with thyroid levels?! I have been having a lot of dizzy spells lately, more than just the feeling when you stand up too quickly and my menstrual cycles are heavier and take me down for a few days. My levels and labs were fine, so I guess it is a mystery. I have not been taking supplements as regularly and looks like my vitamin D could stand to be increased. Thanks for ordering them!

# Questions for Insightful Endocrinologists to Consider

The hypothalamic–pituitary–thyroid axis, hypothalamic–pituitary–adrenal axis, hypothalamic–pituitary–gonadal axis, hypothalamic–pituitary–GH–liver–IGF1 axis, calcium–PTH–Vitamin D homeostasis, total body–energy balance, and overall nutrient metabolism and distribution are all highly complex systems. Hormone synthesis, secretion, transport through the circulation and other fluids, receptor binding, second messenger generation, gene expression, post-transcriptional modification, ultimate hormone action, and feedback regulation are all discreet processes that are unique and critical components of each individual hormonal and metabolic system.

Most of us delighted in learning about the intricacies of homeostatic regulation within these systems. We have diligently pursued further understanding how disease processes can affect these systems and how our static and dynamic endocrine tests and imaging modalities can dissect apart the individual components of the systems to pinpoint where the pathology exists so that the best possible treatments can be developed for endocrine and metabolic disorders. As a result of the work of dedicated scientists and devoted clinicians, we have developed testing platforms that are remarkably accurate and treatment strategies that are safe and highly effective.

Nonetheless, all of us who are involved in caring for patients with known or possible endocrine disorders must continue to be innovative thinkers, who are eager to make, understand, and apply new discoveries that will push our knowledge, diagnostic skills, and treatment options to even higher levels. So, we must ask: Based on our current clinical endocrine testing and imaging capabilities, do we really understand, without a doubt, every aspect of the function and dysfunction of the very complex endocrine and metabolic processes within our patients? Is it possible that some symptoms a patient suffers could result from inherited or acquired abnormalities (genetic, epigenetic, or other) at any of these multiple steps of hormone and metabolic physiology for which we currently do not have adequate tests?

Are we ready to declare that we now know everything there is to know about hormone secretion, transport, and action, that our tests can evaluate every aspect of endocrine and metabolic function, and that there is no need for improvement in the options we currently offer patients to treat their endocrine diseases? Should we not acknowledge instead that we don't know everything and that we eagerly await new research discoveries to help us take better care of our patients?

I am not suggesting that all or even many patients with "pseudo-endocrine" disorders have an actual endocrine or metabolic disorder and that, if we just order enough tests, we will identify them; nor do I believe that when additional tests of the endocrine system become available, all or most of these patients will be found to have a previously undiagnosed endocrine disorder. However, I do believe we should acknowledge our current diagnostic and therapeutic limitations and support innovative research to overcome these limitations. We should practice evidence-based medicine but be open to novel ideas when they are based on solid science, and that we should always strive to develop compassionate and supportive relationships with all of our patients, regardless of whether or not they prove to have identifiable endocrine or metabolic disorders.

## Additional Important Considerations

Endocrinologists are the acknowledged experts in the diagnosis and treatment of disorders of hormone secretion, transport, and action and of numerous metabolic diseases. It is an honor that a person respects our expertise and entrusts their healthcare to us. Every patient deserves our respect and compassion. When patients say, "Fix my thyroid, adrenal, pituitary, or metabolic condition," what they are really saying is "Please help me." The patient's quality of life is poor, and she/he is frustrated. Can we play a role in improving this patient's quality of life? Can we help this patient even if there is no apparent endocrine disorder? We should consider it an honor and privilege that he/she entrusts us with an opportunity to help her/him. Therefore, we should listen attentively, examine our patient, offer additional testing if appropriate, admit that current testing options have some limitations and always provide honesty, encouragement, and compassion.

It's an exciting time to be an endocrinologist. There is still so much to learn, and so many people we may be able to help.

# Suggested Reading

1. Garber J, et al. Clinical practice guidelines for hypothyroidism in adults: cosponsored by the American Association of Clinical Endocrinologists and the American Thyroid Association. Endocr Pract. 2012;18(6):988–1028. Thyroid. 2012;22(12):1200–35.
2. Jonklaas J, Bianco AC, Bauer AJ, Burman KD, Cappola AR, Celi FS, Cooper DS, American Thyroid Association Task Force on Thyroid Hormone Replacement, et al. Guidelines for the treatment of hypothyroidism: prepared by the American Thyroid Association Task Force on thyroid hormone replacement. Thyroid. 2014;24(12):1670–751.
3. Guglielmi R, Frasoldati A, Zini M, Grimaldi F, Gharib H, Garber JR, Papini E. Italian Association of Clinical Endocrinologists Statement-Replacement Therapy for primary hypothyroidism: a brief guide for clinical practice. Endocr Pract. 2016;22(11):1319–26.
4. Bornstein SR, Allolio B, Arlt W, et al. Diagnosis and treatment of primary adrenal insufficiency: an endocrine society clinical practice guideline. J Clin Endocrinol Metab. 2016;101:364–89.
5. Fleseriu M, Hashim IA, Karavitaki N, et al. Hormonal replacement in hypopituitarism in adults: an endocrine society clinical practice guideline. J Clin Endocrinol Metab. 2016;101:3888–921.
6. Molitch ME, Clemmons DR, Malozowski S, Merriam GR, Vance ML. Evaluation and treatment of adult growth hormone deficiency: an endocrine society clinical practice guideline. J Clin Endocrinol Metab. 2011;96:1587–609.
7. Bollerslev J, Rejnmark L, Marcocci C, Shoback DM, Sitges-Serra A, van Biesen W, Dekkers OM, European Society of Endocrinology. European Society of Endocrinology Clinical Guideline: treatment of chronic hypoparathyroidism in adults. Eur J Endocrinol. 2015;173(2):G1–20.

8. Jerant A, Fenton JJ, Kravitz RL, et al. Association of clinical denial of patient requests with patient satisfaction. JAMA Intern Med 2018 Jan 1;178(1):85–91. Published Online November 27, 2017.
9. Pryor L. How to counter the circus of pseudoscience. New York Times, Jan 5, 2018.
10. Seaborg E. The myth of adrenal fatigue. Endocrine News, Sept 2017. p. 29–32.
11. Schaffer R. In age of internet diagnoses, endocrinologists confront myth of "adrenal fatigue". Endocrine Today, April 2018. p. 1–12.
12. Hormone Health Network adrenal fatigue fact sheet: www.hormone.org/diseases-and-conditions/adrenal/adrenal-fatigue.
13. Hormone Foundation (Endocrine Society) website – adrenal fatigue: https://www.hormone.org/-/media/hormone/files/myth-vs-fact/mfsadrenalfatigue-520.pdf?la=en.
14. Mayo Clinic website – adrenal fatigue: https://www.mayoclinic.org/diseases-conditions/addisons-disease/expert-answers/adrenal-fatigue/faq-20057906.
15. Akturk HD, Chindris AM, Hines JM, Singh RJ, Bernet VJ. Over-the-counter "adrenal support" supplements contain thyroid and steroid-based adrenal hormones. Mayo Clin Proc. 2018;93(3):284–90.
16. Donegan D, Bancos I. Opioid-induced adrenal insufficiency. Mayo Clin Proc. 2018;93(7):937–44.
17. Wilson's Syndrome website: http://www.wilsonssyndrome.com/meet-dr-wilson/.
18. Wikipedia – Wilson's Syndrome: https://en.wikipedia.org/wiki/Wilson%27s_temperature_syndrome.
19. American Thyroid Association (ATA) website – search for Wilson's Syndrome: www.Thyroid.Org.
20. State of Florida, Department of Health. Final order number: DPR9200039ME – Ruling against Wilson's Syndrome, Feb 12, 1992.
21. Reverse T3 Syndrome website: www.stopthethyroidmadness.com.
22. Baillargeon J, Kuo YF, Westra JR, Urban RJ, Goodwin JS. Testosterone prescribing in the United States, 2002–2016. JAMA. 2018;320(2):200–2.
23. Layton JB, Kim Y, Alexander GC, Emery SL. Association between direct-to-consumer advertising and testosterone testing and initiation in the United States, 2009–2013. JAMA. 2017;317(11):1159–66.
24. Schwartz LM, Woloshin S. Low "T" as in "Template": How to sell disease. JAMA Intern Med. 2013;173(15):1460–2.

25. Gomes-Lima C, Burman KD. Reverse T3 or perverse T3? Still puzzling after 40 years. Cleve Clin J Med. 2018;85(6):450–5.
26. Schmidt RL, LoPresti JS, McDermott MT, Zick SM, Straseski JA. Is reverse triiodothyronine ordered appropriately? Data from reference lab shows wide practice variation in orders for reverse triiodothyronine. Thyroid. 2018;28(7):842–8.
27. Muller RS. Making a difference in adrenal fatigue. Endocr Pract. 2018;24(12):1103–5.
28. Gota CE. What you can do for your fibromyalgia patient. Cleve Clin J Med. 2018;85(5):367–76.
29. Warraich H. Dr Google is a liar. New York Times, Dec 16, 2018; Page A19 of the New York Edition.
30. Hellmuth J, Rabinovici GD, Miller BL. The rise of pseudomedicine for dementia and brain health. JAMA. 2019;321:543–4.

# Chapter 2
# Pseudo-Endocrine Disorders: My General Approach to Management of the Patient

**Michael T. McDermott**

We all have our own individual approaches to the evaluation and management of patients with challenging medical conditions, including those with pseudo-endocrine disorders. I have discussed this with many seasoned colleagues, including several of the authors of other chapters in this book. These are useful learning experiences for me. Each provider should approach patients with these issues in their own natural way, using their knowledge of Endocrinology, their well-honed personal instincts, and always their highest degree of humanism, respect, and compassion. In the discussion below, I describe the approaches that I have found most useful in providing the best possible care and assistance to patients with pseudo-endocrine disorders.

M. T. McDermott (✉)
University of Colorado Hospital, Aurora, CO, USA
e-mail: michael.mcdermott@cuanschutz.edu

© Springer Nature Switzerland AG 2019
M. T. McDermott (ed.), *Management of Patients with Pseudo-Endocrine Disorders*,
https://doi.org/10.1007/978-3-030-22720-3_2

## Listen Attentively

I ask the patient to describe their symptoms and then listen attentively, without interruption. This helps to validate for the patient that I hear them, that I believe they are having these symptoms and that the symptoms are seriously affecting their quality of life, that I understand their concerns and frustrations, and that I am willing to be part of the solution. I maintain eye contact, if the patient is willing, and avoid typing in the electronic health record as much as possible. If I must type in order to accurately capture and remember key details, I periodically ask the patient to look at my monitor to make sure that I have recorded the details and their concerns accurately. I then ask for clarification of any parts of their description that I did not understand and ask additional questions to probe further into their major concerns. I also ask questions about lifestyle issues, such as their diet, exercise, and sleep habits (including if they snore) and about their use of tobacco, alcohol, marijuana, and other legal or illegal drug use. I carefully ask about their family life and their employment situation and satisfaction. I ask about their level of stress and their coping mechanisms. I rarely use the word "depression" on a first or second visit, unless the patient is forthcoming about this issue, but I get a good idea about this from the discussion described above. I avoid allowing the patient to spend much time describing their frustrations about previous providers and prior evaluations. All of this must be done, of course, within reasonable time constraints because we all have busy practices and our subsequent patients that day also deserve to be seen on time and to have adequate time devoted to their issues and concerns. Therefore, it may be beneficial to have the patient return for a second visit to continue the discussion. My emphasis throughout this time is attentive listening.

## Perform a Thorough Physical Examination

The value of a thorough physical examination cannot be overstated. True endocrine disorders are often associated with distinct physical findings, which can be readily appreciated by the experienced physician. In addition, this further validates that you believe and are concerned about your patient's symptoms and are interested in evaluating them further. Furthermore, the physical contact of an examination can enhance the physician–patient relationship and can also be the first step in therapy. I am amazed at how often patients tell me that their previous provider "never even examined me."

## Review Results of Previous Evaluations

I also ask the patient about previous testing and review the reports if available.

## Order Additional Testing as Needed

Frequently the patient's previous providers, in an attempt to be cost-effective, have ordered a limited number of tests. I find it useful to repeat some of the previously ordered tests if they had borderline results, were done in an unfamiliar laboratory, were done at the wrong time of day or after sleep deprivation, or if there is a question about assay interference by other medications, supplements (especially biotin), or heterophile antibodies. If not yet done, I consider testing for additional disorders that may have been overlooked, such as those for diabetes mellitus, calcium abnormalities, adrenal disorders, hypogonadism, celiac disease, vitamin D deficiency, vitamin B12 deficiency, and sleep apnea. Some may argue that extensive testing is not cost-effective, and I often agree, but I also take into consideration the additional costs that will be incurred by these patients if they continue to visit multiple physicians in the future in search of answers if I do not thoroughly evaluate their complaints.

## Discuss Your Findings with the Patient

I find it useful to explain briefly to the patient, in understandable language, pertinent aspects of endocrine physiology and how and why we use the tests that we order. An acknowledgment that everything is not known about endocrine function and dysfunction and that there could be conditions, yet to be identified, for which we currently do not have diagnostic tests is often helpful. It is important for the patient to understand also that symptoms frequently experienced by many people are nonspecific and could be due to other conditions unrelated to the endocrine system.

## Discuss Treatment Options

Satisfactory outcomes for these patients require a skillful and compassionate approach by the physician. Management advice should include healthy lifestyle measures, starting with a well-balanced diet, regular exercise, adequate sleep, and stress reduction. Treatment of any endocrine and metabolic disorders uncovered during the evaluation should be discussed and implemented. Contributing non-endocrine medical and psychiatric conditions can be discussed but are often more appropriately managed by primary care providers and other specialists.

I always try to convey to the patient that we are partners in the quest to relieve their symptoms and improve their quality of life. I want them to clearly understand that I do care. I find honesty, encouragement, and compassion to be the most effective measures for a successful outcome. My discussion with my patients is appropriately individualized, of course, but most often proceeds along these lines:

**Honesty** "I'm not sure what is causing your symptoms. I have done all the appropriate tests and have not found an Endocrine disorder."

**Encouragement** "While we didn't find a cause for your symptoms, your test results do indicate that you do not have any serious medical conditions."

**Compassion** "I hope that your symptoms will resolve soon with healthy lifestyle measures.

I am certainly willing to repeat some of your tests in 3–6 months if the symptoms persist."

## Important Considerations Again

Repeating my comments from the previous chapter, I consider it an honor that a person respects my expertise and entrusts their healthcare to me. Every patient deserves my respect and compassion. The patient's quality of life is impaired, and she/he is asking for my help. I search for any way I can help to improve the patient's quality of life, even if there is no apparent endocrine disorder. Therefore, I listen attentively, examine my patient, offer additional testing if appropriate, admit that current testing options have some limitations and always provide honesty, encouragement, and compassion.

## Suggested Reading

1. Garber J, et al. Clinical practice guidelines for hypothyroidism in adults: cosponsored by the American Association of Clinical Endocrinologists and the American Thyroid Association. Endocr Pract. 2012;18(6):988–1028. Thyroid. 2012;22(12):1200–35.
2. Jonklaas J, Bianco AC, Bauer AJ, Burman KD, Cappola AR, Celi FS, Cooper DS, American Thyroid Association Task Force on Thyroid Hormone Replacement, et al. Guidelines for the treatment of hypothyroidism: prepared by the American Thyroid Association task force on thyroid hormone replacement. Thyroid. 2014;24(12):1670–751.
3. Guglielmi R, Frasoldati A, Zini M, Grimaldi F, Gharib H, Garber JR, Papini E. Italian Association of Clinical Endocrinologists statement-replacement therapy for primary hypothyroidism: a brief guide for clinical practice. Endocr Pract. 2016;22(11):1319–26.

4. Bornstein SR, Allolio B, Arlt W, et al. Diagnosis and treatment of primary adrenal insufficiency: an Endocrine Society clinical practice guideline. J Clin Endocrinol Metab. 2016;101:364–89.
5. Fleseriu M, Hashim IA, Karavitaki N, et al. Hormonal replacement in hypopituitarism in adults: an Endocrine Society clinical practice guideline. J Clin Endocrinol Metab. 2016;101:3888–921.
6. Molitch ME, Clemmons DR, Malozowski S, Merriam GR, Vance ML. Evaluation and treatment of adult growth hormone deficiency: an Endocrine Society clinical practice guideline. J Clin Endocrinol Metab. 2011;96:1587–609.
7. Bollerslev J, Rejnmark L, Marcocci C, Shoback DM, Sitges-Serra A, van Biesen W, Dekkers OM, European Society of Endocrinology. European Society of endocrinology clinical guideline: treatment of chronic hypoparathyroidism in adults. Eur J Endocrinol. 2015;173(2):G1–20.
8. Jerant A, Fenton JJ, Kravitz RL, et al. Association of Clinical Denial of patient requests with patient satisfaction. JAMA Intern Med 2018 Jan 1;178(1):85–91. Published Online November 27, 2017.
9. Pryor L. How to counter the circus of pseudoscience. New York Times, Jan 5, 2018.
10. Seaborg E. The myth of adrenal fatigue. Endocrine News, 2017. p. 29–32.
11. Schaffer R. In age of internet diagnoses, endocrinologists confront myth of "adrenal fatigue". Endocrine Today, April 2018. p. 1–12.
12. Hormone Health Network adrenal fatigue fact sheet: www.hormone.org/diseases-and-conditions/adrenal/adrenal-fatigue.
13. Hormone Foundation (Endocrine Society) website – adrenal fatigue: https://www.hormone.org/-/media/hormone/files/myth-vs-fact/mfsadrenalfatigue-520.pdf?la=en.
14. Mayo Clinic website – adrenal fatigue: https://www.mayoclinic.org/diseases-conditions/addisons-disease/expert-answers/adrenal-fatigue/faq-20057906.
15. Akturk HD, Chindris AM, Hines JM, Singh RJ, Bernet VJ. Over-the-counter "adrenal support" supplements contain thyroid and steroid-based adrenal hormones. Mayo Clin Proc. 2018;93(3):284–90.
16. Donegan D, Bancos I. Opioid-induced adrenal insufficiency. Mayo Clin Proc. 2018;93(7):937–44.

Chapter 2. Pseudo-Endocrine Disorders: My General... 21

17. Wilson's syndrome website: http://www.wilsonssyndrome.com/meet-dr-wilson/.
18. Wikipedia – Wilson's syndrome: https://en.wikipedia.org/wiki/Wilson%27s_temperature_syndrome.
19. American Thyroid Association (ATA) website – search for Wilson's syndrome: www.Thyroid.Org.
20. State of Florida, Department of Health. Final order number: DPR9200039ME – Ruling against Wilson's syndrome, Feb 12, 1992.
21. Reverse T3 syndrome website: www.stopthethyroidmadness.com.
22. Baillargeon J, Kuo YF, Westra JR, Urban RJ, Goodwin JS. Testosterone prescribing in the United States, 2002–2016. JAMA. 2018;320(2):200–2.
23. Layton JB, Kim Y, Alexander GC, Emery SL. Association between direct-to-consumer advertising and testosterone testing and initiation in the United States, 2009–2013. JAMA. 2017;317(11):1159–66.
24. Schwartz LM, Woloshin S. Low "T" as in "Template". How to sell disease. JAMA Intern Med. 2013;173(15):1460–2.
25. Gomes-Lima C, Burman KD. Reverse T3 or perverse T3? Still puzzling after 40 years. Cleve Clin J Med. 2018;85(6):450–5.
26. Schmidt RL, LoPresti JS, McDermott MT, Zick SM, Straseski JA. Is reverse triiodothyronine ordered appropriately? Data from reference lab shows wide practice variation in orders for reverse triiodothyronine. Thyroid. 2018;28(7):842–8.
27. Muller RS. Making a difference in adrenal fatigue. Endocr Pract. 2018;24(12):1103–5.
28. Gota CE. What you can do for your fibromyalgia patient. Cleve Clin J Med. 2018;85(5):367–76.
29. Warraich H. Dr Google is a liar. New York Times, Dec 16, 2018; Page A19 of the New York Edition.
30. Hellmuth J, Rabinovici GD, Miller BL. The rise of pseudomedicine for dementia and brain health. JAMA. 2019;321:543–4.

# Chapter 3
# Rogue Practitioners and Practices

**Michael T. McDermott**

In recent years, we have seen a disturbing proliferation of print, broadcast, and Internet advertisements concerning fabricated diseases that have no actual scientific or credible clinical evidence for their existence and unproven remedies for these made-up maladies that are openly shilled for profit. We have seen practitioners who proclaim themselves to be experts in hormonal therapy without any formal training and who often promote hormonal treatments without adequate endocrine evaluations. We have seen practitioners who make astonishing promises regarding the benefits of herbal, supplemental, and other unproven therapies that they themselves sell in their offices and/or online. And we have seen what we know to be frankly harmful and even dangerous products that contain animal whole organ (most commonly thyroid and/or adrenal) extracts or hormonal injections that produce highly elevated levels of sex hormones (especially testosterone)

M. T. McDermott (✉)
University of Colorado Hospital, Aurora, CO, USA
e-mail: michael.mcdermott@cuanschutz.edu

without any concern for short-term patient safety or long-term outcomes. And we have heard anecdotal stories from patients who visited these practitioners and had no beneficial results or frankly concerning on-treatment results at a surprisingly high financial cost, even though they had been promised symptom improvement, safety, and full insurance coverage.

We discussed the management of individual patients in the first two chapters of this book, but the issues described in the previous paragraph are of general public health concern. What is our responsibility as individual practitioners in the face of these rogue practitioners and practices? Certainly, we have a primary obligation to protect each of our patients from these unscrupulous, charlatan practitioners and the unproven, costly, and sometimes dangerous treatments they promote. We do this through one-on-one in-person education for our patients. We can also direct them to credible professional websites such as those of the Hormone Foundation (Endocrine Society), American Thyroid Association, and Mayo Clinic, for example; reliable information regarding Adrenal Fatigue and Wilson's Syndrome is available on these sites (see reference list below).

More broadly, however, we should seek opportunities to bring these issues to the attention of the general public. For example, I was able to be interviewed on a local Denver television station about testosterone therapy; during this brief interview, I informed the listeners that low testosterone levels are often just a manifestation of more serious underlying medical conditions or of medications, that treatment of these conditions should be the primary focus of therapy, and that low testosterone levels caused by these conditions are often restored to normal, without a need for lifelong testosterone replacement therapy, if the underlying medical conditions are appropriately managed. Our Division Head, Dr. Bryan Haugen, was also interviewed and was given the opportunity to discuss and warn the community about questionable and unproven thyroid treatment programs offered and advertised by local non-endocrinologist, non-physician practitioners. We can encourage our local and national professional organizations [state medical societies, American Medical Association (AMA), American College of Physicians (ACP), the Endocrine Society, the American Association of Clinical Endocrinologists (AACE), and the American Thyroid Association (ATA)] to publish fact sheets, official statements, and guidelines regarding these types of practices. And we can write editorials and commentaries in our local newspapers. One particularly well-written piece by Dr. Lisa Pryor was published in the *New York Times* (Jan 5, 2018) and was entitled "How to Counter the Circus of Pseudoscience." I highly recommend reading this outstanding article.

Another option is to report rogue practitioners and practices to your local state medical board. A small group of Colorado physicians reported a local physician who was treating patients who complained of fatigue with a combination of high dose prednisone and desiccated thyroid extract without testing for either adrenal insufficiency or hypothyroidism prior to initiating this aggressive therapy. I was asked to testify in court regarding this case. The outcome was removal of his medical license; he subsequently retired.

Dr. Denis Wilson, who declared "Wilson's Syndrome" to be a widespread debilitating but treatable disorder was sanctioned by the Florida Board of Medicine after a 50-year-old woman died of an arrhythmia and heart attack while on excessive amounts of thyroid hormone prescribed by Wilson. In 1992, the Florida Board of Medicine accused him of "fleecing" patients with a "phony diagnosis." The Board of Medicine and Wilson agreed to a 6-month suspension of Wilson's medical license, after which Wilson agreed to attend 100 hours of CME, submit to psychological testing, and pay a $10,000 fine before resuming practice. Wilson also agreed not to prescribe thyroid medication unless the Board of Medicine determined that the medical community had accepted "Wilson's Syndrome" and his treatment (Reference: State of Florida, Department of Health. February 12, 1992. Final Order Number: DPR9200039ME).

In 2012, after the sanctions, Dr. Wilson posted this on his website:

Since I've published my book there has been growing interest in and mention of Reverse T3, and the use of T3 in the treatment of low thyroid symptoms. For example, many thyroid-related health sites, books, fitness trainers, physicians, spokespeople, and businesses, tout the importance of peripheral conversion of T4 to T3 and/or Reverse T3 (RT3) and the usefulness of T3 in the treatment of low thyroid symptoms in patients with normal thyroid blood tests. Over twenty years ago, I received a lot of opposition both from mainstream and alternative medicine circles. Now, it's great to see that my ideas are being embraced and disseminated more and more.
Best regards,
Denis Wilson, MD (June 21, 2012)

As physicians, we have much more influence over these issues than anyone else in our communities. As shown above, the public listens to physicians and what we say makes a difference. Below are two examples of Colorado physicians who want to do something about this and are taking action. The first is a group email sent by an excellent practicing endocrinologist to multiple colleagues throughout Colorado regarding the growing practice of testosterone pellet injections. The second is a personal letter to me from a retired physician who still cares about the quality of health care and wrote to bring to my attention an acupuncture provider who has started a local chapter of "Thyroid Centers of America."

# Two Letters from Concerned Endocrinologists

Hello Endocrine Colleagues.
I am reaching out to many of you, and know that many more are not on this email, to enlist whoever is willing to help fight the escalating Bio-T programs that are infiltrating our patients. I have reached out to CMS and The State Board and was met with same response; no one wants to get involved. I have also reached out to the Endocrine Society for help in addressing this issue and also have not seen a reply. As this program becomes more aggressive in their treatment, we are routinely seeing women with T levels in the 200-600 range. When discussing this with their doctors I am told that men should have levels in the 900-1200 range.
I finally called the FDA to report my concerns and was able to speak with the consumer advocate. I am writing a formal letter in the hopes that we can have the FDA investigate further the

## Chapter 3. Rogue Practitioners and Practices 27

fraudulent claims and management. If you have not visited the Bio-T program website recently, I would encourage you do this. The website makes claims of bio-T pellets treating PTSD, Alzheimer's, diabetes and even Parkinson's disease. The pellets are manufactured and sold by this single company, which in my experience is the predominate force in the Denver area.

There are additional websites claiming how providers can enrich their pockets by $250,000 a year using these programs. We have seen so many women being negatively impacted by these claims
http://www.htcapractitioner.com/benefits/
https://www.biotemedical.com/

If you have cases that you can provide to me, with declassified information, demonstrating these high levels and any adverse claims this will bolster our complaint with the FDA. I don't know if it will take us anywhere, but I for one am saddened to continue to see so many patients be hurt, lose money and am frustrated with the lack of the medical community to help and protect these patients. If you have any additional thoughts that you would like me to include, I would be grateful

Thank you for your time, I know for myself this area has consumed much of my time in re-educating patients.
Linda Buckley MD

Dear Dr. McDermott

Recently, my morning edition of the Denver Post had the enclosed wrap-around ad on the front page. I had never heard of "The Thyroid Centers of America" nor of (name deleted) L.Ac. My local librarian at St. Joseph Hospital informed me that L.Ac. means licensed acupuncturist. Since the Hyatt house is only about 4 miles south of me, I made a reservation to attend.

There were about 25 middle-aged women and 5 men attending. One of the men appeared to be in his late 20s. Later he claimed to be symptom-free and was attending for his mother.

The speaker began by asking "what was the major problem with modern medical care?" The audience agreed that "fragmentation" was a major problem. The speaker went on to explain that his mother had developed Hashimoto's thyroiditis, an autoimmune disease, and once the patient's initial autoimmune disorder is controlled, the body goes on to develop additional autoimmune conditions. His mother developed a total of four. He began devoting his life to finding help for her.

He discovered that our livers are being attacked by halides (chlorides, bromides, etc.). He stated that most European nations do not allow fluoride in their public drinking water (!). And, I later confirmed this via the Internet. Because the liver is poisoned, it cannot produce a necessary substance that allows the intestine to complete conversion of all of T3 to its active form. Thus, thyroid tests may be normal, but active thyroid hormones are lacking. He never mentioned TSH measurements.

His program has 5 steps: 1) detoxify the liver; 2) achieve hormonal balance; 3) exercise; 4) improve nutrition; 5) my notes are blurred but I think it was to bring all of these 4 steps to optimal levels. He never mentioned acupuncture.

At this point he announced that because we had attended this educational lecture, his initial consultation could be had for $47 instead of the usual price of $187. Provided we signed up that evening. Three women hurried to the front desk (? shills) to take advantage of this offer. I departed.

Holistic medicine has a definite appeal and can be practiced honestly and profitably, I believe; but I wonder how he can prescribe hormones as a licensed acupuncturist. Perhaps the detoxifying of the liver brings all of one's hormones into balance.

It used to be that the local medical Society would investigate marginal medical practices and, if found fraudulent, put them out of business. I do not know if that is still true or that we live in a "live and let live" era.

Were you aware of The Thyroid Centers of America? He said there was one in Houston.

Please let me know by letter or phone.

Very truly yours,

Albert F Nibbe MD (retired; age 91)

# Suggested Reading

1. Garber J, et al. Clinical practice guidelines for hypothyroidism in adults: cosponsored by the American Association of Clinical Endocrinologists and the American Thyroid Association. Endocr Pract. 2012;18(6):988–1028. Thyroid. 2012 Dec;22(12):1200–35.
2. Jonklaas J, Bianco AC, Bauer AJ, Burman KD, Cappola AR, Celi FS, Cooper DS, American Thyroid Association Task Force on Thyroid Hormone Replacement, et al. Guidelines for the treatment of hypothyroidism: prepared by the American Thyroid Association task force on thyroid hormone replacement. Thyroid. 2014;24(12):1670–751.
3. Guglielmi R, Frasoldati A, Zini M, Grimaldi F, Gharib H, Garber JR, Papini E. Italian association of clinical endocrinologists statement-replacement therapy for primary hypothyroidism: a brief guide for clinical practice. Endocr Pract. 2016;22(11):1319–26.

4. Bornstein SR, Allolio B, Arlt W, et al. Diagnosis and treatment of primary adrenal insufficiency: an Endocrine Society clinical practice guideline. J Clin Endocrinol Metab. 2016;101:364–89.
5. Fleseriu M, Hashim IA, Karavitaki N, et al. Hormonal replacement in hypopituitarism in adults: an Endocrine Society clinical practice guideline. J Clin Endocrinol Metab. 2016;101:3888–921.
6. Molitch ME, Clemmons DR, Malozowski S, Merriam GR, Vance ML. Evaluation and treatment of adult growth hormone deficiency: an Endocrine Society clinical practice guideline. J Clin Endocrinol Metab. 2011;96:1587–609.
7. Bollerslev J, Rejnmark L, Marcocci C, Shoback DM, Sitges-Serra A, van Biesen W, Dekkers OM, European Society of Endocrinology. European Society of endocrinology clinical guideline: treatment of chronic hypoparathyroidism in adults. Eur J Endocrinol. 2015;173(2):G1–20.
8. Jerant A, Fenton JJ, Kravitz RL, et al. Association of clinical denial of patient requests with patient satisfaction. JAMA Intern Med 2018 Jan 1;178(1):85–91. Published Online November 27, 2017.
9. Pryor L. How to counter the circus of pseudoscience. New York Times, Jan 5, 2018.
10. Seaborg E. The myth of adrenal fatigue. Endocrine News, Sept 2017. p. 29–32.
11. Schaffer R. In age of Internet diagnoses, endocrinologists confront myth of "adrenal fatigue". Endocrine Today, April 2018. p. 1–12.
12. Hormone Health Network adrenal fatigue fact sheet: www.hormone.org/diseases-and-conditions/adrenal/adrenal-fatigue.
13. Hormone Foundation (Endocrine Society) website – adrenal fatigue: https://www.hormone.org/-/media/hormone/files/myth-vs-fact/mfsadrenalfatigue-520.pdf?la=en.
14. Mayo Clinic website – adrenal fatigue: https://www.mayoclinic.org/diseases-conditions/addisons-disease/expert-answers/adrenal-fatigue/faq-20057906.
15. Akturk HD, Chindris AM, Hines JM, Singh RJ, Bernet VJ. Over-the-counter "adrenal support" supplements contain thyroid and steroid-based adrenal hormones. Mayo Clin Proc. 2018;93(3):284–90.
16. Donegan D, Bancos I. Opioid-induced adrenal insufficiency. Mayo Clin Proc. 2018;93(7):937–44.
17. Wilson's syndrome website: http://www.wilsonssyndrome.com/meet-dr-wilson/.

18. Wikipedia – Wilson's syndrome: https://en.wikipedia.org/wiki/Wilson%27s_temperature_syndrome.
19. American Thyroid Association (ATA) website – Search for Wilson's syndrome: www.Thyroid.Org.
20. State of Florida, Department of Health. Final order number: DPR9200039ME – Ruling against Wilson's syndrome, Feb 12, 1992.
21. Reverse T3 syndrome website: www.stopthethyroidmadness.com.
22. Baillargeon J, Kuo YF, Westra JR, Urban RJ, Goodwin JS. Testosterone prescribing in the United States, 2002–2016. JAMA. 2018;320(2):200–2.
23. Layton JB, Kim Y, Alexander GC, Emery SL. Association between direct-to-consumer advertising and testosterone testing and initiation in the United States, 2009–2013. JAMA. 2017;317(11):1159–66.
24. Schwartz LM, Woloshin S. Low "T" as in "Template": How to sell disease. JAMA Intern Med. 2013;173(15):1460–2.
25. Gomes-Lima C, Burman KD. Reverse T3 or perverse T3? Still puzzling after 40 years. Cleve Clin J Med. 2018;85(6):450–5.
26. Schmidt RL, LoPresti JS, McDermott MT, Zick SM, Straseski JA. Is reverse triiodothyronine ordered appropriately? Data from reference lab shows wide practice variation in orders for reverse triiodothyronine. Thyroid. 2018;28(7):842–8.
27. Gota CE. What you can do for your fibromyalgia patient. Cleve Clin J Med. 2018;85(5):367–76.
28. Warraich H. Dr Google is a liar. New York Times, Dec 16, 2018; Page A19 of the New York Edition.
29. Hellmuth J, Rabinovici GD, Miller BL. The rise of pseudomedicine for dementia and brain health. JAMA. 2019;321:543–4.

# Chapter 4
# Influence of the Internet in Endocrinology Practice

**David R. Saxon**

The expanded availability and use of the Internet by patients have greatly altered the landscape of medical care over the past 25 years. Patients and their family members can now much more readily access medical information – both sound and unsound – that undoubtedly impacts the care they seek, the treatment options they choose, and the conversations they have with their physicians. Not surprisingly, many Americans are choosing to obtain health information online. In 2013, the Pew Research Center reported that 59% of U.S. adults had searched online for health information within the past year, 35% had used the Internet to try to figure out what medical condition they or another may have ("online diagnosers"),

---

D. R. Saxon (✉)
University of Colorado School of Medicine, Department of Medicine, Division of Endocrinology, Metabolism and Diabetes, Aurora, CO, USA

Division of Endocrinology, Metabolism and Diabetes, Rocky Mountain Regional Veterans Affairs Medical Center, Aurora, CO, USA
e-mail: David.saxon@ucdenver.edu

© Springer Nature Switzerland AG 2019
M. T. McDermott (ed.), *Management of Patients with Pseudo-Endocrine Disorders*,
https://doi.org/10.1007/978-3-030-22720-3_4

and 53% of online diagnosers talked with a clinician about what they found online [1].

The ability of patients to obtain health information on the Internet has had significant implications for the practice of endocrinology. With the Internet, vague symptoms like fatigue and weight gain often lead patients to online searches that suggest the presence of endocrine disorders such as hypothyroidism, hyperthyroidism, hypercortisolism, adrenal insufficiency, and testosterone deficiency. Armed with a preconceived notion of what endocrine disease they might have, patients now – perhaps commonly – come to endocrine visits looking for the endocrinologist to confirm their suspicions through specific lab testing and there may be a deep disappointment or resentment when certain requested testing is not performed, or results are negative. In a recent survey of endocrine patients, the majority (78%) looked for health information online, and while they generally demonstrated a good understanding of what constitutes trustworthy information, 40% simply relied on the top search engine option as their main criteria for choosing where to obtain information [2]. Unfortunately, at this time, few safeguards are in place to ensure that reputable medical information occupies the top-listed search engine sites.

Social media sites can be of benefit to patients with endocrine disorders, serving as a place to find support, gather medical information, and to express medication and treatment concerns. However, some social media forums undeniably promote pseudo-endocrine disorders that garner the attention of many. On Facebook, as of March 2019, a group named "Adrenal Fatigue and Thyroid Care" has over 54,000 members, whereas the Hormone Health Network, an online educational resource center for endocrine disorders sponsored by the Endocrine Society, has only 13,000 members. Such data suggests that social media dissemination of what most endocrinologists would consider to be sound medical advice and knowledge may lag behind the spread of (pseudo)endocrine-related medical information that is without a strong scientific basis.

Although not extensively studied, celebrity testimonials and popular news stories about specific endocrine and pseudo-endocrine disorders appear to lead to increased online health

## Chapter 4. Influence of the Internet in Endocrinology... 33

information seeking by the general public. For example, in November 2014, the former Fox News pundit Glenn Beck revealed to the public that he had suffered from "adrenal fatigue." This story was covered by a number of major news outlets including *USA Today*, *Washington Post*, *Vanity Fair*, and *Politico*, as well as many local news organizations. By using Google Trends, a website that analyzes the popularity of Google search queries across regions and languages, it appears that there was a spike in searches for the term "adrenal fatigue" during the week that Mr. Beck's story was in the news (see Fig. 4.1). Regional variation in interest in this story was also apparent during that 1-week period with West Virginia, North Dakota, and Vermont having the highest percentage of searches for "adrenal fatigue." Whether this specific or similar national media coverage resulted in an uptick of medical visits by patients concerned that they may have adrenal fatigue is unknown, but one wonders if such media coverage may cause some degree of mass psychogenic illness as has been seen in various cultural contexts after disasters and vaccinations [3, 4].

For practicing endocrinologists, it is easy to become discouraged and cynical about the seemingly widespread availability of fake or inaccurate online information about endocrine disorders. However, Internet use by patients can also be studied to understand the information needs of the general public and of communities of patients with specific endocrine disorders, thereby providing an opportunity to improve care. For example, a recent analysis of WebMD

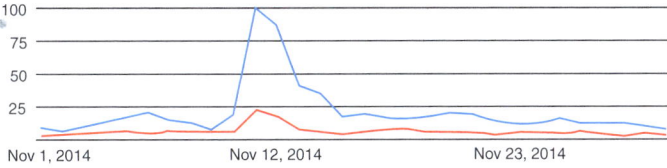

FIGURE 4.1 Google trend of search interest in "Glenn Beck" and "adrenal fatigue" during 11/1/14–11/30/14. Blue = "Glenn Beck" searches. Red = "adrenal fatigue" searches. (https://trends.google.com/trends/explore?date=2014-11-01%202014-11-30&geo=US&q=glenn%20beck,adrenal%20fatigue)

patient reviews of levothyroxine identified six distinct themes of medication concerns and found that these concerns differed depending on patients' age, gender, and treatment duration [5]. The authors suggest that such information has the potential to lead to tailored medication counseling interventions that could improve patient treatment satisfaction.

Patients' use of the Internet to gather information about endocrine and pseudo-endocrine disorders is not going to go away and is likely to expand. Endocrinologists will, therefore, need to develop specific communication techniques and management strategies that address the online medical (mis) information that patients may be exposed to in a head-on manner. One strategy might be to more directly question patients about their online health information seeking behavior and how that information has influenced the type of care they have sought, the treatments they have taken or considered, their adherence to treatment, and their beliefs about their illness. Another strategy could be for physicians to more routinely guide patients to reputable online medical information resources (perhaps through website links attached to lab reports, after visit summaries, and with new prescriptions). While ultimately the spread of medical misinformation on the Internet will continue to frustrate endocrinologists in certain clinical situations, we must continue to be unwavering in our dedication to providing appropriate and comprehensive care to all our patients.

# Bibliography

1. NW 1615 L. St, Washington S 800, Inquiries D 20036 U-419-4300 | M-419-4349 | F-419-4372 | M. Health Online 2013 | Pew Research Center [Internet]. 2013 [cited 2019 Mar 4]. Available from: http://www.pewinternet.org/2013/01/15/health-online-2013-2/.
2. Kyriacou A, Sherratt C. Online health information seeking behavior by patients prior to their outpatient appointments in endocrinology. In: BioScientifica; 2018 [cited 2019 Mar 4]. Available from: https://www.endocrine-abstracts.org/ea/0056/ea0056p618.

3. Bass E, Kaplan-Liss E, Dorf D, Broderick JE. A challenging empirical question: what are the effects of media on psychogenic illness during a community crisis? J Community Med Health Educ. 2012;2(1):118.
4. Clements CJ. Mass psychogenic illness after vaccination. Drug Saf. 2003;26(9):599–604.
5. Park SH, Hong SH. Identification of primary medication concerns regarding thyroid hormone replacement therapy from online patient medication reviews: text mining of social network data. J Med Internet Res. 2018;20(10):e11085.

# Chapter 5
# Debunking Internet Myths: What Is the Best Approach?

**Deirdre Cocks Eschler and Jonathan D. Leffert**

## Introduction

Over 80% of the United States (US) population has access to the Internet [1], and many use it as a resource for medical information. The sevenfold increase in Internet use from 2000 to 2015 [1] has changed the frontier of patient–physician relationships and health care practice.

D. C. Eschler
Renaissance School of Medicine at Stony Brook University, Stony Brook, NY, USA

Health Sciences Center, Level 16, Department of Medicine, Stony Brook, NY, USA

J. D. Leffert (✉)
North Texas Endocrine Center, Dallas, TX, USA
e-mail: jleffert@leffertmail.com

© Springer Nature Switzerland AG 2019
M. T. McDermott (ed.), *Management of Patients with Pseudo-Endocrine Disorders*,
https://doi.org/10.1007/978-3-030-22720-3_5

# Background and Significance of Clinical Problem

Currently, almost 75% of people in developed countries use the Internet as a source of health-related information [2]. Symptom searches are the most common [3]. In 2013, 35% of adults in the U.S. searched the Web to self-diagnose: about 50% of these talked with their doctor about their research and about 40% had their diagnosis confirmed [2]. It is not yet clear from research in this area whether such Internet searching leads to increased patient anxiety and overutilization of health-care resources [3]. There are suggestions that Internet searching may improve a patient's understanding of his/her condition and lead to a more prompt diagnosis (reviewed in [3]). A systematic review showed that it can improve a patient–physician relationship when a patient shares their findings on the Internet, particularly if the physician is responsive and not threatened [4].

In some countries, hundreds of home tests to self-diagnose conditions including diabetes, sexually transmitted diseases, and infections are available to the Internet consumer [5] and patients can self-medicate based on their Internet research (reviewed in [4]). Such self-treating can be dangerous, as one can buy drugs including non-FDA approved, custom-compounded "bioidentical" hormones [6], and anabolic steroids on the Internet without a prescription.

Nonspecific symptoms that include fatigue, weight gain, and other vague complaints will often lead the Internet-searcher to a possible endocrine etiology of their symptoms, such as hypothyroidism, adrenal abnormalities, and testosterone deficiency. Fatigue was listed as number 4 of the top 10 Internet health searches [7]. Patients may subsequently present to primary care doctors and endocrinologists armed with the information from the Internet. Unfortunately, information from the Internet on endocrine diseases is usually unfiltered and inaccurate. It can leave the reader to conclude their fatigue and weight gain have a simple solution of a "thyroid" pill, for example. Furthermore, the confluence of often inaccurate Internet information, easy to use testosterone medications, wide-ranging testosterone assays with biological variability, and the society's high value placed on youth, have resulted in the explosion of patients with "testosterone deficiency." Finally, the last group of patients with imprecise symptoms and lack of biochemical specificity for diagnosis are those with self-diagnosed "adrenal fatigue."

# Thyroid

## Thyroid Case

A 21-year-old female with a history of fatigue and weight gain presented to her naturopath. She had no previous medical or surgical history. On physical exam, her BMI was 19 kg/m$^2$, her thyroid gland was not enlarged, and the rest of her exam was unremarkable. Her thyroid test showed a TSH of 1.4 mU/L and free T4 of 1.2 ng/dL (both in normal range) and an elevated reverse T3. The patient then consulted the Internet regarding the reverse T3 elevation. From this source, it was recommended by her naturopath that she would require further evaluation and consideration of thyroid hormone treatment.

## Thyroid and the Internet

Fatigue is a commonly searched symptom on the Internet and often leads a patient to believe that they have hypothyroidism despite normal TSH values. Additionally, patients are able to purchase thyroid hormone online which can lead to very serious adverse outcomes [8]. Even when the consumer doesn't explicitly desire thyroid hormone, most commercially available thyroid supplements contain T4 and T3, some at doses higher than those used to treat hypothyroidism [9]. Additionally, the Internet offers false information stating that an imbalance in and overactivity of reverse T3, due to excess or deficient cortisol levels, will deplete the body of T3 and lead to hypothyroidism that will go undiagnosed by the medical practitioner [10, 11]. There are also statements that thyroid hormone resistance may contribute to symptoms despite normal labs. Other websites, devoted to people with Hashimoto's hypothyroidism, suggest that diets rich in protein, iodine, iron, selenium, zinc, omega 3 fats, and vitamins A, B, and D will improve thyroid function [12]. In addition, these web sites suggest that one should avoid potential "inflammatory" foods like gluten, dairy, eggs [12], and "toxins" like mercury from dental amalgams [13] and those from our air and drinking water by special high-efficiency particulate air (HEPA) filters and specific water filters [14].

## Thyroid Physiology, Diagnosis, and Treatment of Hypothyroidism

The human thyroid produces predominantly thyroxine (T4) and to a lesser extent triiodothyronine (T3). About 40% of T4 is converted in the tissues to the active metabolite, T3, which can subsequently bind to nuclear receptors in tissues [15], and another 40% is converted to an inactive metabolite reverse T3 (rT3) [16]. Reverse T3 is difficult to measure and is not used to guide clinical practice, with the very rare exception of its possible utility in the differentiation of central hypothyroidism from nonthyroidal illness [17].

The most common symptoms of hypothyroidism are fatigue, muscle cramps, dry skin, voice changes constipation, cold sensitivity, and fatigue [18]. Symptoms of hypothyroidism do not always correlate with biochemical thyroid function [19] and a hypothyroid symptom score is less likely to predict biochemically hypothyroid patients over 60 years old [20]. However, patients with more hypothyroid symptoms present, particularly if they were new in the preceding year, and are more likely to have biochemical hypothyroidism [19, 20]. The American Thyroid Association (ATA) recommends, however, against using a scoring system to diagnose hypothyroidism as they lack sensitivity and specificity [18].

In diagnosing and treating hypothyroidism in the nonpregnant patient, the ATA recommends using the TSH and free

T4 and recommends against the measurement of T3 levels [18]. The ATA strongly recommends against treatment with levothyroxine (LT4) for patients who are biochemically euthyroid (have a normal TSH and free T4) but have symptoms that can overlap with hypothyroidism [15]. In a double-blind, placebo-controlled, crossover study, 22 patients with symptoms similar to hypothyroidism but with normal thyroid function tests and 19 controls were studied. Despite an increase in FT4 and a decrease in TSH on LT4 therapy (thus proving compliance), study patients showed an improvement on psychological testing while on LT4 that was no different from results with placebo; however, they had a lower score for visual memory testing while on LT4 [21]. Furthermore, studies have shown there is no difference in energy metabolism and expenditure and body composition (including fat mass and waist circumference) in euthyroid patients who are treated with LT4 [22]. Treatment was shown to lower resting energy expenditure in one study [23].

## Circling Back to the Patient

In this case, the patient focused on the reverse T3 as a marker of thyroid hormone deficiency that she had "researched" and found to be a significant factor in thyroid function. After a detailed discussion with her regarding the physiology of thyroid metabolism and the lack of significance of an elevated reverse T3 as a biochemical marker for thyroid dysfunction, she understood that she did not need treatment with levothyroxine. We discussed alternative diagnostic possibilities for her symptoms, and suggestions for referral.

# Testosterone

## Case: "Low T"

A 30-year-old male presents for evaluation of "low T." The patient had been seen by a "low T" center initially for fatigue without any symptoms of sexual dysfunction. His initial testosterone level was 280 ng/dL on one sample drawn in the afternoon. He was started on testosterone cypionate 75 mg every week initially and increased to 100 mg every week because of lack of symptomatic improvement. On physical exam, the patient appears plethoric and has decreased testicular size. In addition to weekly testosterone injections, he is also on an aromatase inhibitor to decrease his potential risk of gynecomastia. He presents to discuss the cause of his "low testosterone" and the duration of treatment.

## Testosterone Use and Abuse and Internet Data

From 2000 to 2011, there was a 12-fold increase in testosterone sales worldwide, with the highest increase in prescriptions occurring in Canada (thought to be due to Internet pharmacies being located here) and the second highest in the U.S. [24], a trend that has likely continued. During this time, in the U.S., only ~75% of men new to testosterone had a testosterone level checked within the preceding year [25]. In 2011, over 2% of men in their 40s and almost 4% of men in their 60s were taking androgen replacement therapy in the U.S., most of whom didn't have a clear indication for its use [25] despite the fact that the prevalence of true pathological hypogonadism is estimated at 0.5% [26]. In a recent paper, the market size for hypogonadism in the U.S. includes 6–77% of men, with an up to a fourfold increase in prescriptions in the last 20 years [27]. This increase in use is due to off-label indications and to marketing and advertising direct to consumers with a "high prevalence of misinformation on Internet advertising" [27].

In a recent study assessing the "readability, credibility and quality of patient information for hypogonadism and testosterone replacement therapy on the Internet," the authors concluded that the Internet provides poor-quality information that is difficult for many to understand [28]. In another study, 75 websites found in a Google search of "testosterone replacement" in five of the most populous cities in the U.S. that urologists and endocrinologists comprised only ~15% of providers prescribing testosterone therapy while over one-third of the clinics were managed by nonphysicians [29]. Alarmingly, one does not need a clinic to buy testosterone, a controlled substance, or other anabolic androgenic steroids as they are easily available for purchase online without a prescription with a simple credit card payment [30].

## *Diagnosis and Treatment of Male Hypogonadism*

The Endocrine Society (ES) reports that men with signs and symptoms of testosterone (T) deficiency and with testosterone levels less than 300 ng/dL on at least two occasions are considered hypogonadal [31]. Signs and symptoms specific to T deficiency include delayed or incomplete sexual development, small testis, and loss of axillary and pubic hair. Those suggestive of T deficiency include low libido, erectile (particularly spontaneous) dysfunction, gynecomastia, low sperm count, low BMD, and hot flashes. Nonspecific symptoms include low energy, poor concentration, depressed mood, mild anemia, low muscle bulk [31]. When suspected, the T level should be checked while fasting and in the morning, and if low, repeated as almost one-third of men who initially have a low T, will have a normal value when repeated (reviewed in [31]). Free T should be measured when there may be alterations in sex hormone binding globulin and T levels are in the low normal range [31].

Only after one has discussed risks and benefit of therapy should T therapy be given to symptomatic men with confirmed low T. It should not be given to men with an elevated PSA, prostate or breast cancer, an elevated hematocrit, obstructive sleep apnea, or urinary symptoms that are severe, congestive heart failure that is uncontrolled, a clotting disorder, or a cerebral vascular event or MI in the preceding 6 months [31]. There are potential side effects of testosterone replacement that must be discussed with the patient. Side effects include acne, erythrocytosis, decreased sperm count and subsequent infertility, possibly subclinical prostate cancer, and growth of metastatic prostate cancer. There is weaker evidence to suggest an association of T use with a worsening of obstructive sleep apnea, breast cancer growth, or gynecomastia [31]. The US FDA requires T-producing companies to report warning about a possible increase in cardiovascular (CV) risk with T use. While the data from large randomized controlled trials lack conclusive results, the ES guidelines state that some studies suggest men with low T have increased mortality and CV risk [31]. It is uncertain whether testosterone treatment improved erectile dysfunction in hypogonadal men more than phosphodiesterase inhibitors alone [32, 33].

## Circling Back to the Patient

Discussion of "low testosterone" in healthy young males on high-dose testosterone replacement is always a challenge. These men are most often eugonadal and looking for symptom relief for other underlying psychological or body dysmorphic issues. The practitioner should emphasize the importance of evaluation of the underlying cause of hypogonadism as the initial step in any diagnostic evaluation of a confirmed low testosterone. To accomplish this goal, the patient needs to discontinue the testosterone replacement and return in roughly 3 months for repeat evaluation of their pituitary–gonadal axis. The patient should be aware that testosterone therapy is a lifelong treatment in hypogonadal men and it has potential side effects. This can be a challenging group of patients, with high expectations for treatment benefit.

# Adrenal Fatigue

## "Adrenal Fatigue" Case

A 45-year-old female presents for discussion of exhaustion, mood changes, and muscle aches after seeing a chiropractor. The chiropractor ordered a panel of laboratory testing including a salivary cortisol profile obtained over a period of several hours. The salivary cortisol values were consistent with "adrenal fatigue." Her past medical history and physical exam are unremarkable. She is interested in treatment for "adrenal fatigue."

## *Adrenal Insufficiency Versus the Internet Myth of "Adrenal Fatigue"*

The myth of adrenal fatigue dates back to a naturopathic chiropractor, James Wilson, who coined the term in 1998. Adrenal fatigue falsely claims that chronic stress leads to an exhaustion of adrenal cortisol, resulting in a myriad of nonspecific symptoms including gastrointestinal issues, muscle aches, sleep and memory disturbances, and chronic fatigue. A Google search for "adrenal fatigue" in 2018 provided 629,000 results. When faced with such an online self-diagnosis, the Internet consumer can purchase "adrenal support" supplements easily. However, all of such supplements reviewed by a group at the Mayo Clinic contained a small quantity thyroid hormone and almost all contained at least one steroid hormone [34], both of which can lead to negative consequences in someone with normal thyroid and adrenal function.

Adrenal fatigue is not a true medical diagnosis supported by scientific literature. In a systematic review of 3470 articles, 58 of which met inclusion criteria, there was no data to support the diagnosis of "adrenal fatigue" as a medical disorder [35]. Furthermore, the authors point out that corticosteroids, often recommended as a treatment for adrenal fatigue, have numerous side effects and put one at increased risk for cardiovascular, psychiatric, and bone disease as well as sleep disturbance, glaucoma, and myopathy (reviewed in [35]). Moreover, chronic corticosteroid use and abuse will suppress one's own HPA axis, creating a potential danger in times of increased demand as in illness or trauma or when abruptly stopped.

Primary adrenal insufficiency, on the other hand, is a true medical condition that is quite rare, with an incidence of 4:1,000,000/year in the western world and a prevalence of

100–140 per million [36]. Symptoms of adrenal insufficiency include fatigue, abdominal pain, weight loss, and signs include low blood pressure and darkening of the skin [36]. To make the diagnosis of adrenal insufficiency, a 250 μg ACTH stimulation test is required with a stimulated cortisol greater than 18 μg/dL [36].

## Circling Back to the Patient

It is always difficult to deal with a "disease" entity presumed by patients to be an endocrine disorder which has been promoted by individuals outside of the specialty. This unique situation requires time and patience to explain the underlying physiology of the pituitary–adrenal axis at the patient's educational level. In doing so, the patient will gain the understanding that outside of the disease entity of adrenal insufficiency, "adrenal fatigue" does not exist as a diagnosis. The patient can be referred to the Endocrine Society webpage on adrenal fatigue, www.hormone.org/diseases-and-conditions/adrenal/adrenal-fatigue, for further education. One should explain the underlying paradigm of all medical illness that without a diagnosis, there is not an endocrine treatment. Supplements that have been suggested by the alternative medicine community may contain active thyroid and adrenal hormone and can have significant side effects. While it is important to rule out true primary adrenal insufficiency, this diagnosis is rare, and the patient should be encouraged to seek alternative diagnoses for their symptoms that may include numerous possibilities such as depression, sleep apnea, anemia, or cardiovascular or respiratory problems.

# Summary

The Internet provides a wealth of medical information, though it can sometimes be inaccurate and misleading. When investigating the spread of true versus false news feeds on Twitter, MIT researchers found that false information spreads faster than true information with science-related news categories ranking third in its spread to the most people [37]. The Web, however, can improve a doctor to patient relationship and patient satisfaction, particularly if a provider responds positively to a patient's findings [4].

While the FDA in the U.S. requires prescriptions for medicine to be filled by a licensed practitioner, the online consumer can purchase medication and even controlled substances. There are methods in place to try to curtail the sale of such drugs from unlicensed online pharmacies [38].

Management of the Internet self-diagnosed patient is always challenging. All patients require a rigorous evaluation but patients with Internet self-diagnosis will require added time in the evaluation for education from a professional. These patients are searching desperately for help from an undefined condition that needs both diagnosis and treatment. The patient would like a simple clear-cut diagnosis and treatment plan but often, the answer may be part of a somatic disorder that will require more in-depth psychiatric analysis. Nevertheless, as endocrinologists, we must educate the patient about the scientifically based pathophysiology for the disease process in a confident and understandable way for the layperson. With a calm demeanor and compassion towards the patient, trust is established and allows the physician to make recommendations that the patient will accept. This process will hopefully lead the patient to a practitioner who has the correct background and training to diagnose and treat the individual.

# References

1. Smiths A. What percentage of people in this world have a computer? How many of them are connected to the Internet? How many of them know how to code? 2017 [updated 2017, Sept 13]. Available from: https://www.quora.com/What-percentage-of-people-in-this-world-have-a-computer-How-many-of-them-are-connected-to-the-internet-How-many-of-them-know-how-to-code.
2. Fox S, Duggan M. Health online 2013. Pew Research Center; 2013.

3. Mueller J, Jay C, Harper S, Davies A, Vega J, Todd C. Web use for symptom appraisal of physical health conditions: a systematic review. J Med Internet Res. 2017;19(6):e202.
4. Tan SS, Goonawardene N. Internet health information seeking and the patient-physician relationship: a systematic review. J Med Internet Res. 2017;19(1):e9.
5. Kuecuekbalaban P, Schmidt S, Muehlan H. The offer of medical-diagnostic self-tests on german language websites: results of a systematic internet search. Gesundheitswesen. 2018;80(3):240–6.
6. How do I get bioidentical hormones? Available from: http://bhrtforme.tripod.com/bioidentical-hormones-no-prescription.html.
7. Shmerling R. Dr. Google: the top 10 health searches in 2017. 2017 [updated 2018, Feb 26]. Available from: https://www.health.harvard.edu/blog/google-top-10-health-searches-2017-2018022113300.
8. Neuberg GW, Stephenson KE, Sears DA, McConnell RJ. Internet-enabled thyroid hormone abuse. Ann Intern Med. 2009;150(1):60–1.
9. Kang GY, Parks JR, Fileta B, Chang A, Abdel-Rahim MM, Burch HB, et al. Thyroxine and triiodothyronine content in commercially available thyroid health supplements. Thyroid. 2013;23(10):1233–7.
10. Thyroid health – Understanding reverse T3 2017, Apr 20. Available from: https://www.nahypothyroidism.org/thyroid-health-understanding-reverse-t3/.
11. Bowthorpe J. Reverse T3 (also called Reverse Triiodothyronine) 2009, Jan 7 [cited 2018 May 1]. Available from: https://stopthethyroidmadness.com/reverse-t3/.
12. Osborne P. How diet and nutrition can help your thyroid 2017, July 26 [cited 2018 May 1]. Available from: https://hypothyroidmom.com/how-diet-and-nutrition-can-help-your-thyroid/#more-12325.
13. Hedberg N. Searching for the causes of Hashimoto's disease. The key to healing 2017, Jan 1. Available from: https://hypothyroidmom.com/searching-for-the-causes-of-hashimotos-disease-the-key-to-healing/#more-11526.
14. Fallis J. 13 Things helped this hypothyroid man beat chronic mental illness 2016, Sept 19. Available from: https://hypothyroidmom.com/13-things-helped-this-hypothyroid-man-beat-chronic-mental-illness/#more-10283.
15. Jonklaas J, Bianco AC, Bauer AJ, Burman KD, Cappola AR, Celi FS, et al. Guidelines for the treatment of hypothyroidism: prepared by the American Thyroid Association task force on thyroid hormone replacement. Thyroid. 2014;24(12):1670–751.

16. Engler D, Burger AG. The deiodination of the iodothyronines and of their derivatives in man. Endocr Rev. 1984;5(2):151–84.
17. Schmidt RL, LoPresti JS, McDermott MT, Zick SM, Straseski JA. Does reverse triiodothyronine testing have clinical utility? An analysis of practice variation based on order data from a national reference laboratory. Thyroid. 2018;28(7):842–8.
18. Garber JR, Cobin RH, Gharib H, Hennessey JV, Klein I, Mechanick JI, et al. Clinical practice guidelines for hypothyroidism in adults: cosponsored by the American Association of Clinical Endocrinologists and the American Thyroid Association. Endocr Pract. 2012;18(6):988–1028.
19. Canaris GJ, Steiner JF, Ridgway EC. Do traditional symptoms of hypothyroidism correlate with biochemical disease? J Gen Intern Med. 1997;12(9):544–50.
20. Carle A, Pedersen IB, Knudsen N, Perrild H, Ovesen L, Andersen S, et al. Hypothyroid symptoms fail to predict thyroid insufficiency in old people: a population-based case-control study. Am J Med. 2016;129(10):1082–92.
21. Pollock MA, Sturrock A, Marshall K, Davidson KM, Kelly CJ, McMahon AD, et al. Thyroxine treatment in patients with symptoms of hypothyroidism but thyroid function tests within the reference range: randomized double-blind placebo controlled crossover trial. BMJ. 2001;323(7318):891–5.
22. Dubois S, Abraham P, Rohmer V, Rodien P, Audran M, Dumas JF, et al. Thyroxine therapy in euthyroid patients does not affect body composition or muscular function. Thyroid. 2008;18(1):13–9.
23. Samuels MH, Kolobova I, Smeraglio A, Peters D, Purnell JQ, Schuff KG. Effects of levothyroxine replacement or suppressive therapy on energy expenditure and body composition. Thyroid. 2016;26(3):347–55.
24. Handelsman DJ. Global trends in testosterone prescribing, 2000–2011: expanding the spectrum of prescription drug misuse. Med J Aust. 2013;199(8):548–51.
25. Baillargeon J, Urban RJ, Ottenbacher KJ, Pierson KS, Goodwin JS. Trends in androgen prescribing in the United States, 2001 to 2011. JAMA Intern Med. 2013;173(15):1465–6.
26. Handelsman DJ. Androgen physiology, pharmacology, and abuse. In: DeGroot LJ, Jameson JL, editors. Endocrinology. 6th ed. Philadelphia: Elsevier Saunders; 2010. p. 2469–98.
27. Bandari J, Ayyash OM, Emery SL, Wessel CB, Davies BJ. Marketing and testosterone treatment in the USA: a systematic review. Eur Urol Focus. 2017;3(4–5):395–402.

28. McBride JA, Carson CC, Coward RM. Readability, credibility, and quality of patient information for hypogonadism and testosterone replacement therapy on the Internet. Int J Impot Res. 2017;29(3):110–4.
29. Oberlin DT, Masson P, Brannigan RE. Testosterone replacement therapy and the internet: an assessment of providers' health-related web site information content. Urology. 2015;85(4):814–8.
30. McBride JA, Carson CC 3rd, Coward M. The availability and acquisition of illicit anabolic androgenic steroids and testosterone preparations on the internet. Am J Mens Health. 2018;12:1352–7.
31. Bhasin S, Brito JP, Cunningham GR, Hayes FJ, Hodis HN, Matsumoto AM, et al. Testosterone therapy in men with hypogonadism: an Endocrine Society clinical practice guideline. J Clin Endocrinol Metab. 2018;103:1715–44.
32. Mulhall JP, Valenzuela R, Aviv N, Parker M. Effect of testosterone supplementation on sexual function in hypogonadal men with erectile dysfunction. Urology. 2004;63(2):348–52; discussion 52–3.
33. Spitzer M, Basaria S, Travison TG, Davda MN, Paley A, Cohen B, et al. Effect of testosterone replacement on response to sildenafil citrate in men with erectile dysfunction: a parallel, randomized trial. Ann Intern Med. 2012;157(10):681–91.
34. Akturk HK, Chindris AM, Hines JM, Singh RJ, Bernet VJ. Over-the-counter "adrenal support" supplements contain thyroid and steroid-based adrenal hormones. Mayo Clin Proc. 2018;93(3):284–90.
35. Cadegiani FA, Kater CE. Adrenal fatigue does not exist: a systematic review. BMC Endocr Disord. 2016;16(1):48.
36. Bornstein SR, Allolio B, Arlt W, Barthel A, Don-Wauchope A, Hammer GD, et al. Diagnosis and treatment of primary adrenal insufficiency: an Endocrine Society clinical practice guideline. J Clin Endocrinol Metab. 2016;101(2):364–89.
37. Vosoughi S, Roy D, Aral S. The spread of true and false news online. Science. 2018;359(6380):1146–51.
38. Heymann P. "Keep Internet Neighborhoods Safe" a proposal for preventing the illegal internet sales of controlled substances to minors 2006 July 13. Available from: http://www.law.harvard.edu/programs/criminal-justice/kins-draft.pdf.

# Chapter 6
# Bewildered by Biotin

**Alicia Algeciras-Schimnich and Carol Greenlee**

## Introduction

Over the past few years, biotin has become one of the most popular and widely used over the counter supplements, with claims of improving hair, skin, and nails. While the daily requirement for biotin is around 30–70 mcg, most supplements contain high doses of 5000–20,000 mcg (5–20 mg). These supplements result in blood levels of biotin that can interfere with common laboratory assays, specifically those using biotin–streptavidin chemistry. In the presence of high blood levels of biotin, the assay can lead to abnormally low (such as with TSH and PTH) or abnormally high (such as fT4, fT3, and cortisol) results.

---

A. Algeciras-Schimnich
Department of Laboratory Medicine and Pathology, Mayo Clinic, Rochester, MN, USA

C. Greenlee (✉)
Western Slope Endocrinology, Grand Junction, CO, USA
e-mail: cgreenlee@westslopeendo.com

Reports of biotin interference leading to incorrect biochemical diagnoses in both adults and children have been published previously [1, 2]; however, the upward trend in biotin consumption has increased the chances of biotin interference in certain immunoassays, potentially leading to misdiagnosis and inappropriate treatments of individuals taking these high-dose biotin supplements. For example, six children taking biotin to treat inherited metabolic diseases were erroneously diagnosed with Graves' disease [1]. Some of these children were started on anti-thyroid medications before the biotin interference was detected. At least one patient death has been reported following a falsely low troponin result when a troponin test known to have biotin interference was used [3]. This has resulted in a safety communication by the Food and Drug Administration regarding the importance of reporting biotin use to mitigate the risk of incorrect laboratory test results [3].

In order to be able to identify potential biotin interference, it is important to understand the expected behavior of the laboratory test in the presence of biotin as well as to be aware of confounding clinical factors that might mask a potential interference. In this chapter, we describe the mechanisms of analytical interference in assays utilizing the biotin–streptavidin methodology and present a number of cases of hormonal abnormalities due to biotin consumption.

# Biotin

Biotin, also referred to as Vitamin B7 or Vitamin H, is part of the water-soluble complex of B-vitamins. It is a coenzyme for several carboxylases involved in protein, fat, and carbohydrate metabolism [4]. Biotin is readily available in a variety of animal and plant-based foods such as egg yolk, soybeans, leafy vegetables, pork, and liver [5]. An adequate daily intake of biotin in adults has been proposed to be 30 mcg a day [6]. In the United States (U.S.), biotin deficiency is rare because the daily composition of biotin-containing foods and the production of biotin from intestinal bacteria are sufficient to meet the body's daily requirements [4, 6, 7]. Biotin is completely absorbed achieving peak serum concentrations 1–3 hours post oral ingestion [8, 9]. The main route of biotin clearance is renal excretion with a physiologic half-life in the range of 8–16 hours [8, 9]. In patients with impaired renal function, biotin clearance will be significantly prolonged and, therefore, this needs to be considered when suspecting biotin interference. For example, in a patient with end-stage renal failure, biotin interference in the parathyroid hormone (PTH) assay was still observed up to 15 days after removal of the 10 mg biotin supplement [10].

Biotin is available over the counter in doses ranging from 5000 to 20,000 mcg, amounts that greatly exceed the adequate daily intake of 30 mcg a day. Clinically high doses of biotin therapy are indicated for certain inborn errors of metabolism, including holocarboxylase synthetase deficiency (40,000–80,000 mcg/day), biotinidase deficiency (5000–20,000 mcg/day), and biotin–thiamine-responsive basal ganglia disease (100,000–300,000 mcg/day) [11–13]. High doses of biotin (300,000 mcg/day) are also being investigated for the treatment of progressive multiple sclerosis (MS) and other demyelinating pathologies [14, 15]. Biotin supplementation in MS is hypothesized to activate fatty acid synthesis to support remyelination of demyelinated axons [16]. Although the clinical uses of biotin have remained relatively limited, in recent years, the use of biotin supplements has increased due to its somewhat unfounded beauty benefits claims [17]. Biotin is heavily marketed as an over-the-counter solution for healthy skin, for hair-loss prevention and to improve brittle nails. Given the tolerability and lack of toxicity of these high doses of biotin, many consumers may not list them in their medication history. In the U.S., up to 20% of individuals report consuming biotin-containing supplements [17].

The normal daily intake of biotin results in relatively low serum biotin concentrations (<0.8 ng/mL) that are not expected to interfere with immunoassays [18]. However, the same is not true when high doses of biotin supplements are consumed. A pharmacokinetic study in healthy individuals taking biotin supplements in doses ranging from 5000 to

20,000 mcg/day showed that absorption was rapid with dose-dependent peak serum concentrations achieved in less than 1 hour [19]. Peak concentrations of 41 ng/mL, 91 ng/mL and 184 ng/mL were observed at doses of 5000, 10,000, and 20,000 mcg/day, respectively [19]. The time required for the serum biotin concentration to fall below a specific threshold was also dependent on the initial dose. For example, assuming an assay has a biotin interference threshold of 30 ng/mL or higher, an 8-hour washout period was sufficient to reach a biotin serum concentration below this threshold in individuals taking 10,000 mcg/day; while in individuals taking 20,000 mcg/day, 31 hours were required to reach a biotin serum concentration below this threshold [19]. If biotin interference is observed at a threshold lower than 30 ng/mL, a longer period after the last dose of biotin will be required. Therefore, there is not a single time period that will guarantee interference-free test results; instead, it will be both biotin dose-dependent and assay threshold dependent.

## Mechanism of Biotin Interference

The high-affinity interaction between the biotin and streptavidin has provided an efficient method for separating free from bound antigen in both immunometric and competitive immunoassays over the past 25 years [20, 21]. Today this chemistry is widely used in several fully automated immunoassay platforms. The usual biotin dietary intake is not expected to interfere with these immunoassays; however, the high doses of biotin present in some dietary supplements saturate the biotin binding sites on streptavidin, preventing the capture of the antigen of interest during the reaction. The effect of biotin will be dependent on the type of immunoassay. High concentrations of biotin could lead to falsely elevated results when using biotin–streptavidin competitive immunoassays, whereas in biotin–streptavidin immunometric assays it could lead to falsely low results.

Immunometric (sandwich) assays are used to measure larger molecules such as thyroid-stimulating hormone (TSH), thyroglobulin, and parathyroid hormone (PTH). In the immunometric assay format (Fig. 6.1), the analyte is "sandwiched" between two different antibodies: a biotinylated capture antibody and a detection antibody, which is conjugated with an enzyme or a luminescent or fluorescent compound. Taking TSH as an example, a biotinylated anti-TSH antibody binds to TSH in the patient's sample. This complex is captured by the streptavidin-coated surface while an anti-TSH conjugated antibody reacts with a different antigenic site on the TSH molecule. The amount of signal is directly proportional to the concentration of TSH in the sample. High levels of biotin in serum compete with the biotinylated anti-TSH capture antibody for binding to the streptavidin-coated

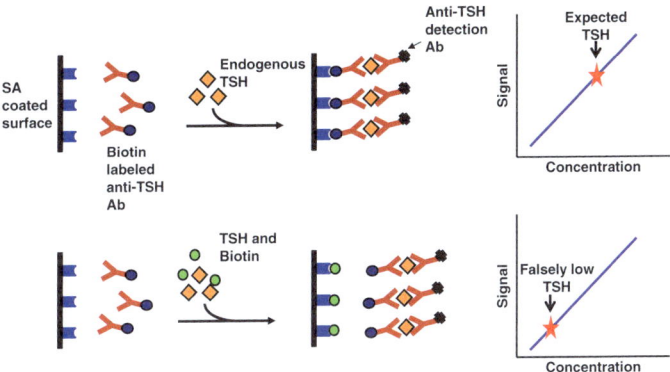

FIGURE 6.1 Mechanism of biotin interference in immunometric assays: TSH example. Serum TSH binds to a biotinylated anti-TSH antibody (Ab). This complex binds to the streptavidin (SA)-coated solid surface, while an anti-TSH detection Ab reacts with a different antigenic site on the TSH molecule. Unbound labeled antibody is washed away. The amount of signal is directly proportional to the concentration of TSH in the sample. High levels of biotin in serum compete with the biotinylated anti-TSH Ab for binding to the SA-coated solid surface. The lack of binding of the TSH–antibody complex to the SA-coated solid surface results in a falsely low TSH concentration

surface. The lack of binding of the TSH/biotinylated anti-TSH antibody complex leads to a falsely decreased TSH concentration.

Competitive immunoassays are used to measure small molecules such as thyroid and steroid hormones. In the competitive assay format (Fig. 6.2), a biotinylated antibody is captured onto a streptavidin-coated surface. A labeled analyte (enzyme or luminescent or fluorescent labeled) competes with the analyte of interest in the patient's sample for binding to the biotinylated antibody. The amount of signal is inversely proportional to the concentration of an analyte in the sample. Taking T4 as an example, T4 in the patient's sample competes with a labeled T4 for binding to a biotinylated anti-T4 antibody. The biotinylated anti-T4 antibody/T4 complex is captured onto a streptavidin-coated surface. The

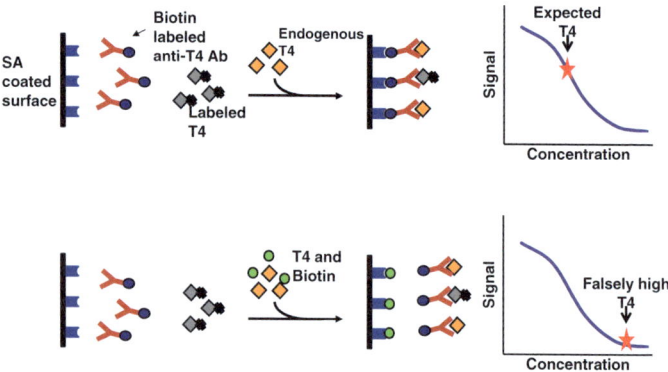

FIGURE 6.2 Mechanism of biotin interference in competitive immunoassays: T4 example. Labeled T4 and endogenous T4 compete for binding to a biotinylated anti-T4 antibody (Ab). The biotinylated anti-T4 Ab: T4 (labeled or endogenous) complexes bind to the streptavidin (SA)-coated solid surface. Unbound T4 (labeled or endogenous) is washed away. The signal is inversely proportional to the concentration of T4 in the sample. High levels of biotin in serum compete with the biotinylated anti-T4 Ab for binding to the SA-coated solid surface. Unbound anti-T4 Ab: labeled T4 complexes are washed assay. Lack of binding of the anti-T4 Ab: labeled T4 results in a low signal. This translates to falsely elevated T4 concentrations

signal generated by the labeled T4 bound to the anti-T4 antibody is inversely proportional to the concentration of T4 in the sample. High levels of biotin in serum bind to the streptavidin-coated surface and prevent binding of the biotinylated anti-T4 antibody, resulting in a signal that is falsely decreased and, therefore, a reported T4 concentration that is falsely increased.

Depending on the design of the immunoassays, both positive and negative analytical errors may occur for the same patient, mimicking a pathological hormonal condition (Table 6.1) [22]. Therefore, a patient taking biotin could present with elevations of both T4 and thyrotropin receptor antibody (TRAb) concentrations and a low TSH concentration, or an elevated cortisol in combination with a suppressed adrenocorticotropic hormone (ACTH) concentration, or an elevated 25-hydroxyvitamin D concentration with a suppressed PTH. In all scenarios, unawareness of biotin consumption and assay interference could lead to inappropriate patient management. It is important to know that not all immunoassay systems use the biotin–streptavidin technology.

Biotin interference can be unpredictable. A study that evaluated 37 biotin-based assays showed that consumption of 10,000 mcg biotin supplements caused interference in several immunoassays but not in other assays for which interference had been predicted. The reason for this observation was not elucidated but might be related to differences in biotin tolerance between assays [23]. Table 6.2 summarizes five widely used immunoassay systems, their use of the biotin–streptavidin complex in their assay design and the biotin threshold for interference provided by the manufacturer [22]. Depending on the assay, different misleading biochemical profiles can be observed. For example, when using the Beckman Coulter assays, the presence of high biotin levels will falsely elevate the FT4 and FT3 values but TSH levels will be unaffected. With the Roche Elecsys assays, the FT4 and FT3 measurements will also be falsely elevated and TSH will be falsely low or suppressed. In addition, biotin interference thresholds differ

TABLE 6.1 Potential errors in hormone testing, due to biotin interference

| Biological presentation | Erroneous diagnosis | Potential risk/ adverse consequence | Already reported |
|---|---|---|---|
| Thyrotropic axis<br>Low TSH<br>High FT3, FT4<br>High antibodies | Hyperthyroidism Graves' disease | Anti-thyroid drug therapy Inappropriate management | Yes |
| Calcium/ phosphate metabolism<br>High 250HD<br>Low PTH | Vitamin D intoxication PTH suppression | Inappropriate explorations Inappropriate stopping of vitamin D supplementation, even in a normocalcemic patient Delay in initiating appropriate therapy | Yes |
| Corticotropic axis<br>High cortisol<br>Low ACTH | Hypercortisolism | Inappropriate exploration Inappropriate management in case of corticotherapy | Yes |
| Gonadotropic axis<br>High testosterone/ estradiol<br>Low FSH, LH | Excessive peripheral secretion of gonadic steroids or occult gonadic steroids intake | Inappropriate examinations | Yes |

TABLE 6.1 (continued)

| Biological presentation | Erroneous diagnosis | Potential risk/ adverse consequence | Already reported |
|---|---|---|---|
| Somatotropic axis<br>  Low IGF1<br>  Low GH | Pituitary GH deficiency | Inappropriate explorations<br>Possible initiation of inappropriate GH treatment in a child with short stature | No |
| Pregnancy<br>  Low hCG | Absence of pregnancy | Delay in pregnancy monitoring | No |
| Glucose metabolism<br>  Low insulin<br>  Low C-peptide | Possible diagnosis of insulin-dependent diabetes in hyperglycemic patients | Inappropriate complementary explorations<br>Possible initiation of inappropriate therapy<br>Missed diagnosis of hyperinsulinism | No |
| Prolactin<br>  Low prolactin | NA | Delayed diagnosis in patients with a true prolactin adenoma | No |

Reprinted with permission from Piketty et al. [22]. Copyright 2018, De Gruyter
*NA* nonapplicable

between assays. For example, the biotin interference threshold for free T4 in the Roche Elecsys assay is 20 ng/mL (82 nmol/L), whereas it is 50 ng/mL (205 nmol/L) in the Siemens Vista assay. Another caveat to consider is that some biotin–streptavidin-based assays are designed with biotin

TABLE 6.2 Examples of five widely used hormone immunoassays using streptavidin–biotin interaction

| Hormone assays | Beckman Coulter (Access, DXi, DxC) | Immuno diagnostic system (Isys) | Ortho Clinical Diagnostic (Vitros) | Roche (Cobas, Elecsys, Modular) | Siemens (Dimension Vista, ExL) |
|---|---|---|---|---|---|
| FT3 | ✓ | | | ✓ (286) | ✓ (205) |
| FT4 | ✓ | | | ✓ (82) | ✓ (205) |
| Total T3 | | | | ✓ (41) | |
| Total T4 | | | | ✓ (409) | |
| TSH | | | ✓ (20.5) | ✓ (102) | ✓ (2050) |
| TRAb | | | | ✓ (41) | |
| SHBG | | | | ✓ (246) | |
| Thyroglobulin | ✓ | | | ✓ (327) | |
| PTH | | ✓ | ✓ (20.5) | ✓ (205) | |
| 25OH vit D | | ✓ (300) | | ✓ (61) | ✓ (286) |
| Cortisol | | | | ✓ (41) | ✓ (123) |
| ACTH | | | | ✓ (246) | |
| Testosterone | | | ✓ (41) | ✓ (123) | |
| Estradiol | | | ✓ (20.5) | ✓ (147) | ✓ |
| FSH | | | ✓ (41) | ✓ (246) | ✓ |
| LH | | | ✓ (20.5) | ✓ (205) | ✓ |
| Prolactin | | | ✓ (41) | ✓ (164) | ✓ |
| IGF1 | | ✓ (300) | | | |
| GH | | ✓ (300) | | | |
| C peptide | | | | ✓ (123) | |
| Insulin | | | | ✓ (246) | |

Reprinted with permission from Piketty [22]. Copyright 2018, De Gruyter
A "✓" mark indicates that the streptavidin–biotin interaction is used as immune complexes separation methodology. Biotin concentrations (nmol/L) above which an erroneous result can happen are indicated for each assay, when information is given in the reagent notices (i.e., concentration leading to bias above ±10% of the target). In theory, the analytes for which erroneous results occur at the lowest biotin concentration are those that will be most frequently impacted facing biotin supraphysiological intake. Dark rectangle, assay nonavailable in the tests menu

pre-bound to streptavidin before the addition of the patient's sample, theoretically making them not susceptible to biotin interference. Due to all of these confounding factors, it is best to consult the laboratory that performed the testing to determine the assay susceptibility to biotin, the threshold for biotin interference, and the necessary wait times after the last biotin dose when suspecting biotin interference.

Some laboratories might have means to troubleshoot and confirm biotin interference as the culprit of the laboratory abnormalities.

There is not a clear solution to resolve the biotin interference problem. The biotin–streptavidin chemistry has been used for many years in immunoassays without significant issues until the recent uptake of excessive biotin consumption. Advantages of using these assays include the increased sensitivity and the superior reproducibility of the automated systems. It is unlikely that all laboratories would move away from these assays. However, laboratories could be proactive by identifying which assays are affected by high doses of biotin and provide this information at the time of ordering or time of result reporting.

Overall, the effect of biotin on laboratory test results can create some interesting pseudo-endocrine conditions due to laboratory aberrations. As discussed above, the particular pseudo-endocrine profile depends on the assays used, the concentration of biotin in the blood, and the timing of phlebotomy for the laboratory specimen in relation to dosing of the biotin supplement. Sometimes the result is a laboratory abnormality without clinical findings, but in other cases, certain clinical signs and symptoms may make the pseudo-endocrinopathy all that much more convincing and/or confusing. We present here an assortment of cases of pseudo-endocrinopathy related to biotin. These illustrate how the laboratory alterations from biotin interference can result in pseudo-thyroid abnormalities, including overt and subclinical Graves' hyperthyroidism, central hyperthyroidism/thyroid hormone resistance, exogenous over-replacement/thyroid excess and central hypothyroidism/hypopituitarism, as well as a smattering of other clinical scenarios, including pseudo-Cushing's Syndrome, pseudo-testosterone excess, and confusing assessment of calcium disorders.

## Pseudo-Thyroid Abnormalities

### Pseudo-Overt Hyperthyroidism Due to Graves' Disease

A 21-year-old woman was referred to endocrinology for a second opinion regarding her recent diagnosis of subclinical hyperthyroidism. Her main complaints were enlargement and swelling of the neck, weight gain over the past 2 months, heat intolerance, and tremors. Laboratory evaluation revealed a slightly suppressed TSH of 0.2 mIU/L (nl: 0.3–4.2) with a normal free T4 of 1.3 ng/mL (nl: 0.9–1.7). At a 1-month follow-up visit, her thyroid function test results had become suggestive of overt hyperthyroidism with further suppressed TSH but now with elevated free T4 and elevated TRAb levels.

| Test | Result | Reference interval |
|---|---|---|
| TSH | 0.1 mIU/L | 0.3–4.2 |
| Free T4 | 1.7 ng/dL | 0.9–1.7 |
| TRAb | 40 IU/L | <1.75 |

After taking methimazole (10 mg daily) for 2 months, her thyroid function tests remained unchanged. Because of her high TRAb, radioactive iodine treatment was being considered. Evaluation of her medication history revealed she had started taking a 5000 mcg (5 mg) biotin capsule daily between the initial and follow-up visits. Investigation of potential biotin interference and measurement of thyroid function tests with an immunoassay that is not affected by biotin revealed a normal TSH of 1.4 mIU/L (nl: 0.3–4.2) with normal free T4 of 1.0 ng/mL (nl: 0.9–1.7). Troubleshooting of the TRAb result by removal of biotin from the patient's serum showed a TRAb concentration of 11 IU/L, still elevated but significantly lower than the result prior to biotin removal. She remained on methimazole with regular follow-up.

This patient had true subclinical hyperthyroidism. The apparent progression from subclinical to overt hyperthyroidism was caused by the introduction of biotin supplements between the initial and follow-up visits. In this case, all immunoassays were affected by the presence of biotin. The TSH assay was an immunometric assay resulting in a falsely low TSH concentration in the presence of biotin, whereas the free T4 and TRAb assays were competitive assays resulting in falsely elevated free T4 and TRAb concentrations. The opposite impact of biotin on these assays would produce a biochemical profile that mimicked overt hyperthyroidism due to Graves' disease.

## Pseudo-Subclinical Hyperthyroidism Due to Graves' Disease

A 65-year-old woman was found by her primary care physician to have an abnormal TSH of "0" mIU/L (0.47–4.68) with normal free T4 of 1.1 ng/mL (nl: 0.8–2.2) and free T3 of 3.36 pg/mL (nl: 2.77–5.27). Her main complaints were of weight gain and hair loss, but she also reported being newly hot-natured and heat intolerant while in the past she had been cold-natured. She denied tachycardia or tremors but was taking atenolol 100 mg daily for hypertension. Her sleep alternated between sound and disrupted. Her bowel function was described as both constipation and diarrhea. She had new complaints of progressive muscle weakness and more frequent falls with activities of daily living. She was referred to endocrinology for further evaluation. An abdominal CT scan with contrast was completed the day prior to endocrine evaluation for her complaint of unexplained weight gain and was abnormal only for mild fatty infiltration of the liver.

Endocrine examination showed the patient to be obese with a BMI 31.1 kg/m$^2$, blood pressure 122/76 and pulse 80. She had thinning scalp hair, no thyroid eye changes, a normal sized, somewhat firm thyroid gland, and warm, moist palms but no tremor. Muscle stretch reflexes were difficult to elicit and there were varicose veins with trace pitting edema. Additional laboratory testing, done 2–3 weeks after the initial abnormal tests were as follow:

| Test | Result | Reference interval |
|---|---|---|
| TSH | 0.06 mIU/L | 0.47–4.68 |
| Total T3 | 170 ng/dL | 80–190 |
| Total T4 | 9.9 mcg/dL | 5.0–12.5 |
| FT4 index | 10.4 mcg/dL | 4.8–12.7 |
| TRAb | 2.76 IU/L | 0–1.75 |
| Anti-Thyroperoxidase Abs | 2.3 IU/mL | <9.0 |

Measuring of thyroid uptake was precluded by the iodine load from the recent IV contrast. A thyroid ultrasound showed the right lobe to measure 5.6 × 1.6 × 1.6 cm and left lobe 5.2 × 1.6 × 1.6 cm, with normal echogenicity except for 2 sub-centimeter cystic nodules in each lobe.

The possibility of subclinical Graves' disease versus a false positive TRAb test was discussed with the patient. She was offered observation versus a trial on anti-thyroid medication. She reported a strong family history of thyroid disease in many family members including her grandfather, siblings, and daughter. That, along with hopes that her hair loss would lessen, her strength would improve and perhaps weight gain, or at least hunger, would lessen, prompted her to opt for a trial on methimazole.

Over the next several months her thyroid levels showed fluctuations, some of which did not seem to make sense (e.g., both fT4 and TSH concentrations were decreasing). The methimazole doses were titrated up and down based on the labs along with the patient's reports of variable changes in her symptoms.

The patient's medication list included 5 mg (5000 mcg) of biotin daily. She was asked to withhold the biotin supplement for a few days. A subsequent TSH measured after a few days without biotin was 7.1 mIU/L andTRAb was negative at <1.00 IU/L. She was instructed to stop the methimazole and thyroid function was monitored. Both fT4 and TSH have remained normal with a TSH 1.7 mIU/L at last check. The initial laboratory abnormalities were due to biotin interference. The assays used in this case consisted of a streptavidin–biotin assay for TSH and TRAb but not for fT4, fT3, total T4, and total T3. The TSH assay was an immunometric assay resulting in a falsely low result in the presence of biotin, whereas the TRAb assay was a competitive assay resulting in a falsely high result in the presence of biotin.

One endocrinologist noted a "run" on subclinical hyperthyroidism due to Graves' disease in her practice. As in the above case, the local laboratories used biotinylated TSH and TRAb assays and non-biotinylated T4 and T3 assays. A common clinical scenario was that a patient began taking biotin supplements after noting hair loss. When the hair loss persisted, the patient underwent further assessment by the primary care clinician, gynecologist or dermatologist with findings of a low to suppressed TSH but normal T4 and T3 levels (free or total). Further evaluation by the endocrinologist then confirmed suppressed TSH, normal T4, and T3 but elevated TRAb levels. Often patients reported additional symptoms such as difficulty sleeping, irritability, dyspnea on exertion, anxiety, and unusual fatigue or restlessness. Many patients opted for a trial on methimazole in hopes of reducing hair loss.

Interestingly, some patients were disappointed to learn that they did not have a thyroid condition causing their complaints but instead had a lab artifact caused by the biotin supplements they were taking. Another concern was whether the now normal TRAb and TSH represented remission after methimazole therapy rather than normalization of the laboratory measurement by excluding biotin interference. Ongoing, more extended monitoring was therefore required for some of these patients to be certain.

Patients with euthyroid multinodular goiter or thyroid nodules can falsely appear to have toxic MNGs or toxic adenomas in the presence of biotin supplements and a biotin sensitive TSH assay. This can also be seen when monitoring patients on exogenous levothyroxine (LT4) therapy. Biotin ingestion can result in falsely low to suppressed TSH levels and make it appear that the patient has exogenous hyperthyroidism, leading to inappropriate reductions of the LT4 dosage. Often, on follow-up, the TSH will remain low or suppressed despite progressive reductions in the dose of LT4 as described in the case below.

## Pseudo-Exogenous Thyroid Excess/Thyrotoxicosis

A 58-year-old woman presented for follow-up evaluation of postsurgical hypothyroidism. She had previously undergone a thyroidectomy, with no subsequent radioactive iodine therapy, for low-risk papillary thyroid cancer. On LT4 125 mcg daily, she had complaints of insomnia and a serum TSH level of <0.02 mIU/L (nl: 0.47–4.68). Her LT4 dose was reduced to 100 mcg daily, but the TSH remained <0.02 mIU/L. Despite allowing time for recovery from suppression and reducing the dose of LT4 further to 88 mcg daily, the TSH rose only to 0.02 mIU/L. After another LT4 dose reduction to 75 mcg daily, the TSH level returned as <0.02 mIU/L. This was especially puzzling since her body weight was nearly 90 kg, giving her an estimated LT4 dose requirement much higher than she was taking and during this time her FT4 level had dropped from 1.62 to 0.91 ng/mL (nl: 0.8–2.2). She was also experiencing progressive symptoms suggestive of hypothyroidism. The laboratory was asked to check for heterophile antibodies interfering with the TSH assay, but none were identified. The TSH level done at the same time as the heterophile antibody test was 0.25 mIU/L. Subsequently, she was asked about biotin supplements. She was taking 20 mg (20,000 mcg) per day but had never mentioned it during medication reconciliation processes for either her primary care clinician or her endocrinologist. After withholding biotin for 2 days, her TSH measured 1.34 mIU/L. Based on this patient's biotin dose, a longer period without biotin consumption would have allowed more complete clearance of biotin and likely an even higher, more accurate TSH result.

The rise in TSH concentration after withholding biotin did indicate that biotin was the cause of the suppressed TSH result. Inconsistent or nonsensical changes in the TSH level, such as decreasing rather than increasing levels after a significant LT4 dose reduction, can serve as a clue to ask about biotin supplementation. One clue to biotin interference with measurement of TSH (and other assays) is unexplained fluctuations in TSH concentrations that might correlate with the timing of biotin consumption. If patients take biotin intermittently and/or get their blood drawn at different times of day (variable time since biotin ingestion resulting in variable blood levels of biotin and thus variable interference with the assay), they can have even more erratic fluctuations in their TSH levels.

## Pseudo-Central Hypothyroidism

A 60-year-old female presented with complaints of fatigue and cold intolerance. Her internist had appropriately checked thyroid function with a resultant serum TSH of 0.01 mIU/L (nl: 0.47–4.68). Repeat testing showed low normal FT4 and FT3 and a persistently low TSH. She had extensive additional testing that showed an inappropriately low FSH of 10 IU/L (postmenopausal range: 16–157) and a low prolactin of 2.0 ng/mL (nl: 4.8–23.3) but normal IGF-1 and cortisol levels. An MRI was read as normal with no imaging abnormality in the region of the hypothalamus or pituitary. The internist was perplexed about these abnormalities and was uncertain about whether to begin treatment for central hypothyroidism to see if her fatigue and cold intolerance would improve. She then learned of the effects that biotin supplements can have on some laboratory assays. The patient acknowledged taking biotin supplements at 10 mg (10,000 mcg) per day. After holding the biotin for a few days, the repeat measurement of TSH and prolactin revealed levels within the normal range and the FSH level was appropriately elevated for postmenopausal status. In contrast to this scenario, if the TSH assay is not biotinylated but the T4 and T3 assays are, central hyperthyroidism or thyroid hormone resistance can be suspected.

## Pseudo-Central Hyperthyroidism/Thyroid Hormone Resistance

A 42-year-old male patient was referred to a university endocrinology service because of markedly elevated FT4 of 2.8 ng/dL (nl: 0.7–1.9) and T3 of 250 ng/dL (nl: 80–180) with a normal TSH of 1.1 mIU/L (nl: 0.3–4.2). This pattern of lab abnormalities had persisted on repeat testing at his local lab. He was referred for endocrine consultation to see if he had thyroid hormone resistance or a TSH-secreting pituitary adenoma. He had no symptoms of thyroid excess nor of coexisting hypopituitarism. Testing at the university lab revealed normal FT4 1.2 ng/dL (nl: 0.8–2.2), total T4 of 8.9 mcg/dL (nl: 6–12), and total T3 of 99 ng/dL (nl: 80–180) with a normal TSH.

The savvy faculty endocrinologist inquired about biotin, learning that the patient was ingesting around 5 mg (5000 mcg) per day. He then confirmed that the testing laboratories used assays for FT4 and T3 that were biotinylated but an assay for TSH that was not.

## Pseudo-Cushing's Syndrome

A 66-year-old woman presented to her new primary care physician with complaints of unexplained weight gain and coronal hair loss with new and increasing facial hair growth, facial redness and peripheral edema over the preceding 1–2 years. Laboratory evaluation revealed marked elevation of a random serum cortisol level of 46 mcg/dL (nl: 7–25) and an elevated total testosterone of 179 ng/dL (nl: 8–60). Based on these results, she was suspected to have adrenal carcinoma and was scheduled for an adrenal CT scan along with an urgent referral to endocrinology.

Additional history obtained by the endocrinologist included a history of hypertension, fibromyalgia, and long-standing coronal hair loss with only more recent facial hair growth and redness. She had struggled with weight control for years but in the past had been more easily able to lose weight. She complained of increasing muscle weakness, fatigue, and edema.

Chapter 6. Bewildered by Biotin 69

Her medication list included amlodipine 5 mg daily, pregabalin 150 mg four times daily, Celecoxib 200 mg twice daily, furosemide 20 mg daily, Klor-con 20 mEq daily, Minoxidil 2% solution 1 drop applied twice daily, glucosamine 750 mg daily, a vitamin B complex, a multivitamin, and biotin 5 mg (5000 mcg) daily. In the past, she had received glucocorticoid injections into her fibromyalgia trigger points but had not had an injection for 2–3 years.

Her physical exam confirmed a BMI of 30.8 kg/m$^2$, blood pressure 150/90, thinning hair on top of the scalp, a round face with a ruddy complexion and thick white hair growth on the upper lip and cheeks. She had a small dorsal fat pad but no supraclavicular fullness. There was abdominal obesity but no striae and no hirsutism on the torso. Extremity exam did reveal 1+ pitting edema but no thinning of the skin. The adrenal CT scan revealed normal adrenal glands bilaterally. Repeat laboratory testing revealed normal laboratory test results as shown below.

| Test | Result | Reference interval |
|---|---|---|
| AM cortisol | 6.7 mcg/dL | 7–25 |
| ACTH | 18 pg/mL | 7.2–63 |
| Total testosterone | 41 ng/dL | 8–60 |
| Free testosterone | 0.6 ng/dL | 0.3–1.9 |
| Salivary cortisol | <50 ng/dL | <50 |

Upon discussion, the patient reported that she had been using minoxidil solution on her scalp for the past couple of years, along with an herbal shampoo, to help reduce the coronal hair loss. For the past year or so, she had added a Biotin 5000 mcg (5 mg) capsule daily along with a B-complex supplement containing 3000 mcg (3 mg) of biotin in hopes of further reducing the hair loss. Many of her Cushingoid signs and symptoms were side effects of the minoxidil (red face, facial hair growth, and edema), with the edema likely exacerbated by amlodipine treatment of hypertension. She had a history of fibromyalgia with weight gain following treatment with pregabalin (Lyrica).

The initial laboratory abnormalities were due to the interference of biotin with both the cortisol and total testosterone assays and the timing of the specimen collection (middle of the day after taking biotin in the morning). The immunoassays used in this case were competitive assays, giving falsely elevated results at the initial visit. Because of the significant increase use of biotin supplements in recent years, assessing patient medication lists for biotin consumption should be the first step in an evaluation prior to ordering additional testing. If biotin interference is suspected, the laboratory could be contacted for troubleshooting. Alternative approaches include asking the patient to abstain from taking biotin for several days or even a week prior to testing or measuring these analytes on an immunoassay or mass spectrometry assay that does not use biotin in the assay design. The follow-up (repeat) blood specimen on this patient was collected fasting prior to her taking any medications or supplements. The salivary cortisol was measured by mass spectrometry which is not susceptible to biotin interference.

## False Negative Pregnancy Testing

It is not difficult to anticipate other situations where clinical signs and symptoms might suggest Cushing's syndrome with the potential for biotin interference with laboratory results to mislead the evaluation. One such situation would be an adolescent female presenting with weight gain, new striae and amenorrhea, and mildly elevated cortisol levels. In the absence of biotin, a positive pregnancy test would yield the correct "diagnosis." However, biotin supplementation can result in a falsely negative pregnancy test and sometimes marked elevations of blood cortisol levels. This can result in a delay in recognizing the underlying pregnancy and lead to further testing, including imaging, which could have adverse effects on the fetus.

## Pseudo-Testosterone Excess

A 72-year-old male with Type 2 diabetes, chronic fatigue syndrome, and hypogonadism was referred to endocrinology for help managing his testosterone replacement therapy. He had an initial low testosterone of 123 ng/dL (nl: 280–1070) with no measurement of LH or FSH. He was taking depot testosterone injections of 200 mg IM every 2 weeks as prescribed by his primary care clinician. His nadir testosterone concentration on treatment was elevated at 1587 ng/dL (nl: 280–1070). He denied taking extra doses of testosterone or having increased the dose of the biweekly injection. He had no polycythemia and a sex hormone binding globulin (SHBG) level was in the low end of the reference interval. Despite reducing the dose of depot testosterone, his testosterone blood concentrations remained elevated at >1200 ng/dL. The testosterone injections were held for 1 month with testosterone concentrations still being high normal. Eventually, it was discovered that he had added a high dose biotin supplement because he had experienced an increase in male-pattern hair loss with the testosterone therapy. Withholding biotin allowed accurate testosterone assessment, management, and monitoring of the hypogonadism and testosterone replacement therapy.

The testosterone immunoassay, in this case, was a competitive assay that resulted in false elevations of serum testosterone. Measurement of his testosterone by mass spectrometry would have helped in troubleshooting the false elevations. Biotin consumption should be ruled out during the initial evaluation of testicular or ovarian function, but also during ongoing monitoring of any replacement therapy or other treatments. This can impact the diagnosis and management of male patients with primary or secondary hypogonadism, women being assessed for hirsutism or monitoring of androgen deprivation therapy for prostate cancer or transgender replacement therapy.

### Pseudo-Non-parathyroid Hypercalcemia

A 56-year-old woman was found to have an elevated serum calcium level of 10.9 mg/dL (nl: 8.6–10.0) on a chemistry panel performed during her annual exam with her primary clinician. Repeat testing confirmed the hypercalcemia with a PTH level near the lower end of the reference interval at 17 pg/mL (nl: 15–65) and a 25-hydroxyvitamin D level slightly above normal. The patient denied taking any vitamin D supplements. She was referred to endocrinology with a diagnosis of hypercalcemia due to possible vitamin D toxicity of unknown source. In an attempt to find a hidden source of vitamin D intake, the patient was asked to bring in all of her medications, including over-the-counter medications and supplements. No exogenous source of vitamin D was found but it was noted that she was taking a "mega-B" supplement as well as a "hair and nail" supplement which together provided 15,000 mcg (15 mg) of biotin daily. After withholding the biotin, repeat testing showed persistent hypercalcemia but this time with a slightly elevated serum PTH value of 78 pg/mL and a low normal serum 25-hydroxyvitamin D level of 30 ng/dL. The correct diagnosis, therefore, was hypercalcemia due to primary hyperparathyroidism. Biotin interference with the PTH assay is similar to its effect on the TSH assay, resulting in falsely low results.

## Conclusions

As can be seen from these cases, biotin interference with laboratory assays can cause a bewildering array of pseudo-endocrine scenarios. Unfortunately, bewilderment is not the only effect of this interference. The misleading laboratory results can lead to clinical errors in diagnosis and/or management with the potential for patient harm. This emphasizes the need to ask about biotin supplements as part of medication reconciliation history to mitigate the risk of clinical errors. However, the biotin content in some supplements with unique names or combination preparations may not be recognized by the patient. In addition, patients can start taking biotin after their initial assessment leading to confusing results on follow-up monitoring, as seen in some of the above cases.

It is unlikely that biotin–streptavidin-based immunoassays will disappear from clinical laboratories in the near future; therefore, preparing an approach to prevent being bewildered by biotin is advised. In addition to asking about biotin ingestion at the time of an office or hospital visit, it is advisable that this be queried at the time of blood sample collection. It is important that biotin be held for an adequate amount of time to allow clearance of the biotin, which will be influenced by the biotin dose and the renal clearance status of the patient. The prevention and detection of biotin-related aberrant results will require open communication between patients and clinicians as well as between clinicians and the clinical laboratory in cases of suspected interference.

# References

1. Kummer S, Hermsen D, Distelmaier F. Biotin treatment mimicking Graves' disease. N Engl J Med. 2016;375(7):704–6.
2. Minkovsky A, Lee MN, Dowlatshahi M, Angell TE, Mahrokhian LS, Petrides AK, et al. High-dose biotin treatment for secondary progressive multiple sclerosis may interfere with thyroid assays. AACE Clin Case Rep. 2016;2(4):e370–e3.
3. US FDA Administration Safety Communication. Biotin (Vitamin B7): may interfere with lab tests. 11/28/2017.
4. McMahon RJ. Biotin in metabolism and molecular biology. Annu Rev Nutr. 2002;22:221–39.
5. Staggs CG, Sealey WM, McCabe BJ, Teague AM, Mock DM. Determination of the biotin content of select foods using accurate and sensitive HPLC/avidin binding. J Food Compos Anal. 2004;17(6):767–76.
6. Zempleni J, Kuroishi T. Biotin. Adv Nutr. 2012;3(2):213–4.
7. Zempleni J, Wijeratne SS, Kuroishi T. Biotin. In: Erdman Jr JW, Macdonald I, Zeisel SH, editors. Present knowledge in nutrition. Washington, DC: International Life Sciences Institute; 2012. p. 587–609.

8. Wijeratne NG, Doery JC, Lu ZX. Positive and negative interference in immunoassays following biotin ingestion: a pharmacokinetic study. Pathology. 2012;44(7):674–5.
9. Peyro Saint Paul L, Debruyne D, Bernard D, Mock DM, Defer GL. Pharmacokinetics and pharmacodynamics of MD1003 (high-dose biotin) in the treatment of progressive multiple sclerosis. Expert Opin Drug Metab Toxicol. 2016;12(3):327–44.
10. Meany DL, Jan de Beur SM, Bill MJ, Sokoll LJ. A case of renal osteodystrophy with unexpected serum intact parathyroid hormone concentrations. Clin Chem. 2009;55(9):1737–9.
11. Suormala T, Fowler B, Duran M, Burtscher A, Fuchshuber A, Tratzmuller R, et al. Five patients with a biotin-responsive defect in holocarboxylase formation: evaluation of responsiveness to biotin therapy in vivo and comparative biochemical studies in vitro. Pediatr Res. 1997;41(5):666–73.
12. Wolf B. Biotinidase deficiency. In: Adam MP, Ardinger HH, Pagon RA, Wallace SE, Bean LJH, Stephens K, et al., editors. GeneReviews. Seattle: University of Washington; 1993–2018.
13. Tabarki B, Al-Hashem A, Alfadhel M. Biotin-thiamine-responsive basal ganglia disease. In: Adam MP, Ardinger HH, Pagon RA, Wallace SE, Bean LJH, Stephens K, et al., editors. GeneReviews. Seattle: University of Washington; 1993–2018.
14. Sedel F, Papeix C, Bellanger A, Touitou V, Lebrun-Frenay C, Galanaud D, et al. High doses of biotin in chronic progressive multiple sclerosis: a pilot study. Mult Scler Relat Disord. 2015;4(2):159–69.
15. Tourbah A, Lebrun-Frenay C, Edan G, Clanet M, Papeix C, Vukusic S, et al. MD1003 (high-dose biotin) for the treatment of progressive multiple sclerosis: a randomized, double-blind, placebo-controlled study. Mult Scler. 2016;22(13):1719–31.
16. Evans E, Piccio L, Cross AH. Use of vitamins and dietary supplements by patients with multiple sclerosis: a review. JAMA Neurol. 2018;75(8):1013–21. https://doi.org/10.1001/jamaneurol.2018.0611.
17. Soleymani T, Lo Sicco K, Shapiro J. The infatuation with biotin supplementation: is there truth behind its rising popularity? A comparative analysis of clinical efficacy versus social popularity. J Drugs Dermatol. 2017;16(5):496–500.
18. Clevidence BA, Marshall MW, Canary JJ. Biotin levels in plasma and urine of healthy adults consuming physiological doses of biotin. Nutr Res. 1988;8(10):1109–18.
19. Grimsey P, Frey N, Bendig G, Zitzler J, Lorenz O, Kasapic D, et al. Population pharmacokinetics of exogenous biotin and the

relationship between biotin serum levels and in vitro immunoassay interference. Int J Pharm. 2017;2(4):247–56.
20. Wilchek M, Bayer EA. Avidin-biotin mediated immunoassays: an overview. Methods Enzymol. 1990;184:467–9.
21. Diamandis EP, Christopoulos TK. The biotin-(strept) avidin system: principles and applications in biotechnology. Clin Chem. 1991;37(5):625–36.
22. Piketty ML, Polak M, Flechtner I, Gonzales-Briceno L, Souberbielle JC. False biochemical diagnosis of hyperthyroidism in streptavidin-biotin-based immunoassays: the problem of biotin intake and related interferences. Clin Chem Lab Med. 2017;55(6):780–8.
23. Li D, Radulescu A, Shrestha RT, Root M, Karger AB, Killeen AA, et al. Association of biotin ingestion with performance of hormone and nonhormone assays in healthy adults. JAMA. 2017;318(12):1150–60.

# Chapter 7
# Help, My Metabolism Is Low!

**Sean J. Iwamoto and Marc-Andre Cornier**

## Case

A 38-year-old woman with a history of hypothyroidism and obesity comes to the primary care clinic for her annual physical exam and exclaims, "Help, my metabolism low!" Her weight has been steadily increasing over the last 20 years. A couple of months ago, her male friend suggested they "get healthy" and try to lose weight together. They are using a mobile application to track calories and physical activity. In

---

S. J. Iwamoto (✉)
Division of Endocrinology, Metabolism & Diabetes, University of Colorado School of Medicine, Anschutz Medical Campus, Aurora, CO, USA

Division of Endocrinology, Rocky Mountain Regional VA Medical Center, VA Eastern Colorado Health Care System,
Aurora, CO, USA
e-mail: sean.iwamoto@cuanschutz.edu

M.-A. Cornier
Division of Endocrinology, Metabolism & Diabetes, University of Colorado School of Medicine, Anschutz Medical Campus, Aurora, CO, USA

CU Anschutz Health and Wellness Center, University of Colorado School of Medicine, Anschutz Medical Campus, Aurora, CO, USA

© Springer Nature Switzerland AG 2019
M. T. McDermott (ed.), *Management of Patients with Pseudo-Endocrine Disorders*,
https://doi.org/10.1007/978-3-030-22720-3_7

the last month, she has focused on portion sizes and eating more low-carb and low-fat foods. She is jogging 30 minutes 3–4 days per week and recently started a weight lifting regimen 2 days per week and barre workouts 1 day per week. Even though the patient and her friend are doing similar activities, her friend has lost 8 lb. (3.6 kg) but she has not lost any weight yet. She is increasingly frustrated with herself and blames her metabolism.

The woman continues to have regular monthly periods. She takes levothyroxine and an oral contraceptive pill daily. She denies taking any supplements or herbs. She has no family history of heart disease, diabetes, or cancer, but both of her parents have obesity.

On physical examination, her weight is 173 lb. (78.5 kg) and height is 62 inches (157.5 cm) (body mass index, BMI = 31.6 kg/m$^2$). She is afebrile with a heart rate of 72 beats/min and blood pressure of 126/78 mmHg. Her abdominal circumference is 36 inches (91.4 cm). She has no thyromegaly or Cushingoid features. The rest of her examination is also unremarkable.

Laboratory test results:

- TSH = 1.6 mIU/L
- Hemoglobin A1c = 5.6%
- Pregnancy test = Negative

# Discussion

## Evaluation

Up to 70% of human obesity and the inter-individual variation in body weight may be inherited predominantly in a polygenic fashion [1, 2]. Secondary causes of obesity are very rare, and a thorough history and physical exam can help raise or lower suspicion for one of those causes. A pregnancy test should be obtained in all females of reproductive age. A list of medications should be examined for the use of any that are associated with weight gain such as glucocorticoids, diabetes medications (e.g., insulin, thiazolidinediones, sulfonylureas), first- and second-generation antipsychotics, antidepressants, other mood stabilizers, and progestins. Aside from measuring a serum TSH, particularly in someone with a history of hypothyroidism and/or taking thyroid hormone replacement, screening for other endocrine disorders (e.g., hypothalamic obesity, Cushing's syndrome, polycystic ovarian syndrome, hypogonadism, growth hormone deficiency or pseudohypoparathyroidism) should only be performed if clinical suspicion is high based on the patient's history and physical exam. On the other hand, evaluation of obesity-related comorbidities or diseases should include fasting glucose and/or hemoglobin A1C for prediabetes and diabetes, liver-associated enzymes for nonalcoholic fatty liver disease, blood pressure for hypertension, and fasting lipids for dyslipidemia [3, 4]. As overweight and obesity are associated with about 40% of all cancers diagnosed and rates are higher among females and those aged ≥50 years, sex- and age-appropriate cancer screenings need to be addressed [5]. Other comorbid conditions, which can be identified by history and physical exam, include obstructive sleep apnea, osteoarthritis, and depression to name a few.

## *"Low Metabolism"*

The observation that many people fail to lose weight despite reports of calorie restriction led to the hypothesis that obesity is related to lower rates of energy expenditure or hypometabolism. However, data from studies analyzing 24-hour energy expenditure measured by indirect calorimetry in the 1980s–1990s were conflicting [6–8]. A review of studies since then sheds light on the concepts that people with obesity, in fact, have higher absolute resting energy expenditure (REE) and total daily energy expenditure (TDEE) compared to those with normal weight, and that controlling for fat-free mass (the metabolically active component) suggests that these values are similar between patients with obesity and normal-weight individuals [9]. A review of studies assessing physical activity-related energy expenditure (PAEE) in people with or without obesity revealed that those with obesity have higher PAEE, but may perform less activity than those without obesity [10]. On the other hand, a small reduced thermic effect of food may be related to obesity-associated insulin resistance and reduced sympathetic nervous system activity [11]. It must also be emphasized, however, that while REE and body mass (fat-free mass [FFM] and fat mass [FM]) are highly correlated in women (FFM $r = 0.65$ and FM $r = 0.63$, both $P < 0.001$) and men (FFM $r = 0.62$ and FM $r = 0.48$, both $P < 0.001$), there is clear variability in REE for a given body mass, with FFM accounting for 60–85% of the inter-individual variability in REE [12].

## Genetics and Epigenetics

As mentioned above, up to 70% of the variation in body weight may be inherited and primarily in a polygenic fashion. Monogenic causes of obesity, on the other hand, account for a very small proportion of obesity and involve single-gene mutations in corticotropin-releasing hormone receptors 1 and 2, G-protein-coupled receptor 24, leptin, leptin receptor, melanocortin 3 and 4 receptors, neurotrophic tyrosine kinase receptor type 2, proopiomelanocortin, proprotein convertase subtilisin/kexin type 1, and single-minded homolog 1 [13]. Large-scale genome-wide association studies (GWAS) have identified over 300 loci for obesity traits including adiposity, BMI, and the waist-to-hip ratio [1]. The *FTO* locus has the largest, but still small, effect on obesity susceptibility; each risk allele increases the risk of obesity by 1.20–1.32-fold, and BMI by 0.37 kg/m$^2$. Nonetheless, all known BMI-associated genetic variants account for <5% of the variation in BMI. More studies are being published about the associative role of epigenetic processes (e.g., DNA methylation, histone modification, and non-coding RNAs that switch genes on/off without changing the DNA sequence) on obesity susceptibility. Future studies may help to clarify if causal roles are uncovered.

Chapter 7. Help, My Metabolism Is Low! 81

## *Energy Balance (or Energy Homeostasis)*

Weight stability occurs when total daily energy intake equals TDEE. Weight gain results from the imbalance (i.e., more energy intake than expenditure) over time of these two components (See Fig. 7.1). TDEE is linearly related to lean body mass, yet people with obesity consume more calories than lean people because high caloric intake is required to maintain the state of obesity. Even though patients, like the one in this case, say they are monitoring calories or eating smaller portions, gaining or remaining the same weight is indicative that they are still having a higher or equal energy intake as compared to their TDEE. Overweight and obesity are associated with significant under-reporting of energy intake which may contribute to the energy imbalance.

Energy intake is regulated by a complex interaction of physiologic inputs from neurologic and endocrine signals, gut microbiota, external stress, emotional factors, and certain

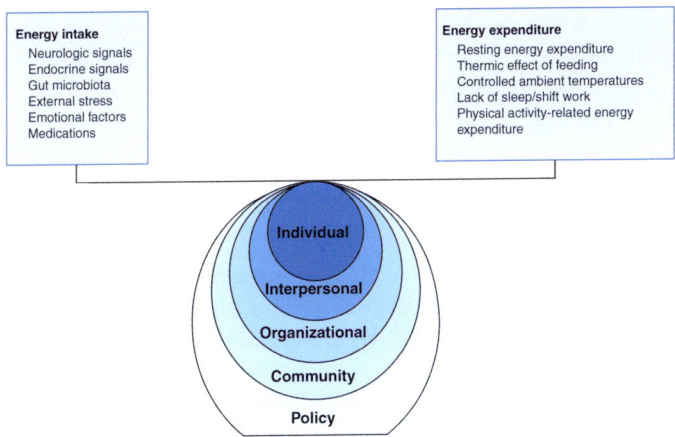

FIGURE 7.1 Using the social-ecological model to demonstrate the complex interrelationship of personal and environmental factors on energy balance. (Adapted with permission: Gonzalez-Muniesa et al. [1]. Publisher: Springer Nature)

medications (e.g., antidepressants and glucocorticoids). Complex molecular signaling allows for communication between adipose tissue, skeletal muscle, the gastrointestinal tract (including the liver and pancreas), and the central nervous system. There appear to be alterations in the physiologic regulation of energy intake in individuals with and at risk of obesity, including resistance to peripheral hormones such as leptin. Energy expenditure is comprised of REE (i.e., basal metabolic rate [BMR]), thermic effect of feeding, controlled ambient temperatures, lack of sleep or shift work, and PAEE. The BMR is the amount of energy required to maintain homeostasis of the body's temperature, electrolytes, and the cardiopulmonary system [14]. The thermic effect of feeding represents about 5–10% of energy expenditure. Physical activity-related energy expenditure is the most variable component of TDEE as it can be 10–20% in sedentary people or up to 60–80% in training athletes. Planned physical activity and activities of daily living will increase PAEE. Reduced PAEE may also increase the risk of obesity by offsetting the energy balance in favor of energy intake. On the contrary, people with obesity do not have reduced BMR or "low metabolism." Their excess caloric intake is stored as adipose tissue, which is the primary source of fuel during periods of energy deficit.

## *Management*

Our patient has obesity as defined by a BMI of $\geq 30.0$ kg/m$^2$ and deserves acknowledgment for her efforts to lose weight and improve her health. Independent of her weight, following a healthy dietary pattern and an active lifestyle is associated with better overall health and wellness. This must be emphasized. It is not productive to simply accuse her of eating more than she thinks, but rather she should be educated on the complexities of how a decrease in energy intake and/or increase in energy expenditure are necessary for weight loss. Primary care approaches to weight loss utilizing motivational interviewing and the "5 A's" framework for behavioral change counseling (i.e., assess, advise, agree, assist, arrange) may help providers maximize their impact on obesity treatment but more controlled studies on outcomes are needed [15, 16]. Recently, a structured "ABCDEF" framework for weight counseling in primary care was proposed: Ask "permission," Be systematic in the clinical workup, Counseling and support, Determine health status, Escalate treatment when appropriate, and Follow up regularly and leverage available resources [17]. As mentioned above, it is advised that cardiovascular disease risk factors and obesity-related comorbidities be evaluated and discussed. Weight loss can be very difficult for patients and it is important for providers to understand patients' motivation for weight loss and support realistic expectations. Health benefits can be seen with 3–5% sustained weight loss and cardiovascular risk reduction can be attributed to 5–10% weight loss. However, these percent weight losses associated with health benefits may feel insignificant to patients when compared to their individual weight loss goals.

Several tools exist to help patients lose weight, including comprehensive lifestyle intervention programs (e.g., Diabetes Prevention Program or MOVE! Weight Management Program [Veterans Health Administration]), commercial weight loss programs, meal replacements, and pharmacotherapy (if BMI $\geq$ 30.0 kg/m$^2$, or a BMI of 27.0–29.9 kg/m$^2$ with at least one obesity-related comorbidity). Bariatric surgery can also be offered (if BMI $\geq$ 40.0 kg/m$^2$, or BMI $\geq$ 35.0 kg/m$^2$ with at least one obesity-related comorbidity, or possibly if BMI is 30.0–34.9 kg/m$^2$ with diabetes or metabolic syndrome) [18]. There are also emerging data on the impact of endoscopic bariatric therapies for weight loss [19].

## *Calorie Restriction and Diet Composition*

To achieve weight loss, a patient needs to create a calorie deficit through dietary modification (i.e., calorie restriction), physical activity, or a combination of the two. Despite tracking calories via mobile applications, it has been previously shown that patients with obesity under-report their caloric intake (and over-report physical activity) [20]. Calorie prescriptions of approximately 1200–1500 kcal/day for women and 1500–1800 kcal/day for men may help some patients achieve their goal of >500 kcal/day deficit for weight loss. Alternatively, the Harris–Benedict equation can estimate TDEE (based on height, weight, age, gender, and activity level) from which a calorie prescription can be developed. Despite trying to eat more low-carb and low-fat foods, our patient needs to realize that a specific macronutrient composition of her diet will not increase her weight loss in the setting of calorie restriction. Additionally, the low-carb and low-fat diets she reports eating may not be getting her to the required calorie deficit for weight loss. It is noteworthy that high rates of weight regain exist in those who achieve even a modest 5–10% weight loss with guideline-recommended caloric restriction and comprehensive behavioral modification.

Alternative dietary interventions such as intermittent fasting (including alternate-day fasting [ADF]) and time restricted feeding (TRF) are being studied for their potential weight loss and overall health benefits. ADF involves the "fast day" (0–25% of caloric needs) alternating with the "fed day" (ad libitum food consumption) and may reduce diabetes and cardiovascular disease risk. TRF consists of restricting feeding to only certain periods of the day. A recent 8-week randomized pilot study in patients with obesity demonstrated that a zero-calorie ADF was safe and, compared to traditional caloric restriction, produced similar weight loss ($-8.2 \pm 0.9$ vs. $-7.1 \pm 1.0$ kg) and was not associated with a significant difference in weight regain at 24 weeks [21]. A 12-week, 8-hr TRF intervention (ad libitum feeding between 10:00 AM and 6:00 PM, water fasting between 6:00 PM and 10:00 AM) demonstrated significant decreases in body weight ($-2.6 \pm 0.5\%$, $P < 0.05$), energy intake and systolic blood pressure compared to matched historical controls [22]. Studies of longer duration are being performed but need to be completed to better understand whether these interventions are viable long-term treatment options.

Guidelines recommend increased aerobic physical activity (e.g., brisk walking) for >150 min/week for weight loss and 200–300 min/week to maintain weight loss or minimize weight regain at 1 year [3]. Although our patient should be advised to increase her amount of aerobic physical activity by an additional 30–60 min/week, dietary modification through calorie restriction will most effectively create the calorie deficit needed for weight loss and should be advised.

## *"Can You Prescribe Something to Boost My Metabolism and Help Me Lose Weight?"*

Even if our patient has a relatively low metabolism, we do not currently have safe treatments to increase the metabolic rate. Although body weight modestly decreases following treatment of hypothyroidism (and increases following treatment for hyperthyroidism), giving thyroid hormone to euthyroid patients with obesity has not been shown to impact weight loss in small, short-term studies of T3 and/or T4 regimens, but may risk causing subclinical hyperthyroidism [23, 24], which can increase the risk of developing atrial fibrillation and osteoporosis. Methylphenidate, classically used to treat attention deficit hyperactivity disorder and narcolepsy, increases REE and postprandial energy expenditure but should not be used in patients without these neuropsychiatric disorders [25].

We have FDA-approved anti-obesity medications (in addition to endoscopic and bariatric procedures) for those who qualify based on BMI ± weight-related comorbidities as discussed above [26]. These should be prescribed when indicated and as an adjunct to behavioral/lifestyle interventions. In this case, our patient could be trialed with anti-obesity pharmacotherapy given her BMI $\geq 30.0$ kg/m$^2$. These medications regulate appetite and energy expenditure through various mechanisms: sympathomimetics (e.g., phentermine,

phentermine-topiramate ER), GABA receptor activation (phentermine-topiramate ER), serotonin (5-HT2C) receptor agonist (e.g., lorcaserin), opioid antagonist + dopamine-norepinephrine reuptake inhibitor (e.g., naltrexone-bupropion), and GLP-1 receptor agonist (e.g., liraglutide). Orlistat, which inhibits pancreatic and gastric lipase, produces more modest weight loss and significant gastrointestinal side effects.

There are non-prescription compounds touted in the lay literature as being "metabolism boosters." Caffeine has been shown to increase energy expenditure and decrease energy intake, but not consistently, and there are suggested sex/gender and BMI-related differences in the metabolism and energy effects of caffeine that need further investigation [27]. A meta-analysis of small, short-term (as few as just a single meal intervention) studies of capsaicinoids (e.g., chili peppers) showed an overall reduction in energy intake, but there was high study heterogeneity and the larger, longer studies of 4–6 weeks duration did not show significant change in energy intake [28].

Patient education and engagement are key to establishing a good provider-patient relationship. Understanding patients' concerns about and overall goals for their weight is important in order to dispel myths and make evidence-based management decisions to balance harms with benefits when it comes to weight loss.

**Take-Home Points**
1. Most of the inter-individual variation in body weight may be inherited (polygenic); monogenic causes of obesity are very rare.
2. People with obesity have higher absolute resting energy expenditure (REE) and total daily energy expenditure (TDEE) compared to those with normal weight but controlling for fat-free mass (the metabolically active component) causes these values to

become similar between patients with obesity and normal-weight individuals. Also, for a given body mass, there is significant variability in REE among individuals.
3. Weight stability occurs when total daily energy intake equals TDEE; weight gain is the result of higher energy intake than expenditure.
4. To achieve weight loss, a patient needs to create a calorie deficit through dietary modification (i.e., calorie restriction), physical activity, or a combination of the two; however, patients often under-report their calorie intake.
5. FDA-approved anti-obesity medications (in addition to endoscopic and bariatric procedures) exist for those who qualify based on BMI ± weight-related comorbidities. Avoid prescribing other medications or over-the-counter supplements ("metabolism boosters") for weight loss, as long-term data on safety and efficacy are lacking.

## References

1. Gonzalez-Muniesa P, et al. Obesity. Nat Rev Dis Primers. 2017;3:17034.
2. Levin BE. Developmental gene x environment interactions affecting systems regulating energy homeostasis and obesity. Front Neuroendocrinol. 2010;31(3):270–83.
3. Jensen MD, et al. 2013 AHA/ACC/TOS guideline for the management of overweight and obesity in adults: a report of the American College of Cardiology/American Heart Association Task Force on Practice Guidelines and The Obesity Society. J Am Coll Cardiol. 2014;63(25 Pt B):2985–3023.
4. Tsai AG, Wadden TA. In the clinic: obesity. Ann Intern Med. 2013;159(5):ITC3–1-ITC3-15; quiz ITC3-16.
5. Steele CB, et al. Vital signs: trends in incidence of cancers associated with overweight and obesity - United States, 2005-2014. MMWR Morb Mortal Wkly Rep. 2017;66(39):1052–8.

6. Ravussin E, et al. Twenty-four-hour energy expenditure and resting metabolic rate in obese, moderately obese, and control subjects. Am J Clin Nutr. 1982;35(3):566–73.
7. Ravussin E, et al. Reduced rate of energy expenditure as a risk factor for body-weight gain. N Engl J Med. 1988;318(8):467–72.
8. Skov AR, et al. Normal levels of energy expenditure in patients with reported "low metabolism". Clin Physiol. 1997;17(3):279–85.
9. Carneiro IP, et al. Is obesity associated with altered energy expenditure. Adv Nutr. 2016;7(3):476–87.
10. Westerterp KR. Impacts of vigorous and non-vigorous activity on daily energy expenditure. Proc Nutr Soc. 2003;62(3):645–50.
11. de Jonge L, Bray GA. The thermic effect of food and obesity: a critical review. Obes Res. 1997;5(6):622–31.
12. Nielsen S, et al. Body composition and resting energy expenditure in humans: role of fat, fat-free mass, and extracellular fluid. Int J Obes Relat Metab Disord. 2000;24(9):1153–7.
13. Rankinen T, et al. The human obesity gene map: the 2005 update. Obesity (Silver Spring). 2006;14(4):529–644.
14. Melmed S, et al. Williams textbook of endocrinology. Philadelphia: Elsevier; 2016. p. xviii, 1916 pages
15. Barnes RD, Ivezaj V. A systematic review of motivational interviewing for weight loss among adults in primary care. Obes Rev. 2015;16(4):304–18.
16. Kahan S, Wilson DK, Sweeney AM. The role of behavioral medicine in the treatment of obesity in primary care. Med Clin North Am. 2018;102(1):125–33.
17. Kahan S., Manson JE. Obesity treatment, beyond the guidelines: practical suggestions for clinical practice. JAMA. 2019;321(14):1349–50.
18. Mechanick JI, et al. Clinical practice guidelines for the perioperative nutritional, metabolic, and nonsurgical support of the bariatric surgery patient--2013 update: cosponsored by American Association of Clinical Endocrinologists, the Obesity Society, and American Society for Metabolic & Bariatric Surgery. Obesity (Silver Spring). 2013;21(Suppl 1):S1–27.
19. Force ABET, et al. ASGE position statement on endoscopic bariatric therapies in clinical practice. Gastrointest Endosc. 2015;82(5):767–72.
20. Lichtman SW, et al. Discrepancy between self-reported and actual caloric intake and exercise in obese subjects. N Engl J Med. 1992;327(27):1893–8.

21. Catenacci VA, et al. A randomized pilot study comparing zero-calorie alternate-day fasting to daily caloric restriction in adults with obesity. Obesity (Silver Spring). 2016;24(9):1874–83.
22. Gabel K, et al. Effects of 8-hour time-restricted feeding on body weight and metabolic disease risk factors in obese adults: a pilot study. Nutr Healthy Aging. 2018;4(4):345–53.
23. Kaptein EM, Beale E, Chan LS. Thyroid hormone therapy for obesity and nonthyroidal illnesses: a systematic review. J Clin Endocrinol Metab. 2009;94(10):3663–75.
24. Pearce EN. Thyroid hormone and obesity. Curr Opin Endocrinol Diabetes Obes. 2012;19(5):408–13.
25. Lorello C, Goldfield GS, Doucet E. Methylphenidate hydrochloride increases energy expenditure in healthy adults. Obesity (Silver Spring). 2008;16(2):470–2.
26. Bessesen DH, Van Gaal LF. Progress and challenges in anti-obesity pharmacotherapy. Lancet Diabetes Endocrinol. 2018;6(3):237–48.
27. Harpaz E, et al. The effect of caffeine on energy balance. J Basic Clin Physiol Pharmacol. 2017;28(1):1–10.
28. Whiting S, Derbyshire EJ, Tiwari B. Could capsaicinoids help to support weight management? A systematic review and meta-analysis of energy intake data. Appetite. 2014;73:183–8.

# Chapter 8
# Idiopathic Postprandial Syndrome

**Helen M. Lawler**

## Case

A 42-year-old woman has been experiencing episodes of tremulousness, palpitations, diaphoresis, headache, and mental fogginess which occur a few hours after meals. She recently had these symptoms about 2 hours after eating watermelon and sugar cookies. A glucometer was given to her and she documented blood glucose readings of 65 mg/dL, 110 mg/dL, and 85 mg/dL during these episodes. She underwent a mixed meal tolerance test that was normal.

---

H. M. Lawler (✉)
University of Colorado School of Medicine, Division of Endocrinology, Metabolism, and Diabetes, Aurora, CO, USA
e-mail: helen.lawler@cuanschutz.edu

PMHx: GERD  Meds: omeprazole, multivitamin

PE:   BP 125/80,  P 85,  Ht 5'5"  Wt 130 lb

   Complete exam – normal

Labs: TSH 1.5 mU/L (nl: 0.45–4.5)

   Normal 24-hour urine fractionated metanephrines and catecholamines

   Normal CMP with glucose of 80 mg/dL

## Questions

- What are typical hypoglycemic symptoms?
- How do we evaluate hypoglycemic symptoms?
- What causes hypoglycemia in nondiabetic individuals?
- How do we help our patient feel better?

## Comments

Hypoglycemia can cause both neurogenic (or autonomic) and neuroglycopenic symptoms. Neurogenic symptoms include adrenergic signs (palpitations, anxiety, tremulousness) and cholinergic signs (diaphoresis, hunger, paresthesias) [1]. Neuroglycopenic symptoms include fatigue, confusion, behavioral change, and loss of consciousness [1]. In healthy individuals, hypoglycemic symptoms often develop at a mean plasma glucose concentration of approximately 55 mg/dL (3.0 mmol/L). Yet, the threshold for experiencing symptoms occurs at lower plasma glucose concentrations in patients with recurrent hypoglycemia. Also, many healthy individuals do not experience symptoms even with lower plasma glucose concentrations. Thus, a diagnosis of hypoglycemia in a nondiabetic individual is defined by the presence of Whipple's triad [2]: (1) Hypoglycemic symptoms, (2) While symptoms are occurring, documented hypoglycemia, (3) Resolution of hypoglycemic symptoms with euglycemia. A normal initial physiologic response to declining blood glucose is a decrease in insulin secretion. Other counter-regulatory hormones, including glucagon and epinephrine, increase in response to hypoglycemia. Although not present acutely, cortisol and growth hormone provide a delayed counter-regulatory response to hypoglycemia.

If unable to capture labs during the outpatient setting, patients who have Whipple's triad should undergo a 72-hour fast to evaluate for an insulinoma which causes hyperinsulinemic hypoglycemia. During a 72-hour fast, plasma glucose is monitored closely and insulin, c-peptide, proinsulin, β-hydroxybutyrate, and a screen for circulating oral hypoglycemic agents are obtained if hypoglycemia occurs. Hyperinsulinemic hypoglycemia is characterized by glucose <55 mg/dL, insulin ≥3 µU/mL, c-peptide ≥0.2 nmol/L, and proinsulin ≥5 pmol/L [3]. If hypoglycemia occurs, before concluding the 72-hour fast, 1 mg of glucagon is given intravenously and glucose is measured 10, 20, and 30 minutes after the injection. If an insulinoma is present, a glucose rise of ≥25 mg/dL (1.4 mmol/L) is anticipated. This is because elevated insulin levels inhibit hepatic glycogenolysis and conserve liver glycogen stores. Administration of glucagon causes the release of glucose from the preserved hepatic glycogen stores [3]. Besides an insulinoma, hyperinsulinemic hypoglycemia can also occur with post-bariatric hypoglycemia (PBH), non-insulinoma pancreatogenous hypoglycemia syndrome (NIPHS), insulin autoimmune hypoglycemia, insulin administration, and sulfonylurea or meglitinide use (Table 8.1) [3]. Yet, patients with PBH and NIPHS usually only experience postprandial hypoglycemia and the 72-hour fast is negative.

Hypoglycemia with low insulin levels can occur with severe liver disease, critical illness, starvation, alcohol use, adrenal insufficiency (due to hypopituitarism, Addison's disease, or congenital adrenal hyperplasia), glycogen storage disease or other hepatic enzyme defects, non-islet cell tumors, or Jamaican vomiting sickness due to consumption of an unripe ackee fruit (Table 8.1) [3]. Certain medications have also been reported to cause hypoglycemia including tramadol, indomethacin, pentamidine, quinolones, quinine, angiotensin-converting enzyme inhibitors, and beta blockers [4, 5].

TABLE 8.1 Causes of hypoglycemia

| Hyperinsulinemic hypoglycemia | Noninsulin-mediated hypoglycemia |
|---|---|
| Insulinoma | Critical illness (sepsis; hepatic, renal, heart failure) |
| Noninsulinoma pancreatogeneous hypoglycemia (NIPHS) | Starvation |
| Post-bariatric hypoglycemia (PBH) | Alcohol |
| Exogenous insulin | Glycogen storage diseases or other hepatic enzyme defects |
| Insulin secretagogue (sulfonylurea, etc.) | Adrenal insufficiency |
| Insulin autoimmune (antibody to insulin or insulin receptor) | Non-islet cell tumors |
| Factitious hypoglycemia (via insulin or insulin secretagogue administration) | Consumption of unripe ackee fruit (Jamaican vomiting sickness) |
| Nondiabetic drugs | Nondiabetic drugs |

Patients with postprandial hypoglycemic symptoms are often told they have reactive hypoglycemia or postprandial hypoglycemia. Yet, reactive or postprandial hypoglycemia is a nonspecific term referring to hypoglycemia (glucose <55 mg/dL) that occurs up to 4 hours after a meal [6]. This terminology is purely a description of the timing of a hypoglycemic event and an evaluation for a possible etiology should be pursued. NIPHS and post-bariatric hypoglycemia occur primarily postprandially. Yet, postprandial hypoglycemia can also occur with insulinoma and the other causes of hypoglycemia listed in Table 8.1 [3]. Thus, the timing of the hypoglycemia in relation to meals is not always a reliable indicator of the etiology.

There are also reports of reactive hypoglycemia occurring as a consequence of upper gastrointestinal surgery including gastrectomy, gastroenterostomy, or vagotomy and pyloroplasty [7]. Yet, many of these studies used the discredited oral glucose tolerance test to diagnose hypoglycemia. An oral glucose tolerance test (OGTT) is not recommended as part of the evaluation for hypoglycemia as hypoglycemia occurs at similar percentages in patients with hypoglycemic symptoms and asymptomatic control patients [8]. In addition, there is speculation that reactive hypoglycemia may occur in patients with early insulin resistance from type 2 diabetes mellitus. The proposed mechanism is that hypoglycemia results from a robust insulin response to a rapid rise in plasma glucose after glucose ingestion. Yet, studies are needed to further investigate this theory.

In patients with a history suggestive of postprandial hypoglycemia, a mixed meal tolerance test (MMTT) is recommended. During the MMTT, the patient consumes a solid or liquid meal that usually provokes symptoms and is then observed for up to 5 hours. Plasma glucose, insulin, proinsulin, and c-peptide levels are obtained at baseline and every 30 minutes for 5 hours.

In conclusion, idiopathic postprandial syndrome refers to hypoglycemic symptoms that occur without chemical evidence of hypoglycemia. Once other etiologies for hypoglycemic symptoms are excluded such as hyperthyroidism, pheochromocytoma, and migraines, then it would be appropriate to identify hypoglycemic symptoms without chemical hypoglycemia (and thus, absent Whipple's triad) as idiopathic postprandial syndrome. This terminology was created to replace the obsolete and confusing "functional hypoglycemia" terminology and to avoid the negative connotation of "pseudohypoglycemia." In addition, "pseudohypoglycemia" has been used in the literature to describe a disparity in actual versus measured plasma or capillary glucose levels [9]. Frequently, underlying anxiety, neuropsychiatric disease, or situational stress reactions are the real culprits of idiopathic postprandial syndrome which the patient characterizes or self-diagnoses as reactive hypoglycemia [10].

## Discussion with Patient

***Honesty*** "Since your blood sugar is normal during these episodes, it is unlikely that your symptoms are due to hypoglycemia. Also, I have completed all of the appropriate tests for other endocrine problems that could cause your symptoms and have not found an endocrine disorder."

***Encouragement*** "While we did not find an endocrine cause for your symptoms, the good news is your test results did not reveal any serious condition. I have had some other patients with similar symptoms have an improvement in their episodes with lifestyle modification."

***Compassion*** "I hope that your symptoms will resolve soon with healthy lifestyle measures. I am certainly willing to pursue further testing if new symptoms develop. We can also repeat testing in the future if indicated."

## Recommendations

Patients with idiopathic postprandial syndrome are often provided with the same recommendations for dietary modifications as those given to patients with reactive hypoglycemia due to gastric bypass surgery. They are advised to eat small frequent meals that are high in protein and fiber and to avoid simple sugars. In addition, regular exercise, adequate sleep, and other lifestyle changes to reduce stress are recommended. Screening for depression with referral for treatment, if present, is also important. Although there is little data to support using an alpha-glucosidase inhibitor such as acarbose in patients with idiopathic postprandial syndrome, a trial could be initiated to see if reducing carbohydrate absorption, and thus, blunting the insulin response to food helps alleviate symptoms [11].

# References

1. Cryer PE. Minimizing hypoglycemia in diabetes. Diabetes Care. 2015;38(3):1583–91.
2. Whipple AO. The surgical therapy of hyperinsulinism. J Int Chir. 1938;3:237.
3. Cryer PE, Axelrod L, Grossman AB, Heller SR, Montori VM, Seaquist ER, Service FJ. Evaluation and management of adult hypoglycemic disorders: an Endocrine Society clinical practice guideline. J Clin Endocrinol Metab. 2009;94(3):709–28.
4. Murad MH, Coto Yglesias F, Wang AT, Mullan RJ, Elamin M, Sheidaee N, Erwin PJ, Montori VM. Drug-induced hypoglycemia: a systematic review. J Clin Endocrinol Metab. 2009;94:741–5.
5. Golightly LK, Simendinger BA, Barber GR, Stolpman NM, Kick SD, McDermott MT. Hypoglycemic effects of tramadol analgesia in hospitalized patients: a case-control study. J Diabetes Metab Disord. 2017;16:30.
6. Brun JF, Fedou C, Mercier J. Postprandial reactive hypoglycemia. Diabetes Metab. 2000;26(5):337–51.
7. Kurihara K, Tamai A, Yoshida Y, Yakushiji Y, Ueno H, Fukumoto M, Hosoi M. Effectiveness of sitagliptin in a patient with late dumping syndrome after total gastrectomy. Diabetes Metab Syndr. 2018;12:203–6.
8. Charles MA, Hofeldt F, Shackelford A, Waldeck N, Dodson LE Jr, Bunker D, Coggins JT, Eichner H. Comparison of oral glucose tolerance tests and mixed meals in patients with apparent idiopathic postabsorptive hypoglycemia: absence of hypoglycemia after meals. Diabetes. 1981;30(6):465–70.
9. Lee KT, Abadir PM. Failure of glucose monitoring in an individual with pseudohypoglycemia. J Am Geriatr Soc. 2015;63(8):1706–8.
10. Berlin I, Grimaldi A, Landault C, Cesselin F, Puech AJ. Suspected postprandial hypoglycemia is associated with beta-adrenergic hypersensitivity and emotional distress. J Clin Endocrinol Metab. 1994;79(5):1428–33.
11. Ozgen AG, Hamulu F, Bayraktar F, Cetínkalp S, Yilmaz C, Túzún M, Kabalak T. Long-term treatment with acarbose for the treatment of reactive hypoglycemia. Eat Weight Disord. 1998;3(3):136.

# Chapter 9
# Pseudohypoglycemia

**Fadi Aboona, Sulmaz Zahedi, and S. Sethu K. Reddy**

The discovery of insulin and other hypoglycemic agents and the ability to measure glucose accurately has led to concern and delineation of hypoglycemic syndromes [1–3]. In this short overview of the clinical phenomenon of pseudohypoglycemia, we hope to provide a framework for approaching these patients.

## Illustrative Cases

*Case 1:* A patient presents with symptoms of fatigue to an ambulatory center. She has documented myasthenia gravis and Raynaud's phenomenon. A capillary glucose level is found to be low at 40 mg/dL. She is then investigated for fasting hypoglycemia. During the fast, capillary glucose levels were checked and found to be in the 35–40 mg/dL range. Of note, venous plasma glucose levels were 80–90 mg/dL. A diagnosis of pseudohypoglycemia secondary to poor peripheral circulation due to the patient's Raynaud's phenomenon was made [4].

*Case 2:* A 24-year-old African-American female comes to the Emergency department complaining of fatigue, lethargy, reduced exercise tolerance, and syncope. She has a history of multiple syncope events throughout her life and these have recently increased. She was advised to keep herself hydrated and was counseled on performing certain maneuvers such as leg crossing and hand gripping to increase blood pressure and reduce the likelihood of syncope. A capillary blood glucose was measured as part of the routine medical evaluation in the Emergency department and was in the 35–40 mg/dL range (normal >70 mg/dL). However, her plasma glucose was found to be in the normal range. She did not experience any symptoms related to hypoglycemia such as sweating, shakiness, and hunger. She was started on a Dextrose 10% infusion. An abnormal ECG led to an echocardiogram demonstrating a left-to-right cardiac shunt confirming the diagnosis of Eisenmenger syndrome. The diagnosis of pseudohypoglycemia secondary to increased capillary extraction of glucose peripherally [5] was made.

*Case 3:* A patient with uncontrolled type 2 diabetes with an HbA1c of 13% is placed on insulin therapy and the blood sugars are now in the 150–250 mg/dL range compared to the baseline range of 250–400 mg/dL. During the follow-up visit in 4 weeks, the patient complains of hunger, sweating, and tachycardia when his glucose levels drop to near 130 mg/dL. Symptoms seem to be resolved with glucose ingestion. The patient is anxious about increasing insulin doses further.

TABLE 9.1 Classification of pseudohypoglycemia

|  | **Pseudohypoglycemia type 1 (PHG-1)** | **Pseudohypoglycemia type 2 (PHG-2)** |
| --- | --- | --- |
| Symptoms of hypoglycemia | Adrenergic > neurogenic | No symptoms |
| Glucose levels | >70 mg/dL | <70 mg/dL |
| Etiologies | Relative hypoglycemia in patients with diabetes mellitus | Poor peripheral circulation |
|  | Postprandial state in some | Increased in vitro glucose consumption |
|  |  | Hyperviscosity |
|  |  | Artifactual glucometer readings |

Pseudohypoglycemia is classically defined as a scenario (similar to Case 3) in which the individual may be displaying symptoms suggestive of hypoglycemia but the plasma glucose levels are greater than 70 mg/dL. We can extend the definition to also include a variation in patients presenting with glucose values below 70 mg/dL but with no symptoms of hypoglycemia. We can title these syndromes as pseudohypoglycemia type 1 (PHG-1) and pseudohypoglycemia type 2 (PHG-2) respectively [6]. See Table 9.1 for clarification of these two subtypes of pseudohypoglycemia.

# Clinical Approach to Patients with Pseudohypoglycemia

The gold standard for hypoglycemia remains the documentation of Whipple's triad (symptoms of hypoglycemia, confirmation of a low blood glucose value, and reversal of the patient's symptoms with glucose administration). Without fulfillment of these criteria, true hypoglycemia is questionable [7].

When should one suspect pseudohypoglycemia [8]? What clinical scenarios have been described in which pseudohypoglycemia is the diagnosis [9]?

With pseudohypoglycemia type 1 (PHG-1), patients may present with nonspecific symptoms such as fatigue, headache, visual disturbances, and lightheadedness. They also may have tremors, increased diaphoresis, or increased heart rate. Some patients may present with neuroglycopenia and complain of slurred speech, confusion, and, rarely, seizures, in which case further workup is required. Since the glucose levels are normal in PHG-1, then true neuroglycopenia should be very unlikely [10]. For patients with PHG-1, the clinician should patiently, gradually reduce the blood glucose levels, giving the body ample time to acclimatize to normal blood glucose levels.

Patients with diabetes can present with primarily adrenergic symptoms of hypoglycemia at relatively higher serum glucose levels during periods of aggressive glucose control [11, 12]. For example, a patient may be accustomed to having hyperglycemia over 300 mg/dL but when the glucose levels improve to approximately 150 mg/dL range, the patient may experience anxiety and adrenergic symptoms [13]. The chronic hyperglycemia alters the "set point" at which hypoglycemic symptoms become apparent. There is no danger of true neuroglycopenia, and the patient's symptoms are relieved with glucose ingestion. As the body acclimatizes to lower blood glucose levels, the patient stops experiencing these symptoms at these relatively high blood glucose levels. This phenomenon is referred to as "pseudohypoglycemia" because the serum glucose may be within normal range despite symptom presentation.

In pseudohypoglycemia type 2 (PHG-2), there are typically no or only vague symptoms. For PHG-2, one must always rule out technical/methodological errors first. Increased glucose utilization or extraction peripherally via erythrocytes or leucocytes must also be considered.

The most common causes are glucose monitoring analytic errors [14]:

1. Decreased capillary flow resulting in increased local extraction and metabolism of glucose: Raynaud phenomena [15],

Acrocyanosis [16], Peripheral vascular disease, Eisenmenger syndrome, Circulatory shock.
2. Increased glycolysis by leucocytes [17] and red blood cells (RBC) when there is a delay in analyzing the blood sample or separating plasma from the blood sample. Blood samples are collected for a variety of reasons and may need to be transported to an outside laboratory. Delays in transportation can lead to biases between glucose meters and laboratory methods due to glycolysis. Erythrocytes metabolize glucose, reducing the glucose concentration in a sample at a rate of 5–7% per hour as long as the serum/plasma remains in contact with the RBC. The rate of glycolysis by leucocytes is even higher, thus having a more dramatic effect on lower values of glucose. Polycythemia can also lower whole blood glucose readings. Normally the RBC glucose is 30% lower than the plasma glucose level. Thus, if the plasma glucose level is 100 mg/dL, and RBC glucose is 70 mg/dL, then the whole blood glucose would be 88 mg/dL. If there is significant erythrocytosis and RBCs make up a larger percentage of the whole blood volume, then the whole blood glucose would be artificially lower.
3. Hyperviscosity syndromes, such as Waldenstrom's macroglobulinemia and monoclonal gammopathies [18], have also been reported to artifactually lead to lower glucose values. One mechanism may be antibody activity of the monoclonal protein against an antigen in the hexokinase reagents. Hyperviscosity may also lead to an altered aqueous component of plasma volume affecting the functional volume and the calculated concentration of glucose [1].
4. Interfering substances on glucose measurement by different glucose meters [19].

   (a) Ascorbic acid (especially high doses used in cancer therapy). High ascorbic acid levels can consume hydrogen peroxide, which can lead to erroneously low glucose readings. On the other hand, ascorbic acid itself can be oxidized at the electrodes leading to a higher glucose reading on meters that use the glucose oxidase method. Understanding this type of interfer-

ence, one should be attentive to inappropriate antihyperglycemic therapy dosing and rely on meters using the hexokinase method.
(b) Vasopressors may reduce peripheral circulation while improving central blood flow and thus lead to falsely lower capillary glucose readings [20].
(c) Mannitol has also been shown to adversely affect capillary glucose measurement and lead to falsely lower values [21].
(d) Acetaminophen is also thought to consume hydrogen peroxide which can lead to falsely lower readings on meters. In contrast, for continuous glucose monitoring (CGM) devices, acetaminophen has been shown to give falsely elevated readings.
(e) High uric acid levels can cause artifactually low glucose readings on meters that use the glucose oxidase method.

Affected patients are often asymptomatic but occasionally may present with nonspecific symptoms such as fatigue, headache, visual disturbances, and lightheadedness. Other patients may present with typical symptoms of neuroglycopenia like slurred speech, confusion, and, rarely, seizures and coma, in which case further workup is required. Clinical correlation and judgment become of utmost importance in such circumstances.

Recommended Evaluation:

- Distinguish between PHG-1 versus PHG-2.
  - Evaluate comorbid conditions that might interfere with capillary glucose readings.
  - Ascertain glucose values from an intravenous sample and compare to a capillary glucose at the same time.
- Evaluate for potential drugs that might interfere with glucose testing.
- Confirm glucose measurement in capillary blood or in venous blood collected in tubes with antiglycolytic agents like sodium fluoride.
- Prompt serum separation and refrigeration of blood samples.

A careful history will determine the etiology of the apparent hypoglycemia in most presentations. Future workup of pseudohypoglycemia will likely involve measurement of interstitial glucose levels with the use of CGM [22–24], which will give the patient added security [25] and for PHG-2, which will not be affected by compromised hand circulation.

# References

1. Macleod JJR. The control of carbohydrate metabolism. Bull Johns Hopkins Hosp. 1934;54:79–139.
2. Cannon WB, Mclver MA, Bliss SW. Studies on the conditions of activity in endocrine glands. XIII. A sympathetic and adrenal mechanism for mobilizing sugar in hypoglycemia. Am J Physiol. 1924;69:46–66.
3. Himwich HE. A review of hypoglycemia, its physiology and pathology, symptomatology, and treatment. Am J Dig Dis. 1944;11(1):1.
4. Dalal BI, Brigden ML. Factitious biochemical measurements resulting from hematologic conditions. Am J Clin Pathol. 2009;131(2):195–204.
5. Theofilogiannakos EK, Giannakoulas G, Ziakas A, Karvounis HI, Styliadis IH. Pseudohypoglycemia in a patient with the Eisenmenger syndrome. Ann Intern Med. 2010;152(6):407.
6. Wang EY, Patrick L, Connor DM. Blind obedience and an unnecessary workup for hypoglycemia: a teachable moment. JAMA Intern Med. 2018;178(2):279–80.
7. Klonoff DC, Alexander Fleming G, Muchmore DB, Frier BM. Hypoglycemia evaluation and reporting in diabetes: importance for the development of new therapies. Diabetes Metab Res Rev. 2017;33(5):e2883.
8. Shaefer C, Hinnen D, Sadler C. Hypoglycemia and diabetes: increased need for awareness. Curr Med Res Opin. 2016;32(9):1479–86.
9. Rushakoff RJ, Lewis SB. Case of pseudohypoglycemia. Diabetes Care. 2001;24(12):2157–8.
10. Khoury M, Yousuf F, Martin V, Cohen R. Pseudohypoglycemia: a cause for unreliable finger-stick glucose measurements. Endocr Pract. 2008;14(3):337–9.

11. Fanelli CG, Lucidi P, Bolli GB, Porcellati F. Hypoglycemia. In: Diabetes complications, comorbidities, and related disorders. Cham: Springer; 2018. p. 617–54.
12. Spanakis EK, Cryer PE, Davis SN. Hypoglycemia during therapy of diabetes. In: Feingold KR, Anawalt B, Boyce A, et al., editors. Endotext [Internet]. South Dartmouth (MA): MDText.com, Inc; 2018.
13. Fabrykant M. Pseudohypoglycemic reactions in insulin-treated diabetics: etiology, laboratory aids and therapy. J Am Geriatr Soc. 1964;12(3):221–38.
14. Tonyushkina K, Nichols JH. Glucose meters: a review of technical challenges to obtaining accurate results. J Diabetes Sci Technol. 2009;3(4):971–80. Published 2009.
15. Kadhem S, Ebrahem R, Ahmed B, Mortada R. Unreliable fingerstick glucose measurement in systemic sclerosis. AACE Clin Case Rep. 2016;2(4):e367–9.
16. Crevel E, Ardigo S, Perrenoud L, Vischer UM. Acrocyanosis as a cause of pseudohypoglycemia. J Am Geriatr Soc. 2009;57(8):1519–20.
17. Kagawa D, Ando S, Ueda T, Nakamura T, Domae N, Uchino H. A case of chronic myelogenous leukemia with pseudohypoglycemia: correlation between leukocyte counts and blood glucose levels. [Rinsho ketsueki] Jpn J Clin Hematol. 1987;28(10):1790–4.
18. Wenk RE, Yoho S, Bengzon A. Pseudohypoglycemia with monoclonal immunoglobulin M. Arch Pathol Lab Med. 2005;129(4):454–5.
19. Ginsberg BH. Factors affecting blood glucose monitoring: sources of errors in measurement. J Diabetes Sci Technol. 2009;3(4):903–13. Published 2009.
20. Liang Y, Rice MJ. Assessing glucose meter accuracy: the details matter! Anesthesiology. 2018;128(5):1044–5.
21. Thabit H, Hovorka R. Bridging technology and clinical practice: innovating inpatient hyperglycemia management in non-critical care settings. Diabet Med. 2018;35(4):460–71.
22. Li M, Zhou J, Bao YQ, Lu W, Jia WP. Prediction of nocturnal hypoglycemia with bedtime glucose level during continuous subcutaneous insulin infusion in type 2 diabetics. Zhonghua Yi Xue Za Zhi. 2010;90:2962–6.
23. Ma XJ, Zhou J. Using continuous glucose monitoring for patients with hypoglycemia. In: Continuous glucose monitoring. Singapore: Springer; 2018. p. 121–8.

24. Peyser TA, Nakamura K, Price D, Bohnett LC, Hirsch IB, Balo A. Hypoglycemic accuracy and improved low glucose alerts of the latest Dexcom G4 Platinum continuous glucose monitoring system. Diabetes Technol Ther. 2015;17:548–54.
25. Wentholt IM, Maran A, Masurel N, Heine RJ, Hoekstra JB, DeVries JH. Nocturnal hypoglycemia in Type 1 diabetic patients, assessed with continuous glucose monitoring: frequency, duration, and associations. Diabet Med. 2007;24:527–32.

# Chapter 10
## Chronic Fatigue

**Margaret A Eagan**

## Case Presentation

SJ is a 39-year-old patient referred to me for possible perimenopause and/or hypothyroidism. The patient complains of chronic fatigue, hair loss, heat intolerance, menstrual problems, memory loss that is affecting her job, mood swings, neck pain, numbness, palpitations, skin rash, sleep problems, and inability to lose weight. She states her symptoms have been present for at least 6 months.

She has been followed by a personal trainer/nutritionist (not a registered dietician) for 8 months and was placed on a very controlled diet of 2200 calories/day. SJ is unsure of the percentage of carbohydrates, protein, and fat. She was told by the nutritionist to do only strength training and no cardiovascular exercise in order to increase muscle mass. She works out (weightlifting) 1 hour 5×/week. She has a very sedentary job

M. A. Eagan (✉)
Anschutz Health and Wellness Center, University of Colorado, Aurora, CO, USA
e-mail: Margaret.eagan@ucdenver.edu

© Springer Nature Switzerland AG 2019
M. T. McDermott (ed.), *Management of Patients with Pseudo-Endocrine Disorders*,
https://doi.org/10.1007/978-3-030-22720-3_10

that she doesn't enjoy. Other history includes participating in bodybuilding competitions in 2006 and 2007 and following a very restrictive diet during this time. Even with the restrictive diet, she was never able to get her body fat <18%. She believes she damaged her metabolism during this time.

Her PMH and PSH are negative. Her FH is positive for type 2 diabetes in her mother. She does not have a specific bedtime. It can vary from 10 PM to midnight. She has difficulty falling asleep but once asleep she stays asleep. She wakes up at 6 AM and leaves for work at 7 AM without eating breakfast. She describes her mood swings as mostly being "down, unmotivated, lack of energy."

Her PE is normal. BMI 29.

**Initial Labs**
- TSH 3.32mIU/L (0.34–5.60 mIU/L)
- HbA1C 6.0 mg/dL (4.0–6.0%)
- Vit D25OH 35 ng/mL (13–62 ng/mL)
- Vit B12 376 pg/mL (180–914 pg/mL

**Diagnoses**
1. Subclinical depression
2. Prediabetes
3. Insomnia
4. Overweight

**Treatments Discussed**
1. Subclinical Depression
    Levothyroxine 75 mcg/day in attempts to decrease her TSH to 0.5–1.5 mIU/L.
    Citalopram 10 mg at bedtime.
    Vitamin D3 2000 IU/day for a goal Vitamin D 25 OH level of high 40s.
    Look into an MBSR program to help with stress and anxiety.
2. Prediabetes
    Metformin ER 500 mg/day.
    Vitamin B12 500 mcg/day.
3. Insomnia
    Sleep habit: calming regimen from 9 PM to 10 PM; take Citalopram at 9:30 PM and lights out by 10 PM. Continue with getting out of bed at 6 AM.

4. Weight
>Cardiovascular activity of a brisk walk 10 minutes/day. Decrease calories from 2200 to 2000 calories/day with an eventual goal of 1800 calories/day. Do a food log with MyFitnessPal app for 2 weeks with goal macronutrients of 40% carbohydrates/30% protein/30% fat.
>Drink a protein drink on her way to work.
>Set an alarm on her phone to remind herself to eat a snack/meal of carbohydrates/ protein and/ or fat every 4 hours.

**Treatments Decided by SJ**
- Levothyroxine and Citalopram
- Daily brisk walk
- Food log

The patient returned for follow up in 6 weeks. Her energy had increased from a 3/10 to 7/10. She had a marked improvement in her mood. She developed a sleep routine from 10 PM to 6 AM. She had dropped two sizes in clothes. She accepted a job transfer to England and was leaving in 5 days.

**Plan**
- Start Vitamin D3
- Start the Metformin ER once she was in England
- Continue to follow up with me through email while living abroad.

# Chronic Fatigue in an Otherwise Healthy Person

When we look at our schedule for the day and see a chief complaint of chronic fatigue the initial reaction is most likely one of dread and a belief that we will be unable to help. We perceive it as one of the most difficult and time-consuming complaints to treat as healthcare providers. It is correct that there is no quick fix for chronic fatigue and even with all of our good intentions about 30% of these clients will have no improvement [1–4].

Improvement, and sometimes remission of chronic fatigue, is possible though with time and patience. Time, however is what we are very short of as providers. Hopefully, this chapter will serve as a guide that will make the evaluation and treatment more efficient and rewarding.

Fatigue by itself is a subjective *symptom,* not a syndrome. It is defined as feelings of tiredness and perception of generalized weakness. Easy fatigability is a decreased capacity for physical activity. Mental fatigue is a difficulty with concentration, memory, and/or emotional stability [2].

Chronic fatigue [2] does not exist in a vacuum. It is multidimensional and multifactorial. Symptoms associated with chronic fatigue are varied and numerous. Your patient's review of systems will usually have more positive than negative symptoms. Common symptoms are constitutional symptoms such as lethargy, weight gain/weight loss, and anorexia; psychological symptoms such as depression, anxiety, mood swings, loss of motivation, poor mental concentration, and sleep problems; respiratory symptoms such as frequent upper respiratory tract infections (URI) and dyspnea; musculoskeletal symptoms such as myalgias and arthralgias; and gastrointestinal symptoms such as abdominal distention, bloating, constipation, and diarrhea.

# Causes of Chronic Fatigue

According to the literature [2], there are four major categories: physiologic, psychologic, biochemical, and idiopathic. Physiological causes can be due to cardiopulmonary, endocrinologic, gastroenterologic, hematologic, immunologic, and infectious or rheumatological abnormalities Fig. 10.1. These usually are the easiest to diagnose and treat. Psychological causes most commonly include depression and anxiety, somatization, and panic disorder. Biochemical causes include alcohol or drug addictions, chronic use of muscle relaxants, hypnotics, antidepressants, antihistamines, and Beta blockers to name a few. Idiopathic fatigue is a diagnosis of exclusion and accounts for approximately 30% of patients. The rest of this chapter will focus on idiopathic chronic fatigue.

**Major causes of chronic fatigue**

| Psychologic | Infectious |
| --- | --- |
| Depression | Endocarditis |
| Anxiety | Tuberculosis |
| Somatization disorder | Mononucleosis |
| Malnutrition or drug addiction | Hepatitis |
| **Pharmacologic** | Parasitic disease |
| Hypnotics | HIV infection |
| Antihypertensives | Cytomegalovirus |
| Antidepressants | **Cardiopulmonary** |
| Drug abuse and drug withdrawal | Chronic heart failure |
| **Endocrine-metabolic** | Chronic obstructive pulmonary disease |
| Hypothyroidism | **Connective tissue disease** |
| Diabetes mellitus | Rheumatoid disease |
| Apathetic hyperthyroidism | **Disturbed sleep** |
| Pituitary insufficiency | Sleep apnea |
| Hypercalcemia | Esophageal reflux |
| Adrenal insufficiency | Allergic rhinitis |
| Chronic renal failure | Psychologic causes (see above) |
| Hepatic failure | **Idiopathic (diagnosis by exclusion)** |
| **Neoplastic-hematologic** | Idiopathic chronic fatigue |
| Occult malignancy | Chronic fatigue syndrome |
| Severe anemia | Fibromyalgia |

*Adapted from: Gorroll, AH, May, LA, Mulley, AG Jr (Eds), Primary Care Medicine: Office Evaluation and Management of the Adult Patient, 3rd ed, JB Lippincott, Philadelphia, 1995.*

FIGURE 10.1 Major causes of chronic fatigue

Idiopathic chronic fatigue consists of debilitating symptoms for >6 months that do not meet the criteria for chronic fatigue syndrome or fibromyalgia [2]. These are the patients we as health-care providers struggle to treat. We are unable to diagnose an actual disorder, so we are unsure how to help and often want to diagnose a psychological disorder such as depression and refer to a mental health provider. In my clinical experience, a majority of patients with idiopathic chronic fatigue have an imbalance in lifestyle behaviors including sleep, nutrition, movement, and mental or emotional health.

## Evaluation

*History taking* is the most important part of the evaluation [7, 8]. Remember fatigue does not exist in a vacuum. It is only one symptom in a constellation of symptoms. The intensity of these other symptoms may determine their ultimate contribution to the cause of fatigue. For example, awakening unrested, daytime sleepiness, eye redness, and blurry vision could be due to a lack of restful sleep.

*Evaluation of fatigue symptoms* (*Circle all that apply*). Have patients fill out this form **prior** to their visit with you if possible.

1. Onset – abrupt or gradual and when symptoms began _____
2. Course – increasing or decreasing
3. Duration – daily or intermittent, if intermittent, how long in between bouts (days, months, years)
4. What increases it – sleep disturbance, vacation, work, a family member, certain foods (which ones_____ _____), exercise (amount, type_____ _____), support from friends and family (too much, too little), change of seasons, medications (which ones____ _____ _____)
5. What decreases it – good night's sleep, vacation, work, a family member, certain foods (which ones__ _____) exercise (amount, type)_____, support from family and friends (too much, too little), change of seasons, medications (which ones)_____ _____
6. What impact does your symptoms have on your daily life – for example, in relationships at home, work_____ _____ _____
7. What accommodations have you made – change in exercise routine or type_____, change in type or amount of work_____, change in living environment (apartment, house, stairs)_____

_____, change in sleeping environment (bed, chair, separate room)_____
_____, change in clothing (buttons, zippers, elastic waist) _____, change in grooming (bath, shower, haircut) _____.

*Evaluation of lifestyle behaviors* Fig. 10.2 – I recommend patients filling this out before their visit.

## Lifestyle Behaviors Evaluation Form

**1.** What would you like to achieve from your visit today?/What is your goal?

_____
_____
_____
_____

**2.** How important is your goal on a scale of 0 to 10?   0 being not important at all and 10 being the most important thing in your life right now.   Circle one number

0   1   2   3   4   5   6   7   8   9   10

**3.** How confident are you that you can achieve your goal on a scale of 0 to 10? 0 being not important at all and 10 being extremely confident.   Circle one number

0   1   2   3   4   5   6   7   8   9   10

**4.** Why do you want to achieve this goal? Be specific.

_____
_____

**5: Sleep**

How many hours do you usually sleep each night? _____ hours per night

What time is lights out?_____ What time are you out of bed?_____

What time do you leave for work?_____What are your work days?/hours?_____
What is your sleep quality? (Circle One): Poor, Average, Good, Excellent
Are you pleased with the quality of your sleep? (**Circle** one):
**Not at all; Somewhat pleased; Very pleased9. Nutrition**

**6. Nutrition**

I describe my current diet as: (**Circle** all that apply)

| | |
|---|---|
| Healthy 100% of the time | Perfect |
| Healthy 80% of the time | Whatever is put in front of me |
| Healthy 50% of the time | Gourmet |
| Healthy 20% of the time | Preplanned |
| Never or rarely healthy | On the go |
| Lots of junk food | Frozen and microwaved |
| Organic | I eat very little (<1000kcal/day) |

FIGURE 10.2 Lifestyle behaviors evaluation form

| | |
|---|---|
| Processed | Including lots of vegetables |
| Large portions of food | Including lots of fruit |
| Appropriate portions of food | Vegetarian |
| Small portions of food | Gluten free |
| Lots of fast food and restaurant meals | High in protein |
| Family friendly | High in fat |
| High in sugar | High in salt |

What do you drink? (**Circle** all that could apply)
Regular sugar soda, water, juices, diet beverages, tea coffee, skim milk, low-fat milk, whole milk

**True or False:**

I believe my diet could be better. True or False
I get very hungry when I limit my food intake/diet. True or False
I crave sweet foods. True or False
I eat more when I am stressed. True or False
I am an emotional eater. True or False

### 7. Movement

My activity level is (**Circle** one)

    Very low - no planned activity, sitting most of the day

    Low - some walking in my daily life

    Average - lots of walking and some planned activity

    High - lots of walking and daily planned activity > 30 minutes/day

    Very High - lots of walking and lots of planned activity > 60 minutes/day

I do the following planned activity:

_____
_____
_____


I could do more activity? (Circle one) True or False
My activity is limited by the following:

_____
_____

### 8. Mental Health

                **Stress**

What is your stress level on a scale of 0 to 10? 0 being none and 10 being extremely high.

    **0 1 2 3 4 5 6 7 8 9 10**

FIGURE 10.2 (continued)

What is your energy level on a scale of 0 to 10? 0 being very low and 10 being very high.

**0 1 2 3 4 5 6 7 8 9 10**

### Mood

During the past month have you felt depressed, sad or blue? Y  N

During the past month have you felt little pleasure or interest in doing things? Y  N

How many times today did you feel in a rush? (**Circle** one):
Three or more;  One to Two;  None

How much do you worry?(circle one)

A lot;  Some but it is under control;  Very little;  It is a waste of time.

### Brain Activity

How many days last week did you learn something new or do something you have never done before? (Circle one)
None; One to two; Three or more

### Social Connectedness

How many people did you share a face to face conversation today that lasted longer than two minutes? (Circle One)
**None; One to two; Three or more**
How long has it been since you last interacted with a child? (Circle one)
**Months or years;  Weeks;  Days**

### 9. Emotional Health
#### Laughter

How many times did you laugh today (not just smile, but laugh for longer than two seconds)? (**Circle one**)
**None;  Once;  Twice or more**

#### Being in the Present

How often are you thinking about things other than what you are currently doing? (Circle one) Often;  Sometimes;  Hardly ever

#### Purpose

Are you proud of your answer when someone asks how you spend your day? (Circle one) Not proud;  A little proud;  Very proud

FIGURE 10.2 (continued)

*Physical evaluation* – Will usually be normal in cases of chronic fatigue of unknown causes since the cause is most likely due to lack of self-care habits and/or subclinical depression or anxiety.

*Laboratory evaluation* – Recommended reasonable initial labs are a basic chemistry panel, CBC, TSH, ferritin, CPK (if muscle pain and/or weakness is present), and Hepatitis C if the patient was born between 1945 and 1965. I also recommend Vitamin D and HbA1C if risk factors are present.

*Diagnosis* is one of exclusion. Your history physical exam and labs will reveal most medical causes of fatigue.

Your thorough evaluation of wellness behaviors and preventive health care will reveal many of the remaining causes.

The remainder of this chapter unless otherwise stated will focus on the treatment of chronic fatigue due to lack of healthy lifestyle behaviors.

*Treatment is gradual and sequential and requires a multifactorial approach.* Remember, there is no quick fix. Treatment requires patience from both the provider and the patient. A large part of the treatment is based on clinical experience and intuition. Treatment is also largely based on the doctor and patient relationship [1, 4, 7, 8].

Most people with chronic fatigue feel unheard by their providers. First, acknowledge that the patient's complaints are real and debilitating. Give information that patients are able to understand and connect with their own experiences. Communicate clear expectations of recovery and schedule frequent regular appointments such as once a month.

Work on a maximum of three changes at a time. Once the patient has mastered three changes, then incrementally add other changes. I allow the patient to choose the first three they wish to work on as these are the ones they most likely feel confident about mastering. A small change such as better sleep habits can have a profound impact [6]. Appropriate management of identified stressors and the continual surveillance of other causes of fatigue is important.

The registered *SEEN* acronym is one I developed as an approach to any patient with chronic medical issues.

1. *SUPPORT* – Develop a relationship-centered doctor–patient relationship by asking, "How can I help you?" Then quietly *listen* to your patient and *observe* their body language without thinking of what further questions to ask. The majority of patients will tell their story in about 1 minute. From just 1 minute of your time listening and observing you have already begun to develop a sense of what is truly important to your patient.
2. *EDUCATE* – Means to draw out that that is from within. Give them information they can understand and connect with their own life experiences. People are motivated to change or open to exploring a problem or

change of perspective first through emotions and second through facts.
3. *EMPOWER* – Your patient. They have the ability to change and to take control and responsibility of their life.
4. *NURTURE* – Your patient. They are not on this journey alone. You and the patient are a team. The provider at first is more the teacher and your patient the student towards better health. As you work together your patient will gain knowledge and confidence where you both will be student and teacher.

Why focus on lifestyle behaviors? Besides helping patients with chronic fatigue, 70% of chronic medical diseases can be prevented or controlled with good lifestyle choices. Lifestyle choices consist of sleep, nutrition, movement, mental health, and emotional health.

## Putting It All Together

1. *Sleep* [6]: A sufficient amount of sleep consists of at least 7 consecutive hours Fig. 10.3. It is essential for optimal physical health, mental health, immune function, and cognition. Sleep is a habit. It takes at least 3 weeks to develop a habit.

Have patients keep a sleep diary for 2 weeks. They can use their fitness trackers, but research shows that these consistently overestimate sleep duration.

Have patients develop a nighttime routine (sleep hygiene). Think CALM-see below

- Consistent bedtime (weekday or weekend).
- Calming regimen starting at least 30 minutes prior to lights out.
- Conducive sleep environment of approximately 60–67 °F.
- Comfortable mattress and pillows.
- Caffeine, nicotine, and heavy meals avoid in the evening or at least 4 hours prior to lights out.
- Activity (physical) every day.
- Light and bright environment at your wake-up time either artificially or naturally.
- Medications such as melatonin 1 hour prior to lights out.

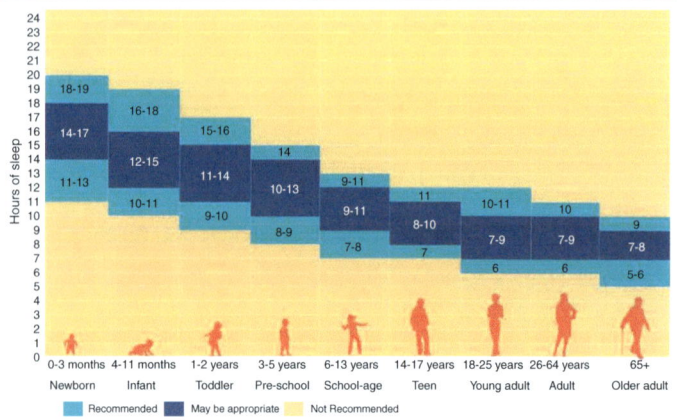

Sleep duration recommendations by age from the National Sleep Foundation*

* These recommendations are very similar, but not identical to those from the American Academy of Sleep Medicine (AASM).[1,2]

1. Paruthi S, Brooks LJ, D'Ambrosio C, et al. Recommended amount of sleep for pediatric population: A statement of the American Academy of sleep medicine. J Clin Sleep Med 2016; 12:785.
2. Consensus Conference panel, Watson NF, Badr MS, et al. Recommended amount of sleep for a healthy adult: A joint Consensus Statement of the american Academy of Sleep Medicine and Sleep research Society. J Clin Sleep Med 2015; 11:591
Republished with permission of National Sleep Foundation, 2016; permission conveyed through Copyright Clearance Center, Inc.

Figure 10.3 Sleep duration recommendations by age from the national sleep foundation

2. *Nutrition*: Education on appropriate macronutrients (protein, carbohydrates, and fat) and their food sources is paramount. Focus on macronutrient percentages more than calories and on the development of healthy lifestyle behaviors. For example, if a patient asks if they should follow a paleo or keto diet, redirect them back to macronutrients. I use the word nutrition or healthy eating rather than diet as much as possible.

Have your patient do a food log for 2 weeks. Ask them to eat their normal diet. Evaluate the average daily percentages of macronutrients. There will be better compliance with electronic food logs such as the MyFitnessPal app. In individuals with normal kidney and liver function, enter percentages of 40% carbohydrates, 30% protein, and 30% fat. Enter calories of 1200–1500/day in the average 40-year-old and older woman (inactive–active) and 1500–1800 calories/day in the average 40-year-old or older male (inactive–active). By maintaining a food log, patients will begin to educate themselves on macronutrients and their food sources and on how to read food labels. Review their food log and make minor adjustments towards achieving the percentages stated above for macronutrients. Look up products and alternatives on the internet during their visit so you learn together. Dieticians are also a wonderful resource, but their services are not usually covered by insurance.

Educate patients about the different macronutrients. Keep it simple. Carbohydrates are our fuel, our energy source. Too many grams or not enough cause fatigue, cognitive difficulties, and emotional liabilities. Proteins are the building blocks of muscle. Good protein sources are meats, fish, beans, dairy products, nuts, and seeds. Too much protein grams can cause kidney damage and not enough can lead to loss of muscle mass. Fats are the building blocks of hormones. Focus on eating polyunsaturated (nuts, avocadoes) rather than saturated fats (butter, fried foods). Excess fat intake can lead to cardiovascular disease. Insufficient fat intake can lead to vitamin malabsorption, an increase in cancer risk especially colon, prostate, and breast cancer, and depression.

3. *Movement* [2]: This consists of formal and informal activity.

Ask your patient the type, frequency, and length of their formal exercise routines. Confirm their routine. Often patients list what they hope to be doing not what they are actually doing.

Have your patient do a **movement** log by wearing a pedometer for at least 2 weeks. I take the total number of steps over 7 days and divide that number by 7 to account for exercise and non-exercise days. The goal is to have on average of at least 10,000 steps/day according to the American Heart Association.

Propose a formal exercise routine that is a mixture of cardiovascular and strength activities. Strength includes flexibility, core, balance, and strength. Research recommends 30 minutes of moderate activity every day [2, 5]. My recommendations are based on the physical condition of my patient. For those who are very deconditioned, I recommend graded exercise therapy beginning with a referral to physical therapy for physical deconditioning. For those who are otherwise healthy but have never exercised I ask if they can commit to a 10-minute brisk walk every day. I explain to them that it is not the time that is important. The important part is walking every day even when they do not feel like it. Once they have accomplished this goal, I add 20 minutes of strength training 3×/week. A good beginner's resource is the NIH Go4life. The goal is to eventually have patients engaging in 3 days of cardiovascular activity consisting of two long steady sessions (40 minutes each) and one short interval session (20 minutes) along with 3 days of strength training for at least 20 minutes. Proper alignment is important to prevent injuries. In an inexperienced exerciser, you might recommend a few (4) sessions with a reputable personal trainer to develop a strength training program for your patient and ensure proper form while exercising.

By informal activity I mean to be in perpetual motion like a child. As we grow older, we become more sedentary. We need to be aware of this and add activity all through our day such as moving 5 minutes/hour, balancing while putting on your socks or brushing your teeth, doing squats while waiting for your lunch to heat up or standing on your toes while waiting in line.

4. *Mental Health*: Behavioral therapy with a licensed clinical professional can help treat anxiety, depression, and other mental health disorders; but how do we treat those who suffer from subclinical depression and anxiety?

Subclinical depression [3] is defined as having clinically relevant depressive or anxiety symptoms without having major depression or anxiety. This can formally be evaluated with the PHQ9 form or more commonly by clinical intuition, experience, and your intake form.

There are no widely accepted guidelines for treatment. I recommend a combination of pharmacologic (prescription and over-the-counter) and nonpharmacologic modalities. Pharmacologic recommendations consist of a low dose SSRI such as Citalopram or Sertraline taken at bedtime. These SSRI's can help with depression, anxiety, and insomnia.

Adjunctive treatment or even solitary treatment with levothyroxine to obtain a low normal TSH level. The majority of studies [9, 10], however, were done in major depression with T3 supplementation only and the majority of studies have been inconclusive. I, however, have had good results with my patients. I recommend monitoring the TSH every 6 weeks until the level is 0.5–1.5 mIU/L. Maintain your patient at this low normal level for 3 months. If there has been no improvement in their symptoms at 3 months, then discontinue the levothyroxine.

Vitamin D supplementation is also controversial [11]. The Vitamin D receptor and 1-alpha-hydroxylase are expressed in the human brain. Low Vitamin D 25OH levels (<20 ng/mL) are frequently found in patients with depression. The recommendation is to supplement with Vitamin D to maintain levels of Vitamin 25OH > 20 ng/mL. However, from personal experience, I have found a Vitamin D 25OH level of approximately 45 ng/dL (13–62 ng/mL) has the best results for mood elevation.

Nonpharmacologic treatments include formal cognitive or dialectical behavioral therapy (CBT, DBT) or mindfulness training (see emotional health below) individually or in groups [12].

5. *Emotional Health*: Emotional health is a state of positive psychological functioning. It is resilience, the ability to bend without breaking. Resilience is the ability to prevent, withstand, and bounce back from adversity. Resilience allows us to take on challenges rather than getting overwhelmed; to have a sense of control and to find meaning in what we are doing. Acceptance, happiness, and gratitude are the main components of resilience [13]. But how does one accomplish these things? It is through mindfulness.

There are numerous formal mindfulness programs/practices. One well-known program is mindfulness-based stress reduction (MBSR) created by Dr. Jon Kabat Zin, a molecular biologist from the University of Massachusetts [14]. His book titled *Full Catastrophe Living* [15] guides you through the formal 8-week MBSR program.

Informal or self-guided practices consist of apps such as calm, mindfi, insight timer and headspace. GoNoodle app is geared more towards children and is an excellent bonding opportunity for parents and children. Another resource is Dr. Amit Sood's *The Mayo Clinic Handbook for Happiness* [16]. It is his suggestions regarding acceptance, happiness, and gratitude that follow:

> "**Acceptance** of life's challenges, finding meaning and making the best of situations. Setbacks are opportunities for growth. **Happiness** is a state of positive emotions, choice and a habit. Choose daily to see the positive around you and to see the positive within the negative. Happiness does not occur naturally for some people and takes practice to become a habit. **Gratitude** is acknowledging and appreciating your blessings" [13].

Three practices to try [13, 16]:

1. Upon awakening bring three people into your mind and send them a blessing or positive thought.
2. When you pass someone on the street send them a silent message of "Be well." Try this also in a work meeting that is going poorly.
3. At the end of the day, upon arriving home, be fully present to your family, pets, plants, or just your home, your sanctuary for 3 minutes.

Mindfulness has been proven to decrease chronic pain, depression, and self-defeating emotional habits. It is not easy, nor does it come naturally to most. It takes practice. Think of it as an exercise for mental fitness. First, we must learn to focus, to be present. Mindfulness is just one technique to strengthen our state of attention (focus). I think of practicing the three things we learned as children. Stay calm. Pay attention. Say thank you. For more information, I strongly recommend the resources above.

I know this seems overwhelming to accomplish with your patients who complain of chronic fatigue but use this as a template. Identify together what areas they would like to concentrate on and, if applicable admit your lack of confidence or experience in certain treatment modalities and refer to a certified Lifestyle Medicine provider.

# References

1. Weil A. How to really help people make healthy lifestyle choices. Global Wellness Summit. 2017.
2. Fosnocht K, Ende J, Elmore J, Kunins L. Approach to the adult patient with fatigue: UptoDate; 2019.
3. Lyness J, Roy-Byrne P, Solomon D. Unipolar minor depression in adults: Management: UptoDate; 2019.
4. Okon T, Arnold R, Givens J. Overview of comprehensive patient assessment in palliative care: UptoDate.
5. Halson S, O'Connor F, Grayzel J. Overtraining syndrome in athletes: UptoDate; 2019.
6. Maski K, Scammell T, Eischler A. Insufficient sleep evaluation and management: UptoDate; 2019.
7. Beach MC, et al. Relationship centered care a constuctive reframing. Perspectives. 2005. JGIM s3-7.
8. Robert Cloninger C. Person centered health promotion in chronic disease. Int J Pers Cent Med. 2013;3(1):5–12.
9. Duncan TJ, Soh SB. Use and misuse of thyroid hormone. Singap Med J. 2013;54(7):406–10.
10. Hage MP, Azar ST. The link between thyroid function and depression. J Thyroid Res. 2012;2012:590648.
11. Li D, Wei G, et al. Vitamin D and depression. A systematic review. J Clin Endocrinol Metab. 2014;99(3):757–67.
12. Lord J, McLaren K, Levy M, Roy-Byrne P, Solomon D. Unipolar depression in adults: supportive psychotherapy: UptoDate; 2019.
13. Sood A. The mayo clinic guide to stress-free living; 2013. p. 1–282.
14. "Mindfulness Based Stress Reduction" course. Center for Courageous Living LLC. 2016.
15. Kabat-Zin J. Full catastrophe living: using the wisdom of your body and mind to face stress, pain and illness; 2013. p. 1–609.
16. Sood A. The mayo clinic handbook for happiness: a 4-step plan for resilient living; 2013. p. 229.

# Chapter 11
## Adrenal Fatigue

**Michael T. McDermott**

## Case

A 47-year-old woman has been experiencing fatigue for about 15 years but complains of "total exhaustion" progressively over the past year. She does not sleep well but does not snore. Her appetite is poor. She only eats full meals occasionally but snacks frequently throughout the day. Mild weight gain (5 lb.) has occurred in the past year. She cannot exercise due to fatigue. She requests to be treated for adrenal fatigue for which she has tested positive.

M. T. McDermott (✉)
University of Colorado Hospital, Aurora, CO, USA
e-mail: michael.mcdermott@cuanschutz.edu

| | |
|---|---|
| PMH: Mononucleosis at age 18 | Meds: Occasional prescription pain medication |
| PE: BP 128/70  P 80  Ht 5'8" | Wt 157 lb. (Orthostatic vitals negative) |

Complete exam normal

Lab: Full-day salivary cortisol profile – Interpreted as "adrenal fatigue"

## Discussion

### True Adrenal Insufficiency

*Primary adrenal insufficiency* develops as a result of disease of or damage to the adrenal glands [1]. The most common cause of primary adrenal insufficiency in the U.S. is autoimmune adrenalitis (Addison's disease). Other, less common, causes include infections (tuberculosis, deep fungal infections, HIV), infiltrative disorders (amyloidosis), intra-adrenal hemorrhage, metastatic cancer, surgical adrenalectomy, and congenital metabolic disorders (adrenoleukodystrophy, adrenomyeloneuropathy). Persons who have primary adrenal insufficiency usually have deficiencies of all three adrenal cortical hormones (cortisol, aldosterone, adrenal androgens).

*Secondary (central) adrenal insufficiency* results from diseases of, damage to, or suppression of the pituitary gland or hypothalamus [1]. This disorder most commonly develops due to the administration of exogenous glucocorticoids ("steroids") to treat systemic or localized inflammatory diseases. Notably, however, central adrenal insufficiency also frequently occurs because of the use (widespread) of opioid narcotics for acute, subacute, or chronic pain management [2, 3]. Other relatively common causes of central adrenal insufficiency include pituitary and parasellar tumors, surgery or radiation therapy in the pituitary–hypothalamic regions, traumatic brain injury (TBI), pituitary infections (syphilis), pituitary hemorrhage/

apoplexy, infiltrative pituitary diseases, metastatic cancer to the pituitary gland, various types of idiopathic pituitary inflammation (hypophysitis – lymphocytic, granulomatous, plasma cell, xanthomatous, and mixed forms), and hypophysitis induced by immune checkpoint inhibitor therapy. Secondary (central) adrenal insufficiency only causes deficient production of cortisol and adrenal androgens; aldosterone secretion remains intact because the renin–angiotensin system, the primary regulator of aldosterone secretion, remains intact.

Symptoms of adrenal insufficiency include fatigue, weakness, myalgias, arthralgias, abdominal pain, nausea, vomiting, headaches, weight loss, postural dizziness, and salt craving. Physical findings most commonly include hypotension and tachycardia; cutaneous hyperpigmentation and vitiligo may be seen but only in primary adrenal insufficiency. Common laboratory features are hyponatremia, hypoglycemia, azotemia, anemia, and eosinophilia; hyperkalemia occurs only in primary adrenal insufficiency (due to aldosterone deficiency).

The best screening test for adrenal insufficiency, according to the current clinical practice guidelines, is a morning serum cortisol level drawn between 8 and 9 AM. An AM serum cortisol level <3 ug/dl is diagnostic of adrenal insufficiency; an AM serum cortisol <5 ug/dl with a plasma ACTH >2 times the upper normal limit is also supportive of the diagnosis. An AM serum cortisol level >15 ug/dl rules out adrenal insufficiency. For those with AM serum cortisol levels between 3 and 15 ug/dl, an ACTH (Cosyntropin 250 mcg) stimulation test is recommended. A peak serum cortisol level <18 ug/dl 30 minutes after ACTH administration is diagnostic of partial adrenal insufficiency [1]. A diagram of the relative cortisol responses to this test in normal subjects and in patients with partial and complete adrenal insufficiency is drawn in Fig. 11.1.

The ACTH stimulation test, however, has some limitations. A meta-analysis of all published and adequate studies determined that the sensitivity of the ACTH stimulation test for detection of primary adrenal insufficiency is 92% (95% confidence interval: 81–94%) but the specificity was not estimable. For detecting secondary adrenal insufficiency, the existing

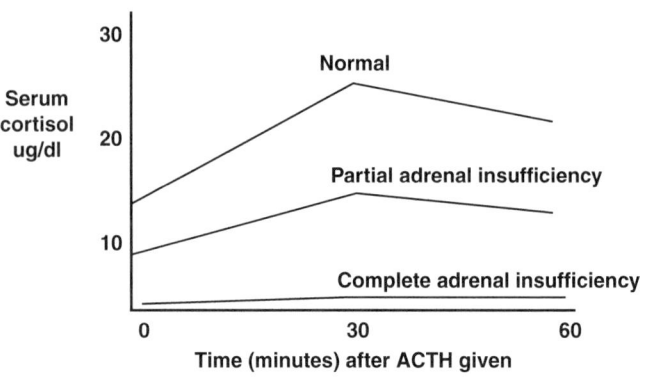

Figure 11.1 Interpretation of the ACTH stimulation test

data were insufficient to estimate either the sensitivity or the specificity of the test [4]. In patients with primary adrenal insufficiency, measurement of anti-adrenal (anti-21-hydroxylase) antibodies will establish the etiology as autoimmune adrenalitis [1].

Impairment of adrenal function occurs gradually in patients with positive anti-adrenal (anti-21-hydroxylase) antibodies. Four stages of progressive adrenal cortical dysfunction have been described (Table 11.1) [5]. Others have suggested that mild plasma ACTH elevations are the first indicator of impending adrenal gland failure [6]. These data emphasize that the diagnosis of early adrenal insufficiency (primary and secondary) may be difficult even with validated tests and requires significant clinical experience and judgment.

Hypothalamic–pituitary–adrenal (HPA) physiology is highly complex. It involves hypothalamic production of corticotrophin-releasing factor (CRF) and vasopressin to regulate the pituitary secretion of corticotropin (ACTH), which stimulates cortisol secretion from the adrenal glands. Cortisol

TABLE 11.1 Proposed stages in the development of overt adrenal insufficiency in patients who have positive serum anti-21-hydroxylase antibodies (Ref. [5])

| Stage | Features |
|---|---|
| 1 | High plasma renin activity (PRA); low/normal plasma aldosterone (PA) |
| 2 | Stage 1 plus a reduced peak cortisol response (<18 ug/dl) to ACTH administration |
| 3 | Stage 2 plus elevated plasma ACTH |
| 4 | Clinically overt adrenal insufficiency (baseline serum cortisol <3 ug/dl) |

is then transported in the bloodstream by binding proteins to peripheral tissues where free (unbound) cortisol crosses cell and nuclear membranes in target cells and binds to nuclear glucocorticoid receptors, where it activates or suppresses transcription of target genes. The resulting messenger RNA (mRNA) is then translated into the cortisol regulated proteins that ultimately mediate tissue cortisol action. This action includes feedback of cortisol at the level of the hypothalamus and pituitary gland to maintain HPA axis homeostasis.

It is certainly possible that some, as yet unrecognized, inherited, or acquired abnormalities may exist at any of these multiple sites of cortisol physiology and may or may not be detectable by our current panel of adrenal axis tests. These exciting possibilities and the implications they have for improving patient care are the reasons endocrine research must be supported and clinicians must stay abreast of the resulting discoveries and their clinical applications.

# The Myth of Adrenal Fatigue

Adrenal fatigue is a proposed condition in which the adrenal glands, while not insufficient by traditional hormone testing, become unable to produce adequate amounts of adrenal hormones to meet the requirements of the body to deal with the daily stresses of life. It is said to occur in patients who are under chronic high stress (mental, emotional, or physical) in their work and/or family life; this chronic stress supposedly exhausts their adrenal glands. It is characterized by nonspecific symptoms such as fatigue, sleep disturbances, difficulty coping, body aches, digestive problems, and dependency on caffeine [7–11]. There are numerous practitioners and websites that promote this pseudo-endocrine condition. Adrenal fatigue was even featured on Dr. Oz on October 22, 2015.

Patients are encouraged to self-diagnose adrenal fatigue based on symptoms alone; scoring systems are suggested. Providers or patients themselves can also order a salivary cortisol profile in which multiple salivary cortisol samples are collected throughout the day and submitted to a lab for analysis (for a price); if the salivary cortisol levels fall below a normative line, the diagnosis of adrenal fatigue is said to be confirmed.

Importantly, adrenal fatigue has never been scientifically proven to exist. Furthermore, salivary cortisol profiles have never been tested scientifically or validated in any way as a tool to evaluate insufficiency of the HPA axis. As clinician-scientists, we must be open to novel ideas and proposals. But rigorous verification by well-designed and well-conducted scientific investigations must still be the standard by which we evaluate and clinically apply new and innovative ideas. It is not sufficient, when patients' health and wellbeing are concerned, to simply propose a hypothesis and then apply it without diligent scientific investigation.

Proposed treatment recommendations start with a healthy well-balanced diet, regular exercise, good sleep habits, stress reduction, and cessation of smoking and alcohol use. Most of us would never object to any of these measures. This is the same advice we give to almost all patients, regardless of the diagnosis. Patients are certainly likely to feel better and have improved quality of life if they follow these recommendations. But adrenal fatigue websites and promoters also suggest that patients take supplements. Once again, there is likely no harm in taking vitamin and mineral supplements as long as some (fat-soluble vitamins A, D, E, and K, for example) are not taken in excess. But adrenal supplements that contain whole adrenal tissue or adrenal extracts are also strongly promoted [12].

The Endocrine Society (Hormone Foundation) has taken the lead in opposing the promotion of adrenal fatigue by practitioners and websites [7–10]. The Hormone Foundation website and its printed literature provide patients with the following clear warnings: "No scientific proof exists to support adrenal fatigue as a true medical condition." "Doctors are concerned that if you are told you have this condition, the real cause of your symptoms may not be found and treated correctly." "Doctors urge you not to waste precious time accepting an unproven diagnosis such as 'adrenal fatigue' if you feel tired, weak, or depressed. If you have these symptoms, you may have adrenal insufficiency, depression, obstructive sleep apnea, or other health problems. Getting a real diagnosis is very important to help you feel better and overcome your health problem." And finally, "If you take adrenal hormone supplements when you don't need them, your adrenal glands may stop working and become unable to make the hormones you need when you are under physical stress. When these supplements are stopped, a person's adrenal glands can remain 'asleep' for months. People with this problem may be in danger of developing a life-threatening condition called adrenal crisis."

The Mayo Clinic website also has the following strong statements [11]: "The term often shows up in popular health books and on alternative medicine websites, but it isn't an accepted medical diagnosis." And, "It's frustrating to have persistent symptoms your doctor can't readily explain. But accepting a medically unrecognized diagnosis from an unqualified practitioner could be worse. Unproven remedies for so-called adrenal fatigue may leave you feeling sicker, while the real cause – such as depression or fibromyalgia – continues to take its toll."

Despite this public criticism, proponents of adrenal fatigue continue to advertise and promote (and financially benefit from) this fabricated disorder. Websites openly display sleeping men and women, young people who are so completely exhausted (from adrenal fatigue) that they have fallen asleep on their couches, at their desks, and on logs out in the forest. They promote symptom scores and the unvalidated salivary cortisol profile to make the diagnosis. And they entice vulnerable patients with online access (for a price) to unproven and potentially dangerous products labeled as "Made from raw, cold-processed bovine glandular tissue"; "Raw Adrenal Glandular Concentrate"; "Natural glandular"; "Blend of glandulars, herbs, vitamins, and more" [12]. This type of pseudo-science circus is well described and denounced as fraudulent and harmful by Dr. Lisa Pryor in her excellent article in the *New York Times* (Jan 5, 2018) [13].

## Back to Our Patient

This patient has severe fatigue and poor quality of life. She is not responsible for the misinformation she has received or believed about adrenal fatigue from other practitioners or the Internet. She has just come to ask for help. She deserves respect, honesty, and compassion like all other patients. We should listen carefully to her symptoms, concerns, and frustrations and assure her that we are committed to helping her find relief for her symptoms. A complete and skillful physical examination is always an important component of the evaluation. We should then review previous lab tests and order additional lab tests, if appropriate, especially if the prior labs showed equivocal results, were done at the wrong time of day, were run in an unfamiliar laboratory, or if there is any question about possible assay interference from supplements. An ACTH stimulation test (see above) may be considered. If not already done, testing for other endocrine-related and metabolic conditions, such as diabetes mellitus, calcium abnormalities, hypogonadism, celiac disease, vitamin D deficiency, vitamin B12 deficiency, sleep apnea, and depression can be considered. Some testing may be more appropriately done by the patient's primary care provider.

Regardless of the diagnosis, we should always emphasize the importance of healthy lifestyle measures to include good nutrition, regular exercise, good sleep habits, smoking cessation, moderation or cessation of alcohol consumption, stress reduction and stress management, and treatment of other coexisting illnesses (endocrine, general medical, psychiatric), if present. Management of non-endocrine related conditions by the primary care provider should be strongly encouraged.

We should also educate patients regarding medical information they find on the Internet and that they should always verify the source of the information in order to evaluate its credibility. This patient should be informed, but not lectured, that adrenal fatigue is not a real disorder and that salivary cortisol profiles have never been validated as a tool to evaluate adrenal insufficiency, whether they are ordered by another practitioner or are self-ordered from a website. And she should be advised that there is no credible evidence that adrenal supplements are beneficial. Furthermore, those products that contain whole adrenal glands or adrenal extracts actually contain steroid hormones that can suppress their own natural adrenal function and can also, depending on the amount of steroid hormones present, lead to steroid-related complications such as diabetes mellitus, osteoporosis, hypertension, hyperlipidemia, peptic ulcer disease, and glaucoma. We should respect the patient's initiative to investigate and implement measures to improve her/his quality of life but must emphasize our core value of practicing evidence-based medicine and the ethical responsibility we have to recommend tests and treatments that have proven efficacy and safety.

Consistent with these views, Dr. Rashmi Mullur published an excellent commentary on the management of adrenal fatigue in 2018 [14]. Stemming from her own experiences, she advises against lengthy or detailed explanations of adrenal physiology and the absence of evidence for the existence of adrenal fatigue and focusing instead on the actual needs of the patient with compassionate listening, an emphasis on healthy lifestyle measures and discussion of alternative approaches to reduce stress and mitigate the lingering effects of past emotional and/or physical trauma [14].

Satisfactory outcomes for these patients are clearly facilitated by the development of an honest, respectful, supportive, and compassionate relationship with their physician. As I have emphasized before, it is an honor that patients entrust their health to us and value our expertise. In return, our goal should be to do our best to improve their quality of life, even if there is no apparent endocrine disorder. This doesn't mean that we should take over the management of areas that are more appropriate for their primary care provider or other specialists. But it does mean that we should make it clear that we believe they are struggling with their symptoms, that we are concerned about their health and welfare, that we would like to be part of the solution if their condition is endocrine based, and that, while we strongly believe in innovative and individualized solutions, we have an obligation to provide them with the best evidence-based advice possible.

# References

1. Bornstein SR, Allolio B, Arlt W, et al. Diagnosis and treatment of primary adrenal insufficiency: an Endocrine Society clinical practice guideline. J Clin Endocrinol Metab. 2016;101:364–89.
2. Oltmanns KM, Fehm HL, Peters A. Chronic fentanyl application induces adrenocortical insufficiency. J Intern Med. 2005;257:478–80.
3. Donegan D, Bancos I. Opioid-induced adrenal insufficiency. Mayo Clin Proc. 2018;93(7):937–44.
4. Ospina NS, Nofal AA, Bancos I, et al. ACTH stimulation tests for the diagnosis of adrenal insufficiency: systematic review and meta-analysis. J Clin Endocrinol Metab. 2016;101:427–34.
5. De Bellis A, Bizzaro A, Rossi R, et al. Remission of subclinical adrenocortical failure in subjects with adrenal autoantibodies. J Clin Endocrinol Metab. 1993;76:1002–7.
6. Baker PR, Nanduri P, Gottlieb PA, et al. Predicting the onset of Addison's disease: ACTH, renin, cortisol and 21-hydroxylase autoantibodies. Clin Endocrinol. 2012;76(5):617–24.

7. Hormone Foundation (Endocrine Society) Website – Adrenal Fatigue. https://www.hormone.org/-/media/hormone/files/myth-vs-fact/mfsadrenalfatigue-520.pdf?la=en.
8. Hormone Health Network Adrenal Fatigue Fact Sheet. www.hormone.org/diseases-and-conditions/adrenal/adrenal-fatigue.
9. Schaffer R. In age of Internet diagnoses, endocrinologists confront myth of "adrenal fatigue". Endocrine Today, April 2018:1–12.
10. Seaborg E. The myth of adrenal fatigue. Endocrine News, Sept 2017: 29–32.
11. Mayo Clinic Website – Adrenal Fatigue. https://www.mayoclinic.org/diseases-conditions/addisons-disease/expert-answers/adrenal-fatigue/faq-20057906.
12. Akturk HD, Chindris AM, Hines JM, Singh RJ, Bernet VJ. Over-the-counter "adrenal support" supplements contain thyroid and steroid-based adrenal hormones. Mayo Clin Proc. 2018;93(3):284–90.
13. Pryor L. How to counter the circus of pseudoscience. New York Times, Jan 5, 2018.
14. Muller RS. Making a difference in adrenal fatigue. Endocr Pract. 2018;24(12):1103–5.

# Chapter 12
## Adrenal Insufficiency, "Relative Adrenal Insufficiency," or None of the Above?

**Maria Vamvini and James V. Hennessey**

While adrenal dysfunction is frequently reported in acutely ill patients and patients with liver cirrhosis, studies have shown that assessing adrenal function in this patient population can be extremely challenging and complex [1, 2]. In this chapter we are presenting a clinical case of an acutely ill middle-aged man with liver cirrhosis that was evaluated by the inpatient endocrine service for possible adrenal insufficiency (AI). Navigating through this case, we will review current evidence on adrenal function and evaluation for AI during acute illness and in patients with liver disease.

Case: A 59-year-old man presented to an outside community hospital complaining of dyspnea and abdominal pain. He had a history of hepatitis C and alcoholic liver disease and

M. Vamvini (✉) · J. V. Hennessey
Division of Endocrinology, Diabetes and Metabolism, Beth Israel Deaconess Medical Center, Harvard Medical School,
Boston, MA, USA
e-mail: mvamvini@bidmc.harvard.edu; jhenness@bidmc.harvard.edu

© Springer Nature Switzerland AG 2019
M. T. McDermott (ed.), *Management of Patients with Pseudo-Endocrine Disorders*,
https://doi.org/10.1007/978-3-030-22720-3_12

cirrhosis (Child's class C), chronic obstructive pulmonary disease (COPD), remote history of Guillain-Barre syndrome, neuropathy, and mood disorder. His home medications included two inhalers (budesonide-formoterol 160 mcg–4.5 mcg/actuation twice a day and as needed albuterol-ipratropium nebulizers), gabapentin, amitriptyline, and quetiapine. He was initially diagnosed with an acute exacerbation of COPD and treated with prednisone 40 mg a day for 5 days along with albuterol-ipratropium nebulizers. His dyspnea subsequently improved, but his abdominal pain persisted, having episodes of nausea and vomiting. His abdominal x-ray revealed distal bowel obstruction for which he was treated with bowel rest and a nasogastric tube for decompression. A flexible sigmoidoscopy and colonoscopy did not reveal any underlying structural pathology. The gastroenterologist raised concern that his bowel obstruction was related to his advanced liver disease and hypoalbuminemia which could be the cause of significant intestinal edema and bowel obstruction. During this acute illness, his liver disease decompensated. He developed diuretic refractory ascites and underwent two large-volume paracenteses with concomitant albumin infusions. His hospital course was further complicated with fever, hepatic encephalopathy, and hypotension, and he was subsequently transferred to our institution for further management in the intensive care unit.

His physical exam on admission to our institution was notable for blood pressure of 94/59 and hypoxia with oxygen saturation of 90% on 3 liters of oxygen. There was limited air entry in both lung bases; his abdomen was distended and tender with hyperactive bowel sounds. There was significant anasarca. His medications on transfer from the outside hospital were furosemide, spironolactone, thiamine, multivitamins, amitriptyline, gabapentin, quetiapine, budesonide-formoterol inhaler, and pantoprazole. His laboratory evaluation was notable for leukocytosis, normocytic anemia, abnormal coagulation studies, and acute kidney injury (Table 12.1). He had recurrence of bowel obstruction, bacteremia, and spontaneous bacterial peritonitis with worsening hepatic encephalopathy

## Chapter 12. Adrenal Insufficiency, "Relative Adrenal… 141

and was treated with vasopressors, broad-spectrum antibiotics, and further albumin infusions in the medical intensive care unit (MICU). He was eventually weaned off the vasopressors successfully and transferred to the regular medicine floor 2 weeks later.

Upon his transfer to the medical floor, his physical exam was notable again for hypotension and hypoxia with BP 98/60, HR 83, oxygen saturation 98% on 3 liters of oxygen with oxygen supplementation through nasal cannula, a distended but soft and non-tender abdomen with positive fluid wave, and normoactive bowel sounds. There was trace bilateral pedal edema but no asterixis. His skin exam revealed no ulcers or wounds, and there were no hyperpigmented or hypopigmented skin lesions. The laboratory results on the day of his transfer out of the MICU are summarized in Table 12.1. His repeat chemistry showed improved creatinine (1.4 mg/dL) and resolution of bilirubinemia. He continued to receive treatment for his hepatic encephalopathy with three therapeutic paracenteses. He was receiving albumin infusions following each paracentesis with improvement of albumin levels to 3.8 g/dL on the day of transfer to the medicine floor. Due to persistent, albeit mild, hypotension the primary team decided to evaluate him for adrenal insufficiency by measuring a morning total cortisol level.

**We should pause here and think about the factors regulating the hypothalamic-pituitary-adrenal (HPA) axis, cortisol secretion, and measured total cortisol levels** The intricate system of cortisol homeostasis is influenced by the intrinsic pulsatility of hypothalamic corticotropin-releasing hormone (CRH) and pituitary adrenocorticotropic hormone (ACTH)-secreting cells. Activation of the HPA axis is initiated by increased secretion of CRH and arginine vasopressin (AVP) from parvocellular neurons of the hypothalamic paraventricular nucleus (PVN) [3, 4]. CRH and AVP then reach the portal circulation of the anterior pituitary and promote ACTH secretion from pituitary corticotropic cells into the

TABLE 12.1 Laboratory data on the day of transfer from the referring institution to our institution and on the day of transfer from the ICU to the medical floor

| Variable | Reference range | Day of transfer from referring institution | Day of transfer from ICU to medical floor |
|---|---|---|---|
| White blood cell count (WBC) | 4.0–10.0 K/uL | 11.1 | 10.2 |
| Hemoglobin (Hgb) | 13.7–17.5 g/dL | 8.2 | 7.1 |
| Hematocrit (Hct) | 40–51% | 24.4 | 21.6 |
| Platelets | 150–400 K/uL | 154 | 122 |
| MCV | 82–98 fL | 84 | 90 |
| Sodium | 135–147 mEq/L | 134 | 136 |
| Potassium | 3.3–5.1 mEq/L | 3.3 | 3.6 |
| Chloride | 96–108 mEq/L | 95 | 106 |
| Bicarbonate | 22–32 mEq/L | 24 | 18 |
| Anion gap | 10–18 mEq/L | 18 | 16 |
| Blood urea nitrogen (BUN) | 6–20 mg/dL | 29 | 24 |
| Creatinine | 0.5–1.2 mg/dL | 3.2 | 1.4 |
| Glucose | 70–100 mg/dL | 105 | 115 |
| Albumin[a] | 3.5–5.2 g/dL | 4.2 | 3.8 |

TABLE 12.1 (continued)

| Variable | Reference range | Day of transfer from referring institution | Day of transfer from ICU to medical floor |
|---|---|---|---|
| Calcium | 8.4–10.3 mg/dL | 8.3 | 8.0 |
| Magnesium | 1.6–2.6 mg/dL | 2.0 | – |
| INR | 0.9–1.1 | 2.5 | 2.5 |
| PT | 9.4–12.5 s | 28 | 27.8 |
| aPTT | 25.0–36.5 s | 50.5 | 62.5 |
| Total bilirubin | 0–1.5 mg/dL | 2.2 | 1.1 |
| Alanine aminotransferase | 0–40 IU/L | 14 | 10 |
| Aspartate aminotransferase | 0–40 IU/L | 32 | 28 |
| Alkaline phosphatase | 40–130 IU/L | 49 | 40 |
| Morning serum total cortisol | 2–20 ug/dL | | 3.6 |

[a]Following repeat albumin infusions

bloodstream. ACTH then stimulates cortisol synthesis in the zona fasciculata cells of the adrenal cortex. This occurs through activation of protein kinase A (PKA) and increased transcription of the steroidogenic acute regulatory protein (StAR). In turn this initiates a series of enzymatic reactions involving P450 cytochromes resulting in cortisol synthesis using cholesterol as a substrate [5]. A negative feedback loop is completed via increased cortisol levels which negatively regulate the activity of the HPA axis and subsequently its own production. This occurs at the level of the pituitary gland, where cortisol inhibits ACTH release, and at the level of the PVN, where it inhibits synthesis and release of CRH and AVP [6]. In stress-free states cortisol secretion is characterized by both circadian and ultradian rhythms. It is secreted in a pulsatile fashion through a 24-hour cycle with peak levels observed during the awake phase. Physical and psychological stress, inflammation, several medications and genetic factors affecting receptors, binding proteins, and adrenal enzymes also affect the HPA axis and subsequently cortisol secretion [7]. Table 12.2 summarizes the most common causes of altered cortisol-binding globulin (CBG) levels and CBG affinity for cortisol which in turns alters measured serum total cortisol levels [7].

Going back to the clinical case, his morning serum total cortisol level was 3.6 ug/dL. Given the low morning total cortisol level, an ACTH stimulation test was performed that same afternoon and revealed a poor total cortisol response (Table 12.3). The endocrine inpatient service was then consulted to provide further guidance on management and treatment of this patient. *Did he indeed have AI, and, if so, is this primary or secondary AI?* In primary AI there is impaired secretion of adrenal glucocorticoid and mineralocorticoid hormones due to primary destruction or dysfunction of the adrenal glands with characteristic lab findings of elevated plasma ACTH levels and low serum cortisol levels. The adrenal gland dysfunction may be due to an autoimmune process (Addison's disease, polyglandular autoimmune syndrome types 1 and 2), hemorrhage within the adrenal gland, metastasis, infection (tuberculosis, HIV, disseminated fungal infections), or drugs that inhibit cortisol biosynthesis (such as etomidate, ketoconazole, fluconazole) [8]. Our patient did not have an ACTH level checked during the initial ACTH stimulation test, so this information was not available to us at the time. There was no personal or family history of any autoimmune disease. He had undergone several imaging studies of his abdomen including two CT scans that showed normal appearance of both adrenal glands without any evidence of hemorrhage, atrophy, or enlargement (Fig. 12.1). A review of his

TABLE 12.2 Common causes of altered CBG levels and CBG affinity for cortisol

| Increased CBG concentration | Decreased CBG concentration | Increased CBG affinity | Decreased CBG affinity |
|---|---|---|---|
| Oral contraceptives | Cirrhosis | Glycosylation | Inflammation |
| Pregnancy | Ethanol | | Fever |
| Selective estrogen-receptor modulator | Inflammation/Sepsis | | Ethanol |
| Mitotane | Obesity/Insulin resistance | | SERPINA6 mutations |
| | IGF-1 | | |
| | Hyperthyroidism | | |
| | Exogenous glucocorticoids | | |
| | Cushing's syndrome | | |
| | Nephrotic syndrome | | |
| | SERPINA6 mutations | | |
| | Neutrophil elastase | | |

TABLE 12.3 Cosyntropin stimulation test on our patient the day of transfer from the MICU to medical floor

| Endocrine test | ACTH pg/ml | Total cortisol ug/dL | Aldosterone ng/dL |
|---|---|---|---|
| Baseline (04:20 PM) | Not checked | 2.3 | Not checked |
| 30 min (04:50 PM) | | 6.6 | |
| 60 min (05:20 PM) | | 7.4[a] | |

[a]322% increase from baseline

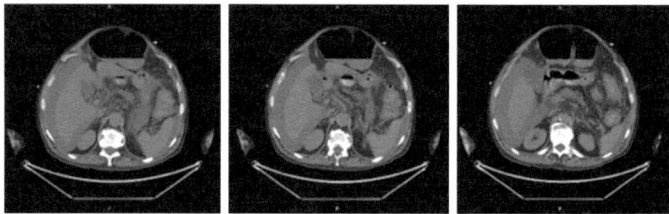

FIGURE 12.1 Abdominal CT without contrast. Adrenal glands both appeared normal

drug history prior to and during his hospitalization confirmed that he had not been exposed to any of the drugs that could lead to primary adrenal insufficiency. His exam did not reveal any skin hyperpigmentation, which is commonly seen in primary AI. He had chronic hyponatremia, but there was no hyperkalemia in his chemistry labs. Taking into consideration the above data, we considered his risk for primary AI to be low. What about his risks for secondary AI? There was no available pituitary imaging, and, therefore, a pituitary mass causing secondary AI could not be excluded. Apart from the brief use of prednisone at the outside hospital, there was no prior history of oral glucocorticoid use. He was, however, on a glucocorticoid inhaler, budesonide160 mcg/actuation twice a day, which could potentially lead to HPA axis suppression and secondary AI [9, 10]. Woods et al. reported that in patients using inhaled glucocorticoids without additional glucocorticoid therapy, 20.5% had abnormal ACTH stimulation test results. The ACTH stimulation test failure rates were 21.2% for patients taking fluticasone, 16.7% for beclomethasone, and 19.1% for budesonide [10]. According to this data, one of his risks for secondary AI was the use of an inhaled glucocorticoid. We should also take into consideration that he was critically ill. *Is it possible that critical illness* per se *could be the cause of AI?*

**Before addressing this question, we should first review the effect of critical illness on the HPA axis and cortisol secretion** During critical illness, there is stress-induced activation of the HPA axis with subsequent increases in cortisol secretion. There is extensive medical literature on AI observed during critical illness, a condition also known as critical illness-related corticosteroid insufficiency (CIRCI). This clinical entity was first described in 1946 by Dr. Hans Selye, a pioneering Austrian-Canadian endocrinologist of Hungarian origin, who was the first to demonstrate the existence of biological stress and conducted studies on the hypothetical nonspecific response of an organism to stressors. Although he did not describe all of the many aspects of glucocorticoid action, he was aware of their role in the stress response [11]. Later, a distinction was made between "absolute" and "relative" adrenal insufficiency in the critically ill. Absolute adrenal insufficiency is well-characterized and understood and refers to an unequivocal failure of cortisol production; it is divided into primary, secondary, and iatrogenic adrenal insufficiency, depending on the etiology [12, 13]. In contrast, "relative adrenal insufficiency" (RAI) is a highly controversial term that refers to an apparent functional deficiency acquired during critical illness and implies an insufficiently activated adrenal cortex relative to the degree of stress, even when plasma cortisol levels are higher than during the healthy non-stressed state [14].

**What are the mechanisms that might lead to adrenal insufficiency during acute illness and sepsis?** In many acutely ill or septic patients, a "dissociation" between ACTH and cortisol concentrations is observed, with low plasma ACTH levels and normal or elevated serum cortisol concentrations. Underlying mechanisms leading to this hormonal dysregulation during acute illness are poorly understood [15]. Based on evidence from experimental studies, HPA axis dysregulation was considered to be due to the negative effect of cytokines such as TNF and IL-1β on CRH-stimulated ACTH release [16]. Different sets of data are suggestive of increased free (not total) serum cortisol levels during acute illness as well as reduced cortisol clearance due to diminished expression and activity of cortisol-metabolizing enzymes. Both lead to elevated cortisol levels and, in turn, to suppression of ACTH secretion [11]. Moving away from the hypothalamus and pituitary, AI in acutely ill patients with sepsis may be caused by structural damage to the adrenal glands due to hemorrhage or infarction as it is known that certain pathogens show specific tropism to the adrenal glands. Lastly, a functional impairment of glucocorticoid synthesis and tissue resistance has been described in sepsis; it is postulated that this "glucocorticoid resistance" could explain the increased size of adrenal glands in patients with prolonged sepsis. It has been reported that increased adrenal gland volume positively correlates with the survival rate of critically ill patients, and consequently the size of the adrenal glands has been suggested as a predictor of sepsis outcome [17].

CIRCI and RAI remain controversial clinical entities, and possible mechanisms continue to be debated. The diagnosis of AI and identification of those critically ill patients with AI who may potentially benefit from glucocorticoid therapy have differed significantly in the published literature, depending on the population of patients studied and the diagnostic criteria used [11, 18]. Various studies have recommended different diagnostic criteria for RAI [19]. For example, Annane et al. proposed that a subnormal serum cortisol incremental response (<9 μg/dL) to exogenous ACTH administration, regardless of the baseline cortisol concentration, is suggestive of RAI [20]. Other studies recommend that a random serum total cortisol <10 μg/dL during critical illness is diagnostic of the presence of AI [18]. Despite a large body of literature, there is no consensus today about how to assess adrenal function in the critically ill patient. The use of the ACTH stimulation test, measuring serum total cortisol to predict the need for glucocorticoid therapy, is no longer recommended in patients with acute illness [18, 21, 22].

Studies have shown that during an acute illness, there is an immediate fall in the circulating levels of the binding proteins, cortisol-binding globulin (CBG), and albumin. CBG binding affinity is also acutely altered in the presence of elevated body temperature (febrile illness) and cleavage by neutrophil elastase [11]. Are these changes in the binding proteins important? Cortisol is a lipophilic molecule transported in the circulation bound to CBG and albumin. CBG binds 80–90% of circulating cortisol with high affinity and low capacity, whereas albumin binds only 10–15% of cortisol with low affinity. In normal healthy states, only a small fraction (5–10%) of cortisol is unbound, biologically active, and free to enter cells, where it interacts with glucocorticoid receptors, provides feedback inhibition in the hypothalamus and pituitary gland, and is ultimately responsible for its cellular functions. In acute illness, low CBG levels and decreased CBG binding affinity translate into lower-than-anticipated measured total serum cortisol concentrations and can thereby lead to the incorrect conclusion that adrenal function is impaired in critical illness [1].

**How would you interpret an ACTH stimulation test in a patient who is acutely ill with sepsis and decompensated liver disease? Would you recommend treatment with glucocorticoids based on the current available data?** Assessing adrenal function in patients who are chronically ill with an acute decompensation in their health status is extremely challenging and complex. As discussed earlier, it is suggested that measured levels of serum total cortisol and the cortisol response to a cosyntropin stimulation test are not reliable markers of adrenal function in a patient with an acute illness [1]. The same notion applies to patients with liver disease and advanced cirrhosis [23]. Several studies have reported that AI is common in patients with compensated and decompensated liver disease. Based on the same literature, cirrhosis is considered to be one of the risk factors for the development of AI; the term "hepato-adrenal" syndrome has been used to label apparent AI observed in this patient population [24].

The term "hepato-adrenal" syndrome was introduced by Marik et al. in 2005 to describe the presence of AI in patients with advanced liver disease with sepsis and/or other complications [24]. The hypothesis is that AI may be a feature of liver disease per se, but the pathophysiology of the "hepato-adrenal" syndrome remains largely unknown [25]. Similar to acute illness and sepsis, suggested mechanisms of AI in liver disease include increased levels of endotoxins, bacterial translocation of enteric organisms, structural damage to the adrenal glands, glucocorticoid resistance, and decreased serum levels of apoA1, HDL, and LDL cholesterol, which is the substrate for cortisol synthesis. These mechanisms are all hypothetical, and treatment with corticosteroids in this patient population remains controversial [26].

Several groups have studied the prevalence of AI in patients with liver disease, but the prevalence rates vary widely from 10% to 92% [25]. These significant discrepancies in the prevalence of AI in cirrhosis can be explained by differences in testing conditions or formulas used to estimate free cortisol levels as well as different criteria and cutoff levels used for establishing the diagnosis of AI. While the GI community seems convinced that RAI and hepato-adrenal syndrome are clinical entities and characteristic of liver disease, the endocrine community remains skeptical whether these syndromes exist. Serum total cortisol is not a reliable assay in patients with dysproteinemia. Patients with advanced liver disease and pronounced hypoalbuminemia are often misdiagnosed as having AI when the diagnosis is made based on the serum total cortisol levels. The main challenge is to find a reliable way to assess adrenal function in states of ill health, such as critical illness, sepsis, cirrhosis, and malnutrition, which are all associated with low serum albumin and CBG levels and compromised cortisol binding to these carrier proteins. Our patient's total cortisol response to ACTH

Chapter 12. Adrenal Insufficiency, "Relative Adrenal... 151

stimulation is difficult to interpret given his significant hypoalbuminemia and dysproteinemia.

Serum free cortisol (SFC) represents a more accurate assessment of adrenal function in patient populations with abnormal levels of binding proteins [2, 27]. Several formulas of variable complexity have been validated for estimation of SFC. The most widely used formulas are the free cortisol index (FCI) and Coolens' equation. The FCI, a ratio of the serum total cortisol level to the CBG level, is the simpler of the two formulas, but it does not take into account the CBG saturability in high-cortisol states and the changes in its binding affinity in certain illnesses. Coolens' formula, which is more complex than the FCI, calculates the free cortisol concentration based on the following equation: "$U2 \times K (1 + N) + U [1 + N + K (G - T)] - T = 0$," where T is total cortisol, G is CBG, U is unbound cortisol, K is the affinity of CBG for cortisol at 37 °C, and N is the ratio of albumin-bound to albumin-unbound cortisol. It is considered to provide a more accurate estimation of SFC levels when CBG is saturated, but it does not account for changes in albumin levels or CBG affinity. Due to the above limitations, this formula has been proven to lack accuracy in patients with sepsis [28]. The limitations of these indirect methods are the oversimplification of a highly complex system as well as the incorporation of multiple sources of error [29].

Given the limitations of estimation formulas, it is recommended that evaluation of adrenal function in cases of dysproteinemia be performed using a direct measurement of SFC levels. This involves first separating cortisol that is bound to CBG or albumin from the SFC, followed by quantification of SFC by immunoassay or liquid chromatography-tandem mass spectrometry (LC-MS/MS). The most common techniques used to separate bound cortisol from free cortisol in the serum are equilibrium dialysis and ultrafiltration. Equilibrium dialysis involves incubating the serum in a compartment with a semipermeable membrane that CBG is not able to cross, while ultrafiltration involves centrifugation of serum samples in a tube fitted with a filter that has pores smaller than CBG molecules [7, 29]. However, these SFC assays are expensive and time-consuming, and the results are usually delayed, making them inconvenient for routine clinical practice and unsuitable for guiding acute clinical decisions. Another limiting factor is the lack of specific criteria for diagnosis of AI using SFC levels [11].

**Are there diagnostic criteria for AI using SFC measurements?** Current standards for defining AI are based on total serum cortisol levels in healthy persons with normal CBG levels. There have been no large studies that have explored the best threshold for identifying patients with or without AI using SFC. Trying to compare the cutoff values previously recommended for SFC is problematic since each study has used different assays and studied different patient populations [23]. The main question is how low should the SFC be to warrant consideration of treatment with glucocorticoids? Rauschecker et al. performed a study aiming to create a normative database of SFC responses to ACTH stimulation (250 mcg) in healthy volunteers and to compare this with the responses of patients with documented primary AI, secondary AI, and cirrhosis (Child-Pugh class A or B) [2]. The authors found that the optimal peak SFC level criterion to correctly diagnose AI patients vs. healthy volunteers was a response of at least 0.9 ug/dL (25 nmol/L) (sensitivity 95% and specificity 100%) [2]. This study did not include patients with more advanced liver disease. Therefore, data regarding normal or abnormal SFC levels and the SFC response to ACTH stimulation remains limited.

Returning to the clinical case, given the initial abnormal serum total cortisol response to ACTH (cosyntropin) stimulation, replacement doses of hydrocortisone (HC) were initiated by the primary team. Prior to initiating HC replacement, the Endocrinology Consult Service recommended a repeat cosyntropin stimulation test measuring serum total cortisol as well as SFC and aldosterone at all three time points (baseline, 30 and 60 min). His baseline ACTH level was also checked this time. Results of the second stimulation test are shown in Table 12.4.

## Chapter 12. Adrenal Insufficiency, "Relative Adrenal... 153

TABLE 12.4 ACTH (cosyntropin) stimulation test results on our patient

| Endocrine test | ACTH pg/ml | Total cortisol ug/dL | Free cortisol ug/dL | Aldosterone ng/dL |
|---|---|---|---|---|
| Baseline (05:43 AM) | 16 | 3.2 | 0.37 | 5 |
| 30 min (06:05 AM) |  | 7.2 | 1.01 | 16 |
| 60 min (06:35 AM) |  | 8.5[a] | 1.33[b] | 19[c] |

[a]266% increase from baseline
[b]360% increase from baseline
[c]380% increase from baseline

His ACTH levels were normal, and there was an appropriate aldosterone response. Based on this data, primary AI was ruled out. His serum total cortisol levels remained low with a persistent suboptimal response to cosyntropin stimulation. His SFC levels, however, peaked at 1.33 ug/dL, which is higher than the recommended cutoff of 0.9 ug/dL [2]. He underwent a pituitary MRI which did not reveal any pituitary structural lesions (Fig. 12.2). He had been on treatment with a glucocorticoid inhaler, which increased the risk of secondary AI based on the study by Woods et al. [10]. Nevertheless, given the threefold increase in his SFC levels with a peak value above the recommended diagnostic threshold, we considered a diagnosis of secondary AI also unlikely. Our biochemical/laboratory diagnosis was confirmed by the lack of symptomatic improvement with glucocorticoid treatment initiated by the primary team; his blood pressure remained in the low to low-normal range even on HC treatment. Based on the above laboratory and clinical data and taking into consideration the high risk for infection while on glucocorticoid treatment, we recommended discontinuation of glucocorticoids. He was monitored off-treatment for 1 week, and it was reassuring that his vital signs improved and he eventually recovered without glucocorticoids.

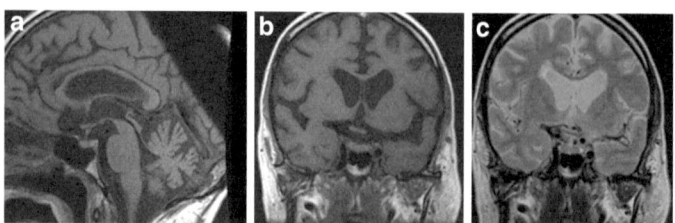

FIGURE 12.2 Pituitary MRI. Normal-appearing pituitary gland (**a**, T1 sagittal; **b**, T1 coronal; **c**, T2 coronal view)

Assessing adrenal function during acute illness or in patients who are chronically ill with an acute decompensation in their health status is extremely challenging and complex. It is suggested that in acute illness, serum total cortisol levels and the response of total cortisol to a cosyntropin stimulation test are not reliable markers of adrenal function due to hypoalbuminemia, low serum CBG levels, and altered CBG affinity for cortisol binding. The same notion applies to patients with liver disease and advanced cirrhosis. Direct measurement of SFC by ultrafiltration followed by LC-MS/MS is the most accurate way to quantify the biologically active free fraction of cortisol and address many of the challenges that we face in the evaluation of the HPA axis in the abovementioned patient population. There is limited data on the best diagnostic criteria for AI using SFC assays. Thus, it is of paramount importance that baseline and post-ACTH stimulation reference ranges be established for SFC using LC-MS/MS. The serum total cortisol level might still be the most cost- and time-effective measurement for evaluating the HPA axis in many clinical situations; total serum cortisol values greater than 18 ug/dL usually rule out significant AI. However, consideration of SFC measurement is useful in more complicated situations when total cortisol levels may be misleading due to dysproteinemia and do not adequately explain the patient's clinical presentation [7].

# References

1. Hamrahian AH, Oseni TS, Arafah BM. Measurements of serum free cortisol in critically ill patients. N Engl J Med. 2004;350(16):1629–38.
2. Rauschecker M, Abraham SB, Abel BS, et al. Cosyntropin-stimulated serum free cortisol in healthy, adrenally insufficient, and mildly cirrhotic populations. J Clin Endocrinol Metab. 2016;101(3):1075–81.
3. Gillies GE, Linton EA, Lowry PJ. Corticotropin releasing activity of the new CRF is potentiated several times by vasopressin. Nature. 1982;299(5881):355–7.
4. Rivier C, Vale W. Interaction of corticotropin-releasing factor and arginine vasopressin on adrenocorticotropin secretion in vivo. Endocrinology. 1983;113(3):939–42.
5. Stocco DM, Wang X, Jo Y, Manna PR. Multiple signaling pathways regulating steroidogenesis and steroidogenic acute regulatory protein expression: more complicated than we thought. Mol Endocrinol. 2005;19(11):2647–59.
6. Kanczkowski W, Sue M, Zacharowski K, Reincke M, Bornstein SR. The role of adrenal gland microenvironment in the HPA axis function and dysfunction during sepsis. Mol Cell Endocrinol. 2015;408:241–8.
7. Verbeeten KC, Ahmet AH. The role of corticosteroid-binding globulin in the evaluation of adrenal insufficiency. J Pediatr Endocrinol Metab. 2018;31(2):107–15.
8. Auron M, Raissouni N. Adrenal insufficiency. Pediatr Rev. 2015;36(3):92–102; quiz 103, 129.
9. Gordon AC, McDonald CF, Thomson SA, Frame MH, Pottage A, Crompton GK. Dose of inhaled budesonide required to produce clinical suppression of plasma cortisol. Eur J Respir Dis. 1987;71(1):10–4.
10. Woods CP, Argese N, Chapman M, et al. Adrenal suppression in patients taking inhaled glucocorticoids is highly prevalent and management can be guided by morning cortisol. Eur J Endocrinol. 2015;173(5):633–42.
11. Boonen E, Van den Berghe G. Mechanisms in endocrinology: new concepts to further unravel adrenal insufficiency during critical illness. Eur J Endocrinol. 2016;175(1):R1–9.

12. Oelkers W. Adrenal insufficiency. N Engl J Med. 1996;335(16):1206–12.
13. Charmandari E, Nicolaides NC, Chrousos GP. Adrenal insufficiency. Lancet. 2014;383(9935):2152–67.
14. Gonzalez H, Nardi O, Annane D. Relative adrenal failure in the ICU: an identifiable problem requiring treatment. Crit Care Clin. 2006;22(1):105–118, vii.
15. Prigent H, Maxime V, Annane D. Science review: mechanisms of impaired adrenal function in sepsis and molecular actions of glucocorticoids. Crit Care. 2004;8(4):243–52.
16. Gaillard RC, Turnill D, Sappino P, Muller AF. Tumor necrosis factor alpha inhibits the hormonal response of the pituitary gland to hypothalamic releasing factors. Endocrinology. 1990;127(1):101–6.
17. Jung B, Nougaret S, Chanques G, et al. The absence of adrenal gland enlargement during septic shock predicts mortality: a computed tomography study of 239 patients. Anesthesiology. 2011;115(2):334–43.
18. Marik PE, Pastores SM, Annane D, et al. Recommendations for the diagnosis and management of corticosteroid insufficiency in critically ill adult patients: consensus statements from an international task force by the American College of Critical Care Medicine. Crit Care Med. 2008;36(6):1937–49.
19. Hamrahian AH, Fleseriu M, Committee AAS. Evaluation and management of adrenal insufficiency in critically ill patients: disease state review. Endocr Pract. 2017;23(6):716–25.
20. Annane D, Sebille V, Charpentier C, et al. Effect of treatment with low doses of hydrocortisone and fludrocortisone on mortality in patients with septic shock. JAMA. 2002;288(7):862–71.
21. Dellinger RP, Levy MM, Rhodes A, et al. Surviving sepsis campaign: international guidelines for management of severe sepsis and septic shock: 2012. Crit Care Med. 2013;41(2):580–637.
22. Sprung CL, Annane D, Keh D, et al. Hydrocortisone therapy for patients with septic shock. N Engl J Med. 2008;358(2):111–24.
23. Thevenot T, Borot S, Remy-Martin A, et al. Assessment of adrenal function in cirrhotic patients using concentration of serum-free and salivary cortisol. Liver Int. 2011;31(3):425–33.
24. Marik PE, Gayowski T, Starzl TE, Hepatic Cortisol R, Adrenal Pathophysiology Study G. The hepatoadrenal syndrome: a common yet unrecognized clinical condition. Crit Care Med. 2005;33(6):1254–9.

25. Trifan A, Chiriac S, Stanciu C. Update on adrenal insufficiency in patients with liver cirrhosis. World J Gastroenterol. 2013;19(4):445–56.
26. Bertino G, Privitera G, Purrello F, et al. Emerging hepatic syndromes: pathophysiology, diagnosis and treatment. Intern Emerg Med. 2016;11(7):905–16.
27. Degand T, Monnet E, Durand F, et al. Assessment of adrenal function in patients with acute hepatitis using serum free and total cortisol. Dig Liver Dis. 2015;47(9):783–9.
28. Coolens JL, Van Baelen H, Heyns W. Clinical use of unbound plasma cortisol as calculated from total cortisol and corticosteroid-binding globulin. J Steroid Biochem. 1987;26(2):197–202.
29. Vogeser M, Groetzner J, Kupper C, Briegel J. Free serum cortisol during the postoperative acute phase response determined by equilibrium dialysis liquid chromatography-tandem mass spectrometry. Clin Chem Lab Med. 2003;41(2):146–51.

# Chapter 13
# Pseudo-Cushing's Syndrome: A Diagnostic Dilemma

**Teresa Brown, Regina Belokovskaya, and Rachel Pessah-Pollack**

## Case Presentation

A 29-year-old female was referred to our institution for transsphenoidal approach (TSA) for presumed Cushing's disease after an outside hospital evaluation showed evidence of hypercortisolism. During the year prior to the referral, she had experienced a 25 pound weight gain, a diagnosis of pre-diabetes, fatigue, and depressed mood. She had a past medical history of obesity but no other relevant conditions.

On review of systems, she endorsed insomnia, increased stress, hirsutism on the chest and chin, facial redness, muscle aches, and headaches. She denied easy bruising or fractures. She was on an estrogen-containing oral contraceptive pill (OCP) and reported regular menstrual cycles. Her OCP had not been discontinued for the biochemical evaluation.

Chart reviewed revealed the following laboratory results: Two urinary free cortisol (UFC) collections were obtained.

T. Brown · R. Belokovskaya · R. Pessah-Pollack (✉)
Icahn School of Medicine at Mount Sinai Medical Center, Division of Endocrinology, Diabetes, & Bone Disease, New York, NY, USA

© Springer Nature Switzerland AG 2019
M. T. McDermott (ed.), *Management of Patients with Pseudo-Endocrine Disorders*,
https://doi.org/10.1007/978-3-030-22720-3_13

The first UFC was 126.8 ug/24 hours (normal <45 ug/24 hours) with a volume of 2300 ml (normal, 700–1600 ml) and a 24-hour urinary creatinine of 3.28 g/volume (normal, 0.63–2.5); the second UFC was 53.2 ug/24 hours with a volume of 1750 cc and a 24-hour urinary creatinine of 1.8 g/volume. Two late-night salivary cortisol levels were within normal range, 0.074 and 0.080 ug/dl (normal <0.112 ug/dl).

Two separate 1 mg dexamethasone suppression tests (DST) revealed inappropriate suppression with serum cortisol levels of 7.2 and 3.1 ug/dl (dexamethasone level = 415 ng/dl; target: 140–295 ng/dl). Plasma ACTH levels were checked with the DSTs and both were <5 pg/ml.

Additional labs on a separate day showed a serum cortisol level of 17 ug/dl, a plasma adrenocorticotropic hormone (ACTH) level of 9 pg/ml (normal, 6–58 pg/ml), and dehydroepiandrosterone sulfate (DHEA-S) of 155 ug/dl (normal, 65–380 ug/dl).

An MRI of her pituitary did not reveal a pituitary adenoma. The etiology of her hypercortisolism was further assessed with inferior petrosal sinus sampling (IPSS) at the outside institution, and results (plasma ACTH levels) were as follows:

| Time | Peripheral | Right central | Left central |
|---|---|---|---|
| 0 | 2.3 | 19.6 | 36.1 |
| 2 | 2.6 | 32.5 | 27.2 |
| 5 | 3.5 | 97.4 | 140.4 |
| 10 | 6 | 193.5 | 221.1 |
| 15 | 4.7 | 73.9 | 110.4 |

In the setting of a central-to-peripheral plasma ACTH gradient ≥2 before CRH administration and ≥3 after CRH, she was referred to our institution for TSA for a presumed pituitary source. Her transsphenoidal surgery was complicated by a cerebrospinal fluid leak and required abdominal graft placement. At the time of surgery, no definite adenoma was seen. Pathology was remarkable for fragments of normal adenohypophysis and neurohypophysis.

Our consult service was requested postoperatively. Vital signs on postoperative day zero upon our consultation were as follows: blood pressure 133/77, T 99.9 F, heart rate 78, respiratory rate 20, weight 90.3 kg, and BMI 30.3. The patient had a full round face with some facial redness and a dorsocervical fat pad. There were no hyperpigmented striae appreciated.

Serum cortisol levels on postoperative days 1, 2, and 3 were 22, 26, and 15 ug/dl, respectively.

Her postoperative course was complicated by a pulmonary embolus, and she was started on rivaroxaban (Xarelto). She was also treated with insulin for hyperglycemia as she could not tolerate metformin and did not want to take oral medications. She also stopped her estrogen-containing OCP.

Two weeks after stopping the estrogen-containing OCP, she was evaluated as an outpatient in our clinic. She had a morning serum cortisol level of 15.2 ug/dl and a plasma ACTH level of 11 pg/ml. She had two late-night salivary cortisol levels of 0.091 and 0.047 ug/dl (normal <0.112 ug/dl). Her initial postoperative UFC was 71.4 ug/24 hours (normal <45 ug/24 hours).

About 6 weeks after stopping the estrogen-containing OCP, her AM cortisol level was 7.6 ug/dl and her UFC was 30 ug/24 hours. A repeat 1 mg dexamethasone suppression test exhibited appropriate suppression.

## *Physiologic Causes of Hypercortisolism (Non-neoplastic)*

Endogenous hypercortisolism can be either physiologic (non-neoplastic) or pathologic (neoplastic). There are many causes of non-neoplastic hypercortisolism, or "pseudo-Cushing's syndrome," which can make neoplastic Cushing's syndrome one of the most challenging diagnoses to make in clinical endocrinology.

A number of stressors have been found to increase hypothalamic pituitary adrenal (HPA) axis activity, and the laboratory findings in these patients can be similar to those with states of pathologic hypercortisolism [1–3]. Subtle activation of the HPA axis may lead to mild increases in cortisol production

Table 13.1 Causes of physiologic hypercortisolism (pseudo-Cushing's syndrome)

| |
|---|
| Alcoholism |
| Alcohol withdrawal |
| Uncontrolled diabetes mellitus |
| Starvation/malnutrition |
| Pregnancy |
| Chronic intense exercise |
| Chronic kidney disease |
| Psychiatric disease |
| Glucocorticoid resistance |

Reference [5]

that can be similar to those found in subclinical Cushing's syndrome [4]. The most common causes of non-neoplastic physiological hypercortisolism, or pseudo-Cushing's syndrome, are alcoholism and alcohol withdrawal, chronic kidney disease, depression or neuropsychiatric disease, pregnancy, uncontrolled diabetes, starvation/malnutrition, chronic intense exercise, and glucocorticoid resistance [5] (see Table 13.1). This chapter will focus on the diagnosis and evaluation of the non-neoplastic etiologies of hypercortisolism that clinicians commonly face in their assessment of Cushing's syndrome.

## *Alcohol-Induced Hypercortisolism*

Alcohol-induced cortisol hypersecretion is a well-known phenomenon. Differentiating pathologic Cushing's syndrome from alcohol-induced hypercortisolism is challenging because of similarities in some of the diagnostic tests and potential limitations in obtaining an accurate history regarding a patient's alcohol consumption. Excessive alcohol intake increases cortisol secretion acutely and chronically [6, 7]. This is primarily mediated through the activation of hypothalamic corticotropin releasing hormone (CRH) secretion into the portal veins, stimulating the anterior pituitary gland to produce excessive ACTH [8, 9]. Vasopressin secretion may also be increased secondary to alcohol and may augment the ACTH response to CRH. Because hepatic dysfunction is also common in alcoholics, impaired peripheral clearance of cortisol may contribute to the elevated serum cortisol levels [10]. Late-night salivary cortisol and UFC measurements may also be increased in patients with alcohol-induced hypercortisolism. Furthermore, the overnight dexamethasone suppression test and dexamethasone-CRH test are often abnormal in the setting of active alcohol consumption and cannot be used to differentiate alcohol-induced hypercortisolism from pathologic Cushing's syndrome [11, 12]. In contrast to true Cushing's disease, however, there may be no ACTH response to stimulation with desmopressin (DDAVP) in alcohol-induced pseudo-Cushing's syndrome (similar to healthy subjects) [13]. Probably the best way to help differentiate between alcohol-induced hypercortisolism and true Cushing's syndrome is to have the patient abstain from alcohol; the clinical features of alcohol-induced pseudo-Cushing's often resolve with alcohol abstinence [14].

## Neuropsychiatric Conditions

Since Cushing's syndrome is often complicated by neuropsychiatric illnesses, proper differentiation of the cause of hypercortisolism becomes challenging in patients with neuropsychiatric conditions. Many of these disorders, especially psychotic depression, have been associated with increases in HPA axis activity [15]. Resistance to cortisol negative feedback can also be caused by decreases in the sensitivity of glucocorticoid and possibly mineralocorticoid receptors [16]. Many patients with underlying neuropsychiatric conditions have abnormal low-dose dexamethasone suppression tests as well as increased late-night salivary cortisol levels and UFC [17]. As the dexamethasone-CRH test can be used in the diagnosis of depression, biochemical discrimination between true pathologic Cushing's syndrome and physiologic stimulation of the HPA axis from neuropsychiatric disorders can be very difficult [18]. Thus, it is often important to obtain psychiatry involvement in the care of these patients to help differentiate the underlying diseases.

## Type 2 Diabetes, Metabolic Syndrome, and Insulin Resistance

Patients with Cushing's syndrome often also have type 2 diabetes mellitus. In fact, since many of the clinical features are similar, these patients may go undiagnosed. The prevalence of Cushing's syndrome in patients with type 2 diabetes has been cited to be as high as 3% [19]. Increased late-night salivary cortisol concentrations have been found in some patients with poorly controlled type 2 diabetes mellitus [20]. However, variations in glucose levels do not have a major correlation with salivary cortisol excretion in diabetes mellitus [21]. It has also been suggested that patients with obesity, metabolic syndrome, and insulin resistance may have "tissue-specific" Cushing's syndrome. One proposed explanation is that increased adipose expression of 11-β-hydroxysteroid dehydrogenase 1 may generate increased tissue cortisol levels [22]. Therefore, subtle abnormalities in HPA axis function in patients with diabetes, especially with poor glycemic control, should be interpreted with caution.

## Pregnancy

Pregnancy is associated with increased levels of serum total cortisol as well as serum free cortisol and salivary cortisol, especially during the third trimester [23–25]. The increase in total cortisol is primarily due to the increases in corticosteroid-binding globulin (CBG) levels as pregnancy progresses, but the increase in free, biologically active cortisol is ACTH-mediated [23, 26]. The increase in plasma ACTH has been attributed to placental secretion of both CRH and ACTH, the increase in progesterone acting as a glucocorticoid antagonist, and a decrease in glucocorticoid negative feedback sensitivity

[23]. CRH-binding protein also increases during pregnancy [27–29]. The diagnosis of Cushing's syndrome in pregnancy, though uncommon, must be based on clinical and biochemical evidence of hypercortisolism [23].

### *Starvation/Eating Disorders*

Starvation-equivalent disorders may be associated with hypercortisolism. Patients in the intensive care unit for long periods of time have significant loss of muscle mass mediated in part by hypercortisolism [30]. Increases in serum cortisol levels have also been observed in healthy women undergoing low-calorie dieting and in women with significant weight loss after bariatric surgery [31]. Starvation associated with some eating disorders activates the HPA axis with varying degrees of hypercortisolism [30, 32]. Patients with anorexia nervosa have an attenuated ACTH response to CRH likely due to negative feedback of cortisol on the corticotrophs of the anterior pituitary [33]. The dexamethasone-CRH test may also be abnormal in patients with anorexia [33], but DDAVP does not stimulate ACTH in these patients, which is similar to healthy subjects [32]. Severity of bone loss and hypothalamic amenorrhea both correlate with the degree of hypercortisolism in these women [34, 35]. While patients with starvation disorders do not fit the typical clinical Cushing's syndrome profile (weight gain, obesity), it is important to be mindful of some of the biochemical changes that are associated with these disorders.

## Tests for Diagnosis of Cushing's Syndrome

The 2008 Endocrine Society guidelines recommend using one or more of three different measures for the initial testing for suspected Cushing's syndrome. These include a 24-hour UFC, an overnight 1 mg dexamethasone suppression test (DST), and late-night salivary cortisol (LNSC) levels [36]. If initial testing is normal, it is unlikely that the patient has Cushing's syndrome; however, if there is high clinical suspicion and normal test results, a referral to an endocrinologist is recommended. If abnormal results are noted on initial testing (e.g., elevated UFC on two occasions, abnormal overnight 1 mg DST, or elevated LNSC levels on two repeat tests), it is important to perform one of the other two tests, if not already performed, and/or repeat the abnormal study and then exclude physiologic causes of hypercortisolism.

It is also essential to note that the assay used can play a role in the reliability of the test. Cortisol metabolites and synthetic glucocorticoids can alter antibody-based immunoassays like RIA and ELISA. Structurally based assays such as high-performance liquid chromatography (HPLC) and liquid chromatography tandem mass spectrometry (LC-MS/MS) are not as likely to be falsely altered, although some drugs, like carbamazepine and fenofibrate, may falsely increase UFC results measured by the structurally based assays [36].

## Urinary Free Cortisol (UFC) Level

There are important considerations in evaluating a UFC level. This test measures unbound cortisol and, therefore, is less likely to be affected by medications and conditions that can alter CBG, such as pregnancy or oral estrogens. The patient should avoid using glucocorticoid-containing substances, such as creams, and should not drink excess fluids >5 L/day on the day of collection as high urine volume can falsely elevate results. Values can be falsely low when a patient's creatinine clearance is <60 ml/min, and levels fall linearly in relationship to the severity of renal disease [37]. It is also important to note that UFC can be normal in some patients with mild Cushing's syndrome [38] and also in those with cyclic disease. The UFC is often less than three times the upper limit of normal in patients with non-pathologic hypercortisolism [39].

## Late-Night Salivary Cortisol (LNSC)

In evaluating a LNSC test, it is important to note that ELISA and LC-MS/MS are the most well-validated assays [40].

In shift workers, patients with depression, and critically ill patients, the circadian rhythm, in which cortisol levels normally begin to rise at 3:00–4:00 AM, reach a peak at 7:00–9:00 AM, and then subsequently fall throughout the rest of the day, may be blunted or absent [41–43]. Noteworthy also is that the salivary glands express 11 B hydroxysteroid dehydrogenase type 2, the enzyme that converts biologically active cortisol to inactive cortisone. In patients who use licorice or chewing tobacco, both of which contain an enzyme called glycyrrhizic acid, an 11B-HSD2 inhibitor, the LNSC, may be falsely elevated. Smokers are known to have higher LNSC levels than non-smokers [44], and, therefore, a patient should be advised not to smoke on the day of collection. Contamination of the collection kit by steroid-containing substances, such as creams, may lead to false-positive results. Patients should also be advised to collect the sample after a quiet evening, as stress can increase salivary cortisol levels [45]. Salivary cortisol measurements are a better choice in patients on estrogen-containing OCPs [39].

## *1 mg Dexamethasone Suppression Test (DST)*

It is important to note that using higher dexamethasone doses of 1.5 or 2.0 mg has not been found to significantly improve the accuracy of the 1 mg DST [46]. Dexamethasone metabolism in individual patients can affect the results of the 1 mg DST. Drugs that induce the hepatic clearance of dexamethasone via the CYP 3A4 enzyme (phenytoin, phenobarbital, carbamazepine, rifampicin, and alcohol) can reduce plasma dexamethasone levels and result in false-positive results. Drugs that impair dexamethasone metabolism via inhibition of CYP 3A4 (aprepitant/fosaprepitant, itraconazole, ritonavir, fluoxetine, diltiazem, and cimetidine) can increase dexamethasone levels and potentially produce false-negative results. Patients with liver or renal failure may also have reduced clearance of dexamethasone. There is also variation in dexamethasone metabolism among healthy individuals with no other medical problems. It is therefore recommended that a serum dexamethasone level be measured along with the cortisol level to ensure that plasma dexamethasone concentrations are appropriate.

**Table 13.2** Drugs that impair interpretation of 1 mg dexamethasone suppression test

| |
|---|
| *Drugs that increase dexamethasone metabolism* |
| Phenobarbital |
| Phenytoin |
| Carbamazepine |
| Primidone |
| Rifampin |
| Rifapentine |
| Ethosuximide |
| Pioglitazone |
| *Drugs that decrease dexamethasone metabolism* |
| Aprepitant/fosaprepitant |
| Itraconazole |
| Ritonavir |
| Fluoxetine |
| Diltiazem |
| Cimetidine |

The 1 mg DST results in false-positive result in up to 50% of females taking oral contraceptive pills [47] (see Table 13.2).

## *Midnight Serum Cortisol Test*

The midnight serum cortisol test can be performed while the patient is awake or asleep. In patients for whom there is high suspicion for Cushing's syndrome but who have a normal UFC and adequate suppression on dexamethasone testing, a sleeping midnight serum cortisol >1.8 ug/dl or awake cortisol value >7.5 ug/dl increases the probability of Cushing's syndrome [48].

When there is lower suspicion but a mildly elevated UFC or lack of suppression on dexamethasone testing, a sleeping cortisol value <1.8 ug/dl excludes Cushing's syndrome [49]. A sleeping cortisol value <1.8 ug/dl excludes Cushing's syndrome in those who fail to suppress on dexamethasone suppression testing due to medications, such as anticonvulsants [49]. To obtain this test, a patient should be admitted to the hospital for more than a 48-hour period to avoid false positives from the stress of hospitalization. Blood should be drawn within 5–10 minutes of waking the patient or from a line (awake or asleep). An awake midnight serum cortisol is significantly easier to obtain and is associated with a normal cutoff value of 7.5 ug/dl [39].

## The 48-Hour 2 mg/day DST and Dex-CRH Tests Are Second-Line Tests Which Can Be Utilized in Certain Situations

In patients with suspected non-neoplastic hypercortisolism from conditions such as psychiatric disease, morbid obesity, alcoholism, and diabetes, the 48-hour, 2 mg/day low-dose DST (LDDST) can be utilized because UFC measurements are less useful in this situation [36]. Two weeks of abstinence from alcohol is necessary to reduce the false-positive rate on this test [44].

The dexamethasone-CRH (Dex-CRH) test is a second-line test consisting of the 48-hour 2 mg/day LDDST (described above) followed by the administration of 1 ug/kg of IV CRH 2 hours after the last dose of dexamethasone. Cortisol is subsequently measured 15 minutes after the CRH is administered. A dexamethasone level should be measured when CRH is administered.

## Inferior Petrosal Sinus Sampling (IPSS): Use and Interpretation

Only after a biochemical diagnosis of pathologic ACTH-dependent Cushing's syndrome has been established should imaging of the pituitary be performed. When the MRI fails to localize the lesion or gives ambiguous results, IPSS should be considered. It is a minimally invasive method that can help identify a pituitary source of excess ACTH to diagnose Cushing's disease. The diagnosis of Cushing's disease is confirmed by a baseline IPSS central/peripheral ratio ≥2 or CRH-stimulated IPSS central/peripheral ratio ≥3 [50].

The use of IPSS for lateralization of corticotroph microadenomas remains controversial and has not yet replaced the thorough examination of the pituitary gland by an experienced neurosurgeon after the diagnosis of Cushing's disease has been made [51].

## Discussion of Our Case

A critical factor to consider in the evaluation of our patient that contributed to her incorrect diagnosis was the use of an estrogen-containing OCP throughout the initial workup period; this likely led to false-positive results on the dexamethasone suppression test. Oral contraceptives increase the serum total cortisol concentration by increasing circulating CBG, while the unbound fraction is not influenced [52]. Therefore, serum total cortisol levels in a 1 mg DST could be elevated despite there being no increased activity of the HPA axis in someone using OCPs.

In a study by Crewther et al., the mean salivary cortisol values in women taking OCPs were similar to those of controls throughout the day, demonstrating that salivary cortisol, as an unbound fraction, is not affected by the OCP-induced increase in CBG [53]. This was confirmed in another study by Manetti et al., who also reported that the mean values of salivary cortisol in women on OCPs were similar to those of controls [54]. Of note, our patient's initial evaluation revealed normal salivary cortisol levels while on an OCP.

Furthermore, Crewther et al., evaluated 24-hour UFC excretion in women on OCPs and found them not to be significantly elevated in any of the subjects [55]. Jung et al., in an earlier study, also reported that 24-hour UFC levels were not significantly elevated in subjects on OCPs [25]. The latter study, however, did demonstrate modestly higher mean UFC levels of 114 +/− 15 nmol/day (41 ug/day) in the OCP group versus 78 +/− 12 nmol/day (28 ug/day) in the control group, but the difference was not statistically significant. They also studied UFC levels in pregnancy and found that UFC levels increased throughout gestation and were statistically significant higher in the pregnant cohort than in the nonpregnant cohort. While there was not a statistical difference in UFC levels between the OCP group and the control group, this study did demonstrate that UFC can rise under the influence of estrogen exposure, even if only slightly. The minimal elevations in our patient's UFC, therefore, may have been confounded by her OCP use.

OCP therapy, therefore, clearly complicates the investigation of possible cortisol excess and the differentiation between Cushing's syndrome and physiological hypercortisolism because of the OCP-induced increase in serum total cortisol; assessing the free cortisol fraction by measuring LNSC levels and the 24-hour UFC can help clarify the distinction between these two conditions. Mudde et al., found that the results of the 1 mg DST performed on the week after cessation of OCPs are accurate in almost all subjects [55]; notably our patient did not have any holiday from her estrogen-containing OCPs during her initial workup. When evaluating a UFC, urinary volume should also be examined; our patient did have increased urinary volumes which may have contributed to her false-positive results.

Studies have also validated the accuracy of LNSC levels in the diagnosis of Cushing's syndrome. The LNSC test has been reported to have superior diagnostic performance compared to UFC in diagnosing Cushing's syndrome [56]. The mean sensitivity and specificity of the salivary cortisol assay were greater than 90% when data was compiled from studies of salivary cortisol assay techniques published between 1998 and 2012 [56]. Furthermore, LNSC levels have been found to establish remission and identify recurrence after transsphenoidal surgery more accurately than 24-hour UFC [57, 58].

Our patient had normal LNSC levels on her initial evaluation; this was a clue that she likely had pseudo-Cushing's syndrome and not true Cushing's disease.

It is also critical to note that, as mentioned above, IPSS should not be done as part of a workup for Cushing's disease until a biochemical diagnosis of Cushing's disease has been established and then only to lateralize a potential lesion when an adenoma has not been clearly identified on dedicated imaging (MRI, CT) of the pituitary gland.

# Conclusions

The diagnosis of neoplastic Cushing's syndrome can be very challenging, and it is important to exclude physiologic (non-neoplastic) causes. A thorough physical exam and history including concurrent medications is necessary to avoid a misdiagnosis of Cushing's syndrome in the setting of confounding factors. Knowledge of common causes of non-neoplastic physiological hypercortisolism is vital in the assessment and correct identification of Cushing's syndrome.

# References

1. Raff H, Findling JW. A physiologic approach to diagnosis of the Cushing syndrome. Ann Intern Med. 2003;138(12):980–91.
2. Raff H, Sharma ST, Nieman LK. Physiological basis for the etiology, diagnosis, and treatment of adrenal disorders: Cushing's syndrome, adrenal insufficiency, and congenital adrenal hyperplasia. Compr Physiol. 2014;4:739–69.
3. Raff H, Carroll T. Cushing's syndrome: from physiological principles to diagnosis and clinical care. J Physiol. 2015;593(3):493–506.
4. Keller-Wood M. Hypothalamic-pituitary-adrenal axis—feedback control. Compr Physiol. 2015;5:1161–82.
5. Findling JW, Raff H. Differentiation of pathologic/neoplastic hypercortisolism (Cushing syndrome) from physiologic/non-neoplastic hypercortisolism (formerly known as Pseudo-Cushing syndrome): response to Letter to the Editor. Eur J Endocrinol. 2018;178(3):L3.

Chapter 13. Pseudo-Cushing's Syndrome: A Diagnostic... 173

6. Inder WJ, Joyce PR, Wells JE, Evans MJ, Ellis MJ, Mattioli L, Donald RA. The acute effects of oral ethanol on the hypothalamic pituitary-adrenal axis in normal human subjects. Clin Endocrinol. 1995;42:65–71.
7. Waltman C, Blevins LS Jr, Boyd G, Wand GS. The effects of mild ethanol intoxication on the hypothalamic-pituitary-adrenal axis in nonalcoholic men. J Clin Endocrinol Metab. 1993;77:518–22.
8. Wand GS, Dobs AS. Alterations in the hypothalamic-pituitary-adrenal axis in actively drinking alcoholics. J Clin Endocrinol Metab. 1991;72:1290–5.
9. Rivier C, Bruhn T, Vale W. Effect of ethanol on the hypothalamic pituitary-adrenal axis in the rat: role of corticotropin-releasing factor (CRF). J Pharmacol Exp Ther. 1984;229:127–31.
10. Lamberts SW, de Jong FH, Birkenhager JC. Biochemical characteristics of alcohol-induced pseudo-Cushing's syndrome [proceedings]. J Endocrinol. 1979;80:62P–3P.
11. Lamberts SW, Klijn JG, de Jong FH, Birkenhager JC. Hormone secretion in alcohol-induced pseudo-Cushing's syndrome. Differential diagnosis with Cushing disease. JAMA. 1979;242:1640–3.
12. Lovallo WR, Dickensheets SL, Myers DA, Thomas TL, Nixon SJ. Blunted stress cortisol response in abstinent alcoholic and polysubstance-abusing men. Alcohol Clin Exp Res. 2000;24:651–8.
13. Coiro V, Volpi R, Capretti L, Caffarri G, Chiodera P. Desmopressin and hexarelin tests in alcohol-induced pseudo-Cushing's syndrome. J Intern Med. 2000;247:667–73.
14. Rees LH, Besser GM, Jeffcoate WJ, Goldie DJ, Marks V. Alcohol-induced pseudo-Cushing's syndrome. Lancet. 1977;1:726–8.
15. Jacobson L. Hypothalamic-pituitary-adrenocortical axis: neuropsychiatric aspects. Compr Physiol. 2014;4:715–38.
16. Pariante CM, Lightman SL. The HPA axis in major depression: classical theories and new developments. Trends Neurosci. 2008;31:464–8.
17. Androulakis II, Kaltsas G, Chrousos G. Pseudo-Cushing's states. In: De Groot LJ, Chrousos G, Dungan K, Grossman A, Hershman JM, Koch C, Korbonits M, McLachlan R, New M, Purnell J, Rebar R, Singer F, Vinik A, editors. Endotext. South Dartmouth: MDText.com, Inc; 2000.
18. Ising M, Kunzel HE, Binder EB, Nickel T, Modell S, Holsboer F. The combined dexamethasone/CRH test as a potential

surrogate marker in depression. Prog Neuro-Psychopharmacol Biol Psychiatry. 2005;29:1085–93.
19. Krarup T, Krarup T, Hagen C. Do patients with type 2 diabetes mellitus have an increased prevalence of Cushing's syndrome? Diabetes Metab Res Rev. 2012;28:219–27.
20. Liu H, Bravata DM, Cabaccan J, Raff H, Ryzen E. Elevated late-night salivary cortisol levels in elderly male type 2 diabetic veterans. Clin Endocrinol. 2005;63:642–9.
21. Bellastella G, Maiorino MI, De BA, Vietri MT, Mosca C, Scappaticcio L, Pasquali D, Esposito K, Giugliano D. Serum but not salivary cortisol levels are influenced by daily glycemic oscillations in type 2 diabetes. Endocrine. 2015;53:220–6.
22. Constantinopoulos P, Michalaki M, Kottorou A, Habeos I, Psyrogiannis A, Kalfarentzos F, Kyriazopoulou V. Cortisol in tissue and systemic level as a contributing factor to the development of metabolic syndrome in severely obese patients. Eur J Endocrinol. 2015;172:69–78.
23. Lindsay JR, Nieman LK. The hypothalamic-pituitary-adrenal axis in pregnancy: challenges in disease detection and treatment. Endocr Rev. 2005;26:775–99.
24. Lopes LM, Francisco RP, Galletta MA, Bronstein MD. Determination of nighttime salivary cortisol during pregnancy: comparison with values in non-pregnancy and Cushing's disease. Pituitary. 2015;19:30–8.
25. Jung C, Ho JT, Torpy DJ, Rogers A, Doogue M, Lewis JG, Czajko RJ, Inder WJ. A longitudinal study of plasma and urinary cortisol in pregnancy and postpartum. J Clin Endocrinol Metab. 2011;96:1533–40.
26. Carr BR, Parker CR Jr, Madden JD, MacDonald PC, Porter JC. Maternal plasma adrenocorticotropin and cortisol relationships throughout human pregnancy. Am J Obstet Gynecol. 1981;139:416–22.
27. Suda T, Iwashita M, Tozawa F, Ushiyama T, Tomori N, Sumitomo T, Nakagami Y, Demura H, Shizume K. Characterization of corticotropin-releasing hormone binding protein in human plasma by chemical cross-linking and its binding during pregnancy. J Clin Endocrinol Metab. 1988;67:1278–83. https://doi.org/10.1210/jcem-67-6-1278.
28. Sasaki A, Shinkawa O, Yoshinaga K. Placental corticotropin-releasing hormone may be a stimulator of maternal pituitary adrenocorticotropic hormone secretion in humans. J Clin Invest. 1989;84:19–2001. https://doi.org/10.1172/jci114390.

29. Thomson M. The physiological roles of placental corticotropin releasing hormone in pregnancy and childbirth. J Physiol Biochem. 2013;69:559–73.
30. Van den Berghe G. Novel insights into the neuroendocrinology of critical illness. Eur J Endocrinol. 2000;143:1–13.
31. Valentine AR, Raff H, Liu H, Ballesteros M, Rose JM, Jossart GH, Cirangle P, Bravata DM. Salivary cortisol increases after bariatric surgery in women. Horm Metab Res. 2011;43:587–90.
32. Miller KK. Endocrine dysregulation in anorexia nervosa update. J Clin Endocrinol Metab. 2011;96:2939–49. https://doi.org/10.1210/jc.2011-1222.
33. Duclos M, Corcuff JB, Roger P, Tabarin A. The dexamethasone-suppressed corticotrophin-releasing hormone stimulation test in anorexia nervosa. Clin Endocrinol. 1999;51:725–31.
34. Lawson EA, Donoho D, Miller KK, Misra M, Meenaghan E, Lydecker J, Wexler T, Herzog DB, Klibanski A. Hypercortisolemia is associated with severity of bone loss and depression in hypothalamic amenorrhea and anorexia nervosa. J Clin Endocrinol Metab. 2009;94:4710–6. https://doi.org/10.1210/jc.2009-1046.
35. Misra M, Miller KK, Almazan C, Ramaswamy K, Lapcharoensap W, Worley M, Neubauer G, Herzog DB, Klibanski A. Alterations in cortisol secretory dynamics in adolescent girls with anorexia nervosa and effects on bone metabolism. J Clin Endocrinol Metab. 2004;89:4972–80.
36. Nieman LK, et al. The diagnosis of Cushing's syndrome: an endocrine society clinical practice guideline. J Clin Endocrinol Metab. 2008;93(5):1526–40.
37. Chan KCA, et al. Diminished urinary free cortisol excretion in patients with moderate and severe renal impairment. Clinical Chemistry. 2004;50(4):757–9.
38. Kidambi S, Raff H, Findling JW. Limitations of nocturnal salivary cortisol and urine free cortisol in the diagnosis of mild Cushing's syndrome. Eur J Endocrinol. 2007;157(6):725–31.
39. Nieman L. Diagnosis of Cushings syndrome in the modern era. Endocrinol Metab Clin. 2018;47(2):259–73.
40. Baid SK, et al. Radioimmunoassay and tandem mass spectrometry measurement of bedtime salivary cortisol levels: a comparison of assays to establish hypercortisolism. J Clin Endocrinol Metab. 2007;92(8):3102–7.
41. Butler PWP, Besser GM. Pituitary-adrenal function in severe depressive illness. Lancet. 1968;291(7554):1234–6.

42. Pfohl B, et al. Pituitary-adrenal axis rhythm disturbances in psychiatric depression. Arch Gen Psychiatry. 1985;42(9):897–903.
43. Ross RJM, et al. Levels of GH binding activity, IGFBP-1, insulin, blood glucose and cortisol in intensive care patients. Clin Endocrinol. 1991;35(4):361–7.
44. Badrick E, Kirschbaum C, Kumari M. The relationship between smoking status and cortisol secretion. J Clin Endocrinol Metabol. 2007;92(3):819–24.
45. Raff H, Raff JL, Findling JW. Late-night salivary cortisol as a screening test for Cushing's syndrome. J Clin Endocrinol Metabol. 1998;83(8):2681–6.
46. Crapo L. Cushing's syndrome: a review of diagnostic tests. Metab Clin Exp. 1979;28(9):955–77.
47. Storr HL, et al. Clinical features, diagnosis, treatment and molecular studies in paediatric Cushing's syndrome due to primary nodular adrenocortical hyperplasia. Clin Endocrinol. 2004;61(5):553–9.
48. Newell-Price J, et al. A single sleeping midnight cortisol has 100% sensitivity for the diagnosis of Cushing's syndrome. Clin Endocrinol. 1995;43(5):545–50.
49. Pecori Giraldi F, et al. The dexamethasone-suppressed corticotropin-releasing hormone stimulation test and the desmopressin test to distinguish Cushing's syndrome from pseudo-Cushing's states. Clin Endocrinol. 2007;66(2):251–7.
50. Yanovski JA, Cutler GB Jr, Doppman JL, Miller DL, Chrousos GP, Oldfield EH, Nieman LK. The limited ability of inferior petrosal sinus sampling with corticotropin-releasing hormone to distinguish Cushing's disease from pseudo-Cushing states or normal physiology. J Clin Endocrinol Metab. 1993;77:503–9.
51. Zampetti B, Grossrubatscher E, Ciaramella PD, Boccardi E, Loli P. Bilateral inferior petrosal sinus sampling. Endocr Connect. 2016;5(4):R12–25.
52. Qureshi AC, Bahri A, Breen LA, et al. The influence of the route of oestrogen administration on serum levels of cortisol-binding globulin and total cortisol. Clin Endocrinol. 2007;66:632–5.
53. Crewther BT, Hamilton D, Casto K, Kilduff LP, Cook CJ. Effects of oral contraceptive use on the salivary testosterone and cortisol responses to training sessions and competitions in elite women athletes. Physiol Behav. 2015;147:84–90.

54. Manetti L, Rossi G, Grasso L, Raffaelli V, Scattina I, Del Sarto S, Cosottini M, Iannelli A, Gasperi M, Bogazzi F, Martino E. Usefulness of salivary cortisol in the diagnosis of hypercortisolism: comparison with serum and urinary cortisol. Eur J Endocrinol. 2012;4:1–25.
55. Vastbinder M, et al. The influence of oral contraceptives on overnight 1 mg dexamethasone suppression test. Neth J Med. 2016;74(4):158–61.
56. Elias PCL, et al. Late-night salivary cortisol has a better performance than urinary free cortisol in the diagnosis of Cushing's syndrome. J Clin Endocrinol Metab. 2014;99(6):2045–51.
57. Carrol TB, Javorsky BR, Findling JW. Postsurgical recurrent Cushing disease: clinical benefit of early intervention in patients with normal urinary free cortisol. Endocr Pract. 2016;22(10):1216–23.
58. Amlash EG, et al. Accuracy of late-night salivary cortisol in evaluating postoperative remission and recurrence in Cushing's disease. J Clin Endocrinol Metab. 2015;100(10):3770–7.

# Chapter 14
## Pseudo-Cushing's Syndrome: Alcohol Abuse, Obesity, and Psychiatric Disorders

Janice M. Kerr

## Case Presentation

A 58-year-old Caucasian female was noted to have progressive weight gain (15 pounds over the past 12 months, BMI = 26) and fatigue (see Fig. 14.1). She also endorsed problems with mild depression and recently reported "falling off the wagon" because of life stressors. She also admitted to drinking half a pint of whiskey/night for the past few months, but was now sober for the last 14 days. She also endorsed previous problems with alcohol withdrawal symptoms, but denied seizures and delirium tremens. Her primary care physician noted central weight gain and proximal muscle wasting. She was also mildly hypertensive (BP = 142/94 mm Hg). A random a.m. cortisol level was normal at 12 mcg/dl (normal 5–22), but her physician was still concerned about possible Cushing's syndrome and requested an endocrine consult.

J. M. Kerr (✉)
University of Colorado, Anschutz Medical Center,
Aurora, CO, USA
e-mail: Janice.Kerr@UCDenver.edu

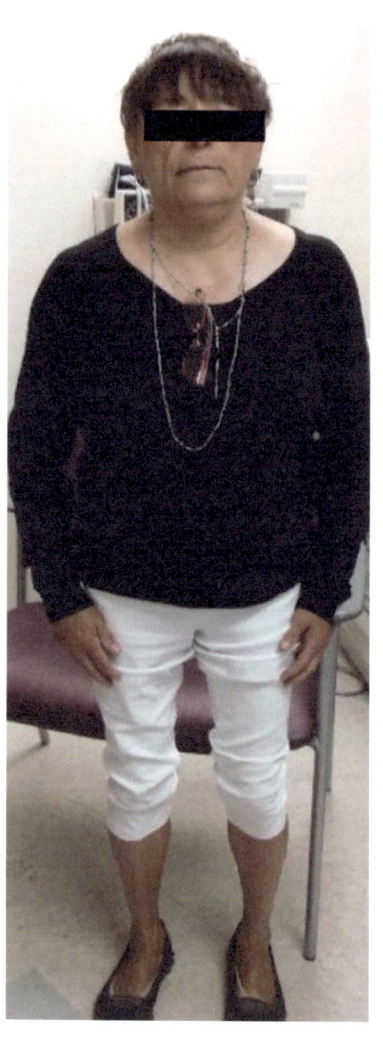

FIGURE 14.1 Pseudo-Cushing's syndrome patient

# Twelve Questions for Health Professionals Considering Hypercortisolism in a Patient

1. *What is hypercortisolism/Cushing's syndrome and what are its main causes?*

    Cushing's syndrome is a "disease complex" from chronically elevated cortisol, and results in multiple dis-

## Chapter 14. Pseudo-Cushing's Syndrome: Alcohol...

turbances in metabolic, endocrinologic, and body composition parameters. The most common cause of hypercortisolism is iatrogenic from prolonged glucocorticoid use. Importantly, *any* steroid exposure of sufficient dose and duration (e.g., injections, oral, inhaled, topical, or rectal preparations) can cause Cushing's syndrome, so it's important to take a detailed medication history before proceeding with further testing. The second most common cause of hypercortisolism is "physiologic-/non-neoplastic-" related, formerly called pseudo-Cushing's syndrome. This is a heterogeneous group of physiological or psychological stressors that can stimulate the hypothalamic-pituitary-adrenal (HPA) axis sufficiently to cause hypercortisolism. Included in these common causes are alcoholism/alcohol withdrawal, neuropsychiatric diseases, poorly-controlled diabetes mellitus (DM), and obstructive sleep apnea. Lastly, pathological/neoplastic causes of hypercortisolism, include an ACTH-secreting pituitary tumor (Cushing's disease, 70% of cases), a cortisol-secreting adrenal adenoma (20% of cases), or an ectopic ACTH-secreting tumor, the least common causes of hypercortisolism [1].

2. *Why is hypercortisolism one of the most challenging pseudo-endocrine conditions?*

   Hypercortisolism is a challenging diagnosis because several of its clinical features are non-specific and common in the general population. In addition, all of the myriad causes of hypercortisolism are potentially clinically and biochemically indistinguishable, particularly in subclinical or mild cases. Ultimately, an inability to correctly identify who should be screened for hypercortisolism, and/or to distinguish physiologic from pathological causes of hypercortisolism, can lead to diagnostic and therapeutic "misadventures," including unnecessary testing and interventions.

3. *What is the prevalence of pathological causes of Cushing's syndrome, and how should that affect your decisions about screening patients?*

Pathological/neoplastic causes of Cushing's syndrome are relatively rare. Specifically, European and US epidemiological studies estimate the incidence of endogenous Cushing's syndrome to be only 75 cases per one million population (or 24,000 affected persons annually in the US) [2]. This is in stark contrast to the high prevalence of disorders that cause physiologic/non-neoplastic hypercortisolism: (1) obesity ~30% or 98 million of the adult US population; (2) alcohol abuse/dependency, 5.5%, or 18 million of the adult US population; and (3) serious mental illness, 4.0%, or 9.8 million of US adults, per year. This broad group of disorders includes: significant depression with psychosis, bipolar disorder, obsessive compulsive disorder (OCD), post-traumatic stress disorder (PTSD), or schizophrenia. The relative rarity of pathological hypercortisolism means that only patients with multiple, progressive, and specific features of Cushing's should be screened.

4. *What are the specific clinical features that should prompt evaluation for possible hypercortisolism in adults?*

Important aspects of diagnosing pathological causes of hypercortisolism include the pace and duration of symptoms and signs. Significant hypercortisolism is usually associated with eventual disease progression, including the development of clinically specific signs and worsening metabolic manifestations (e.g., poorly controlled DM, hypertension, osteoporosis, etc.) [1]. Specific features of Cushing's that should warrant further evaluation include facial plethora/moon facies, supraclavicular fat pads, striae [violaceous and wide (>1 cm) in the abdomen or axilla], proximal muscle weakness (as assessed by asking patients to rise from a chair without using their arms), or atrophic skin changes/ecchymoses (particularly if numerous (>3), large (≥1 cm in size), and not associated with trauma such as venipuncture). A skin fold of <2 mm (over the proximal phalanx of the middle finger, in the nondominant hand) has also recently been demonstrated to be a sensitive predictor for Cushing's syndrome (see Fig. 14.2) [2]. Similarly,

## Chapter 14. Pseudo-Cushing's Syndrome: Alcohol...

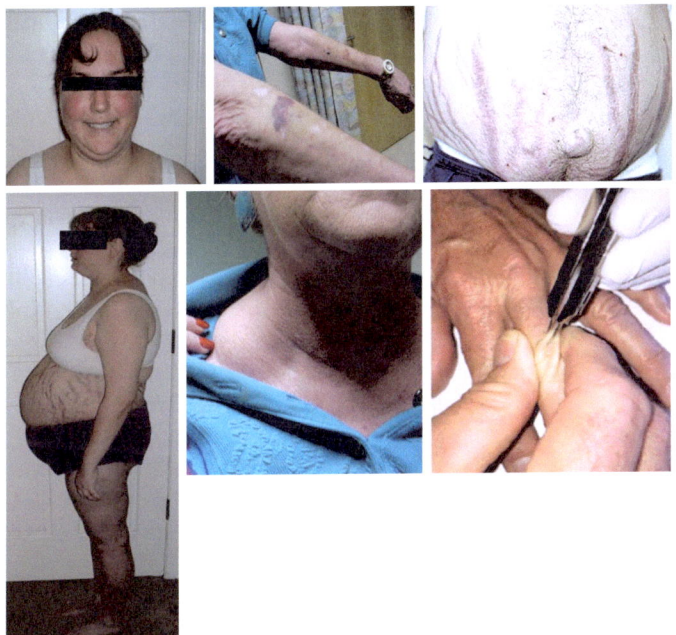

FIGURE 14.2 Specific features of Cushing's syndrome (from left to right): Moon facies and facial plethora, spontaneous ecchymoses and atrophic skin changes, wide (>1 cm) violaceous striae, proximal muscle wasting, supraclavicular fat pads and thin skin folds (<2 mm over the proximal phalanx of the middle finger, in the nondominant hand)

atypical/atraumatic fractures, particularly of the ribs, are concerning for hypercortisolism. Lastly, young patients (<35 years) who develop these clinical features (i.e., atrophic skin changes, spontaneous ecchymoses), atraumatic fractures, or hypertension are more likely to have underlying hypercortisolism and should be screened [3].

*In contrast, non-specific features* for Cushing's syndrome that are common in the general population and should *not* alone prompt screening include (1) *signs* (hirsutism, acne, central obesity, dorsocervical fat pad (buffalo hump), impaired glucose tolerance/diabetes mellitus, metabolic syndrome, hypertension, dyslipidemia, osteopenia/osteoporosis, blood clots, or edema) and (2) *symptoms* (fatigue, depression, decreased libido, menstrual irregularities, back pain, insomnia, impaired memory, irritability, or decreased cognition.)

5. *Is there evidence that obesity or obstructive sleep apnea cause hypercortisolism?*

   Most biochemical studies in obese populations have demonstrated that random serum cortisol levels and dexamethasone suppression tests were normal and not associated with BMI levels. Conversely, there are studies with mixed results in obese patients, showing normal, high-normal or mildly elevated urine free cortisol (UFC), and late-night salivary cortisol levels, which trended with BMI levels. In the studies that correlated increased UFC levels with BMIs, this was attributed to increased cortisol clearance [4–6].

   Obstructive sleep apnea (OSA) is a common disorder, affecting an estimated 2–4% of the general adult population, and is often undiagnosed. Frequent hypoxic episodes and disrupted sleep patterns, from untreated OSA, would be expected to active the HPA axis, although research findings have been inconsistent. Differences in study methodologies, including the Cushing's screening tests used, severity of OSA/obesity, and confounding factors (e.g., depression, mood disorders), likely accounted for some of the discrepant findings. A recent, well-designed study, however, showed that obese and nonobese men and women with OSA had significantly increased 24-hour urinary cortisol excretion and that this hypercortisolism improved with short-term continuous positive airway pressure (CPAP) use [7]. As such, patients at risk for OSA, as assessed by the Epworth Sleepiness Scale or other standardized screening questionnaires, should undergo a sleep study and CPAP treatment, as indicated, before additional Cushing's syndrome evaluation.

6. *Why not just screen all obese patients for hypercortisolism?*

On the basis of prevalence estimates, the likelihood that a person with obesity, hypertension, type 2 diabetes, and dyslipidemia has pathological Cushing's syndrome is only ~1 in 500 (0.2%) [2]. Even in cases of severe obesity (BMI > 45), in the absence of Cushing's-specific clinical features, detection rates for Cushing's syndrome are low (0.7%) [8]. With the high prevalence of obesity in the US population, this is now the least useful feature for diagnosing Cushing's syndrome. Although the pace of weight gain may be helpful, it is more important to focus on the catabolic features of Cushing's syndrome (atrophic skin changes, proximal muscle weakness, atypical fractures, etc.) versus the anabolic features (obesity) [2]. Proposed strategies emphasize the importance of screening only patients with a high pretest probability in order to reduce the number of false-positive results and unnecessary downstream tests, costs, and patient inconvenience.

The potential risk of generalized screening in the obese population was demonstrated by Nieman et al., in a study of 369 obese patients with a median BMI of 54 [9]. No new cases of Cushing's syndrome were identified in this cohort. Importantly, however, nighttime salivary cortisol levels, when assessed by a radioimmunoassay (RIA), had a lower specificity (84%) compared to liquid chromatography-tandem mass spectrometry (95%) and led to unnecessary, additional testing. This highlights the importance of selective screening and supports the general rule that true hypercortisolism should be established by at least two screening tests [10]. Salivary cortisol tests should not be used as a stand-alone, rule-in test [10].

7. *What is the relationship between alcohol abuse and hypercortisolism?*

Excessive alcohol intake, both acute and chronic, may be associated with hypercortisolism [11]. Alcohol-induced hypercortisolism appears to be a centrally-mediated process, via increased corticotropin-releasing hormone (CRH) levels that stimulate pituitary corticotropin (ACTH) secretion and adrenal cortisol overproduction. Clinical features of this physiological hypercortisolism are presumed to be secondary to repeated bouts of hypercortisolism during intoxication, with further increases during subacute/acute withdrawal symptoms [12]. Research studies are limited, however, by small sample sizes, differences in experimental designs, variable alcohol intake/duration, and the cortisol screening methodology. As such, these studies showed mixed results regarding the extent of biochemical abnormalities with chronic alcohol abuse. Specifically some, but not all, studies reported mildly abnormal late-night salivary cortisol levels, failure of a.m. serum cortisol to suppress normally with the late night, 1 mg dexamethasone suppression test (DST), and mildly elevated 24-hour UFC (approximately twofold). In addition, some studies showed that only a small percentage (~20%) of chronic alcoholics had significant clinical or biochemical overlap with Cushing's syndrome, with proximal muscle wasting, hypertension, and central obesity being the most commonly-shared features (see Fig. 14.1) [13]. Cushing's features appear to be independent of liver dysfunction or the presence of cirrhosis, and there is a suspected genetic component to the risk. It is also worth noting that a significant percentage of alcoholics likely have superimposed depression (estimated between 25% and 50%), which may also cause physiologic hypercortisolism.

8. *What is the best way to distinguish physiologic hypercortisolism from pathological etiologies?*

A very detailed history and physical exam are the most important aspects of distinguishing among the various etiologies of hypercortisolism. In cases of potential alcohol abuse, a high index of suspicion is needed, since patients may not be forthcoming with this sensitive information. Ideally, with the help of a trusted primary care physician, a detailed history of the patient's alcohol consumption and potential risk of problematic drinking can be accurately assessed. Since self-reporting is notoriously inaccurate, however, the medical history and physical exam are critical. The following abnormalities should prompt greater consideration for the presence of alcohol-related liver disease: spider angiomas, rhinophyma, transaminitis [aspartate aminotransferase (AST) >alanine aminotransferase (ALT)], hepatomegaly, splenomegaly, cirrhosis/ascites, pancreatitis, gastritis/esophagitis/Mallory-Weiss tears, malnutrition (i.e., thiamine, folate deficiencies), palmar erythema, testicular atrophy/hypogonadism, myopathy, and/or neuropathy.

In cases of suspected neuropsychiatric disorders, the assistance of mental health professionals will often be required for the assessment, classification, and treatment of potential mood disorders. The diagnoses of various neuropsychiatric conditions, including: OCD, bipolar disorder, PTSD, major depression with psychotic features, mania, and schizophrenic disorders, are made all the more challenging by the fact that pathological hypercortisolism can cause and/or exacerbate these conditions. A detailed history and physical exam will be paramount in potentially distinguishing which disorder came first (i.e., mood vs. hypercortisolism), although fortunately a major psychiatric event is a rare initial presentation for Cushing's syndrome.

9. *What are the best screening tests to evaluate for hypercortisolism? Can they distinguish physiological from pathological causes?*

There is no single best screening test for hypercortisolism, and ALL screening tests may be mildly elevated, or abnormal, with physiologic/non-neoplastic hypercortisolism [10]. In general, random serum cortisol levels are insufficient for screening. Instead, the preferred screening strategy for Cushing's syndrome includes: (1) loss of diurnal variation, or abnormal late-night nadir cortisol levels (between 11 p.m. and 12 midnight), using a late-night salivary cortisol test (LNSC); (2) loss of normal, negative feedback inhibition, via a failed suppression of the morning serum cortisol level on the late-night 1 mg DST; and (3) excess cortisol production, as determined by an increased 24-hour UFC excretion. One caveat, however, is that a marked elevation of UFC (3–4 times the upper limit of normal) is more suggestive of pathological causes of hypercortisolism [10].

The relative sensitivities of these Cushing's screening tests are as follows: LNSC >1 mg DST >24-hour UFC. Therefore, normal LNSC levels plus a normal 1 mg DST test result (serum cortisol ≤1.8 mcg/dl) exclude hypercortisolism with a very high negative predictive value (>95%). Conversely, in equivocal cases of hypercortisolism, particularly if associated with suspected physiological etiologies or discordant screening tests, reassessment at periodic intervals (~6 months) can be considered. The general evaluation for hypercortisolism is as detailed in Fig. 14.3. In particularly challenging cases, additional confirmatory/secondary tests, such as the 2 mg, 2-day low-dose dexamethasone test (LDDST), or a dexamethasone-CRH (Dex-CRH) test can be considered. Importantly, however, these tests have not been well-validated in physiologic/non-neoplastic causes of hypercortisolism. The latter test also has limited practicality because of restricted CRH availability, its high

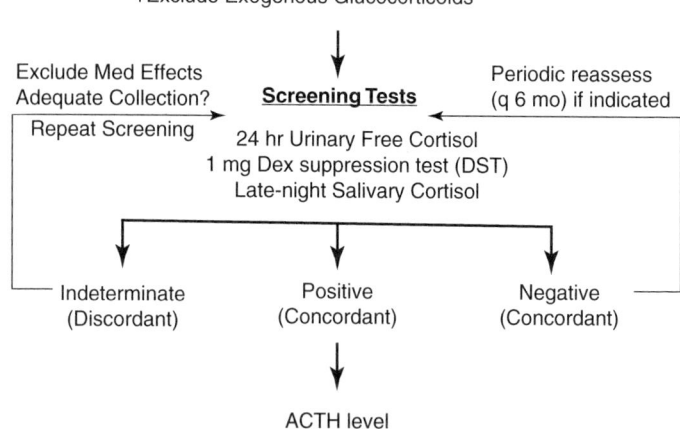

FIGURE 14.3 Algorithm for hypercortisolism evaluation

cost, and the need for exact timing of CRH administration and ACTH and cortisol testing. Furthermore, some researchers have demonstrated that a higher cortisol cutoff (3.4 mcg/dl instead of the standard 1.8 mcg/dl) is needed for high sensitivity (94%) and specificity (100%) in cases of suspected alcohol-related hypercortisolism [14]. Generally, repeat biochemical screening at a later time, and if still clinically indicated, is recommended instead of secondary tests.

*CAVEATS-* It is generally best to perform Cushing's screening tests on an outpatient basis, and not during a hospitalization. Acute illnesses and other stressors (e.g., pain, altered sleep-wake cycles, infection, etc.) can causes false-positive screening results. In addition, these screening tests are predicated on a normal 24-hour diurnal cortisol pattern; therefore, patients with disrupted sleep cycles (e.g., shift workers or patients with primary circadian disorders) should not be screened with standard late-night salivary cortisol or 1 mg DST tests.

10. *Are there any imaging or interventional studies that can distinguish physiologic from pathological causes of hypercortisolism?*

    No. It is generally not useful to perform imaging studies (e.g., pituitary or abdominal imaging) to distinguish physiologic versus pathological causes of hypercortisolism because of the relatively common finding of "incidentalomas" (<1 cm pituitary or adrenal tumors) in these endocrine glands (10–20%, based on age). Similarly, an interventional study, such as a bilateral inferior petrosal sinus sampling (IPSS), may give a false-positive result in patients with physiological hypercortisolism.

11. *What about cyclic Cushing's Syndrome?*

    Cyclic Cushing's syndrome/disease is defined as intermittent periods of biochemical/clinical hypercortisolism followed by biochemical/clinical quiescence that spans variable time periods (from weeks to years). The pathophysiology of this phenomenon remains poorly understood. It is reported to occur in upward of 15% of patients with pathological/neoplastic Cushing's syndrome and obviously makes an already challenging diagnosis even more difficult [15].

When considering cyclic Cushing's syndrome, it's important to exclude incorrectly performed or timed screening tests, and/or non-specific complaints attributable to hypercortisolism, as these are more common explanations for this phenomenon. It is recommended to rescreen patients with discrepant Cushing's screening tests, as clinically indicated, and during times of "symptomatic" hypercortisolemic episodes. Repeat normal salivary cortisol tests exclude hypercortisolism with a high negative predictive value (>95%) and preclude the need for subsequent additional testing.

12. *How should patients with suspected physiologic causes of hypercortisolism be assessed/followed?*

Based on ongoing assessments (history, physical exam, test results), further screening tests should be repeated only after potential causes of physiological hypercortisolism have been adequately addressed. For alcoholic patients, cortisol abnormalities usually normalize after ~1–4 months of abstinence from alcohol [16]. For patients with OSA, a 3-month course of CPAP treatment is generally adequate for normalization of the hypercortisolism. Lastly, for patients with underlying neuropsychiatric disorders, physicians should discuss with them, and/or their treating physicians, the adequacy of psychiatric disease control before potentially performing any additional Cushing's syndrome evaluations. In general, a tincture of time is all that is needed, as these patients typically do not show progression of Cushing's signs and symptoms, and their mildly elevated cortisol levels usually remit with treatment of the underlying disorder.

## Back to Case Presentation

The patient abstained from alcohol, with the help of Antabuse™. Her blood pressure and proximal muscle weakness improved, and her central weight gain stabilized. No additional screening test for Cushing's syndrome was performed.

# References

1. Findling JW, Raff H. Differentiation of pathological/neoplastic hypercortisolism (Cushing's syndrome) from physiologic/non-neoplastic hypercortisolism (formerly known as pseudo-Cushing's syndrome). Eur J Endocrinol. 2017;176:R205–16.
2. Loriaux DL. Diagnosis and differential diagnosis of Cushing's Syndrome. N Engl J Med. 2017;376:1451–9.
3. Nieman LK. Recent updates on the diagnosis and management of Cushing's Syndrome. Endocrinol Metab. 2018;33:139–46.
4. Abraham SB, Rubino D, Sinaii N, Ramsey S, Nieman LK. Cortisol, obesity, and the metabolic syndrome: a cross-sectional study of obese subjects and review of the literature. Obesity. 2013;21:E105–17.
5. Purnell JQ, Brandon DD, Isabell LM, et al. Association of 24-hour cortisol production rates, cortisol-binding globulin, and plasma-free cortisol levels with body composition, leptin levels and aging in men and women. J Clin Endocrinol Metab. 2004;89:281–7.
6. Strain GW, Zumoff B, Strain JJ, et al. Cortisol production in obesity. Metabolism. 1980;29:980–5.
7. Kritilou I, Basta M, Vgontzas AN, et al. Sleep apnea and the hypothalamic-pituitary-adrenal axis in men and women: effects of continuous positive airway pressure. Eur Respir J. 2016;47:531–40.
8. Lammert A, Nikkita S, Otto M, et al. Performance of the 1 mg dexamethasone suppression test in patients with severe obesity. Obesity. 2016;24:850–5.
9. Baid SK, Rubino D, Sinaii N, et al. Specificity of screening tests for Cushing's syndrome in an overweight and obese population. J Clin Endocrinol Metab. 2009;94:3857–64.
10. Nieman LK, Biller BM, Findling JW, Newell-Price J, et al. The diagnosis of Cushing's syndrome: an Endocrine Society clinical practice guidelines. J Clin Endocrinol Metab. 2008;93:1526–40.
11. Groote Veldman R, Meinders AE. On the mechanism of alcohol-induced pseudo-Cushing's syndrome. Endocr Rev. 1996;17:262–8.
12. Besemer F, Pereira AM, Smit JW. Alcohol-induced Cushing syndrome. Neth J Med. 2011;69:318–23.
13. Kirkman S, Nelson DH. Alcohol-induced pseudo-Cushing's disease: a study of prevalence with review of the literature. Metabolism. 1988;37:390–4.

14. Alwani RA, Schmidt-Jongblood LW, de Jong FH, et al. Differentiating between Cushing's disease and pseudo-Cushing's syndrome: comparison of four tests. Eur J Endocrinol. 2014;170:477–86.
15. Alexandraki KI, Kaltsas GA, Isidori AM, et al. The prevalence and characteristic features of cyclicity and variability in Cushing's disease. Eur J Endocrinol. 2009;160:1011–8.
16. Romanholi DJ, Salgado LR. Pseudo-Cushing state. Arq Bras Endocrinol Metabol. 2007;51:1303–13.

# Chapter 15
# Pseudopheochromocytoma

**David R. Saxon and Lauren Fishbein**

*Case* A 54-year-old woman presents to the endocrinology clinic for follow-up 5 years after resection of a right adrenal pheochromocytoma. At the time of the initial pheochromocytoma diagnosis, she presented with paroxysmal hypertension, fatigue, tremors, night sweats, insomnia, and appetite loss. Biochemical evaluation revealed elevated catecholamines; a right adrenal mass with high Hounsfield units (HU) of 15 consistent with a pheochromocytoma was found on a noncontrast computed tomography (CT) scan. She received perioperative alpha blockade, and the mass was resected without complications. Postoperative biochemical evaluation showed normalization of catecholamine levels. She

D. R. Saxon (✉) · L. Fishbein
University of Colorado School of Medicine, Department of Medicine, Division of Endocrinology, Metabolism and Diabetes, Aurora, CO, USA

Rocky Mountain VA Medical Center, Division of Endocrinology, Aurora, CO, USA
e-mail: David.saxon@ucdenver.edu

was then referred for clinical genetic testing and had no known susceptibility gene mutation. Two years after that resection, she began experiencing recurrence of hypertensive episodes and the symptoms that preceded the previous pheochromocytoma diagnosis in addition to an extensive list of new symptoms that included abdominal discomfort, numbness and tingling in her arms and legs, and passive suicidal thoughts. For the next 3 years, extensive testing for recurrent pheochromocytoma was conducted with consistently negative results, including plasma metanephrines, urinary catecholamines, and multiple CT scans of the abdomen and chest and I-123 MIBG imaging. She also had normal thyroid testing. She works closely with a mental health professional as she has been diagnosed with anxiety and depression, but she does not take antidepressants because of previous "horrible reactions" to selective serotonin reuptake inhibitors (SSRIs). She presents today for another opinion. She endorses a great deal of stress in her personal life resulting from a sick child who requires around-the-clock home care. She requests an antianxiety medication but is resistant to the idea of trialing an antidepressant again. She is convinced that her pheochromocytoma has recurred and states that she has read on Internet message boards that many other patients with pheochromocytoma have experienced a recurrence despite negative workups. She is insistent that repeat adrenal imaging is needed.

## Questions

- How is pheochromocytoma typically diagnosed?
- What other conditions can mimic a pheochromocytoma?
- What pathophysiologic mechanisms may be underlying cases of pseudopheochromocytoma?
- How can pseudopheochromocytoma be managed?

## Comments

Pheochromocytomas and paragangliomas are rare catecholamine-producing neuroendocrine tumors within the adrenal gland or extra-adrenal ganglia, respectively, which have a variable clinical presentation. Symptoms typically include episodic or labile hypertension, headaches, profuse sweating, and palpitations. Other presenting symptoms may include anxiety, tremulousness, abdominal pain, chest pain, nausea, vomiting, weakness, fatigue, and dizziness, and interestingly, some patients have no symptoms.

Screening for pheochromocytoma and paraganglioma with plasma free metanephrines and/or 24-hour fractionated urine metanephrines and catecholamines should be done in patients with suspected secondary hypertension (i.e., young age at diagnosis or refractory hypertension) and in patients with symptoms of headaches, palpitations, diaphoresis, and anxiety along with their high blood pressure. Although outside the scope of this chapter, screening should also be done in patients with adrenal incidentalomas or in patients with a known susceptibility gene mutation. Overall, pheochromocytomas and paragangliomas are rare, occurring in 2–8 per million people, and they account for only 0.2–0.6% of all patients with hypertension [1]. Biochemical testing is considered positive when the 24-hour urine tests are at least 3× the upper limit of normal and the plasma tests are at least 2× the upper limit of normal. In these cases, cross-sectional imaging of the abdomen/pelvis should be the next step in the evaluation as 85% of pheochromocytomas and paragangliomas will be in this region, with the majority inside the adrenal glands. There are rare thoracic paragangliomas. Head and neck paragangliomas are most often non-secreting (~96%), although some secrete dopamine which has not been shown to contribute to hypertensive surges. Slightly elevated metanephrines and catecholamines, not reaching the diagnostic cutoff levels, can result from low secreting tumors in rare cases but much more often are due to interfering medications or to drugs or condi-

TABLE 15.1 Interfering substances

Tricyclic antidepressants

Decongestants (i.e., ephedrine)

Certain beta- and alpha-adrenergic medications

Dopaminergic medications (i.e., levodopa)

Selective serotonin reuptake inhibitors (SSRI)
Serotonin norepinephrine reuptake inhibitors (SNRI)

Monoamine oxidase inhibitors (MAOI)

Acetaminophen

Alcohol

Caffeine

Cigarettes

Marijuana

Cocaine

Bananas

Supplements (look for ingredients that may interfere)

tions that mimic pheochromocytoma. If the biochemical testing is normal, other conditions should be sought as the sensitivity of both plasma and urine metanephrines and catecholamines is more than 90% [2].

The most common reasons for indeterminate levels of metanephrines and catecholamines are medications, foods, or drugs that interfere in the assays (Table 15.1). Patients must also be asked about over-the-counter supplements; if the ingredients in supplements are not known, these should be investigated further online or by calling the company. For example, some over-the-counter energy booster supplements contain bovine (or other) adrenal glands and can lead to elevated metanephrines and contribute to symptoms of pheochromocytoma.

If catecholamine levels are still indeterminate after excluding all interfering substances, then cross-sectional imaging

TABLE 15.2 Conditions that mimic state of catecholamine excess

| Labile hypertension | Drugs of abuse (cocaine, amphetamine) |
|---|---|
| CNS lesions (stroke, tumor) | Coronary ischemia |
| Cluster or migraine headaches | Medications |
| Seizures | Baroreflex failure |
| Carcinoid syndrome | Panic disorder |
| Hyperthyroidism | Anxiety disorder |
| Mastocytosis | Posttraumatic stress disorder |
| Renal artery stenosis | Alcohol withdrawal |

may be warranted. Of note, patients with pseudopheochromocytoma usually have normal metanephrine and catecholamine levels or have very mild elevations that are significantly below the cutoffs for diagnosis.

Once pheochromocytoma/paraganglioma is ruled out, the differential diagnosis includes many other conditions (Table 15.2). Disorders that cause excess levels of other hormones can also increase sympathetic nervous system responses. For example, hyperthyroidism is associated with palpitations, weight loss, tremors, and anxiety; carcinoid syndrome is associated with facial flushing without sweating and multiple daily episodes of diarrhea and is usually caused by other types of neuroendocrine tumors. Baroreflex dysfunction can occur in patients with a prior history of a mass in the neck or treatment such as radiation or surgery of the neck resulting in disruption of the carotid body and the baroreceptors. Baroreceptors usually help to minimize blood pressure fluctuations, and, when damaged, patients can have marked and frequent fluctuations in blood pressure [3]. Untreated severe obstructive sleep apnea has been shown to cause mild elevations in catecholamine levels due to intermittent hypoxia, intrathoracic pressure swings, and recurrent arousals [4]. Other conditions in the differential diagnosis are listed in Table 15.2. A thorough history and physical exam can help direct the workup for this differential diagnosis which may require referral to the appropriate specialist providers.

The term "pseudopheochromocytoma" is a diagnosis of exclusion used for those patients with paroxysmal severe hypertension and typical symptoms of catecholamine excess but who lack biochemical and anatomical evidence of pheochromocytoma or have another known cause. In many of these patients, physical symptoms can be debilitating and have a significant negative impact on their quality of life. The exact pathophysiologic mechanism underlying pseudopheochromocytoma is not known, but activation of the sympathetic nervous system leading to increased secretion of catecholamines and their metabolites has been variably identified in patients with the condition. In one study, evaluation of sympathoadrenal function in 11 patients with pseudopheochromocytoma in comparison to 14 age-matched controls was performed [5]. Compared to controls, patients with pseudopheochromocytoma had statistically significantly higher concentrations of baseline epinephrine (120% higher) and metanephrine (80% higher); however, although the authors did not provide normal ranges, all levels appeared to still be within typical normal ranges. In addition, this study showed that patients with pseudopheochromocytoma had exaggerated responses to sympathetic nervous system stimuli from various compounds; for example, plasma epinephrine after glucagon administration was sixfold higher compared with controls [5].

Often a psychological basis for pseudopheochromocytoma can be found. Panic disorder may be present in as many as 40% of patients with the condition [6]. In a case series summarizing the clinical course of 21 patients with pseudopheochromocytoma, psychosocial interviewing revealed that most patients had previous emotional trauma and sometimes even suppressed events that they were unaware of and that likely were contributing to their symptoms [7]. Treatment based on recognition of emotional distress as the underlying cause of the symptomatic paroxysmal hypertension resulted in cessation of paroxysms in 13 (62%) of the patients. Therefore, recommending counseling and medical therapy can be useful. Anxiolytics may be helpful in certain patients given the association with panic attacks. Antidepressants such as SSRIs and even tricyclics also may be useful.

When pseudopheochromocytoma is suspected or considered, better characterization of hypertensive episodes can be elucidated with 24-hour ambulatory blood pressure monitoring. Patients with pseudopheochromocytoma often have normal or only mildly elevated blood pressure between episodes. Therefore, medical treatment of the episodes may be challenging. To treat and prevent the blood pressure surges, medications such as clonidine or alpha-adrenergic blockers (prazosin, doxazosin) with or without beta blockers (metoprolol, atenolol) are best. Typical antihypertensive medications, such as angiotensin-converting enzyme inhibitors (ACEI) or angiotensin receptor blockers (ARB), may not prevent the blood pressure surges and can lead to hypotension between episodes.

## Discussion with Patient

For patients with pseudopheochromocytoma, discussing the normal biochemical evaluation is most often not sufficient to reassure these patients and does not serve to mitigate the symptoms or hypertensive surges. For such patients, we must reassure them of the normal workup which ruled out the tumor (pheochromocytoma), express belief that the symptoms and signs they are experiencing are real and disrupting their lives, and thoroughly investigate other causes for their symptoms.

During the evaluation to rule out all other causes, we often suggest a visit with a therapist or counselor. Patients with pseudopheochromocytoma may not recognize the emotional stressors that may be triggering the symptoms. Suggesting referral to a therapist or counselor may or may not be well-received by the patient, and patients should not be forced to comply. Our approach is to suggest that a therapist or counselor may be helpful given the stress associated with having a condition for which the medical providers cannot find a precise diagnosis. We explain the strong mind-body connection, whether the condition is causing emotional stress or the emotional stress contributes to the condition or both. Yoga or other mindfulness techniques may also be beneficial to the patient whether they want to see a therapist or not. If the patient is open to medical treatment for mental health, offering antidepressants or anxiolytics may be appropriate. If hypertensive surges are confirmed, we offer medical treatment as described above usually with clonidine or alpha blockers to help prevent these surges.

The diagnosis of pseudopheochromocytoma is a difficult one and can be frustrating for both patients and providers. We often do not use the word pseudopheochromocytoma to describe the condition to patients, as the term "pseudo" in this context can be interpreted as being derogatory. Instead, we recommend reviewing with the patient the following points: (1) discuss all the other diagnoses which were ruled out; (2) discuss the good news that no severe conditions were identified; and (3) discuss that the absence of other identifiable conditions suggests that the diagnosis is likely an abnormal activation of the sympathetic nervous system, which can be treated with the methods described above.

## Summary Recommendations

1. Believe the symptoms and signs the patient tells you.
2. Rule out all conditions on the differential diagnosis.
3. Suggest a therapist or counselor to help with the anxiety and stress of not having a diagnosis for the symptoms they are experiencing and/or to deal with an emotional stressor the patient tells you about.
4. Treat the symptoms of sympathetic nervous system activation.

# References

1. Fishbein L. Pheochromocytoma and paraganglioma: genetics, diagnosis, and treatment. Hematol Oncol Clin North Am. 2016;30(1):135–50.
2. Lenders JWM, Duh Q-Y, Eisenhofer G, Gimenez-Roqueplo A-P, Grebe SKG, Murad MH, et al. Pheochromocytoma and paraganglioma: an endocrine society clinical practice guideline. J Clin Endocrinol Metab. 2014;99(6):1915–42.
3. Zar T, Peixoto AJ. Paroxysmal hypertension due to baroreflex failure. Kidney Int. 2008;74(1):126–31.
4. Jullian-Desayes I, Joyeux-Faure M, Tamisier R, Launois S, Borel A-L, Levy P, et al. Impact of obstructive sleep apnea treatment by continuous positive airway pressure on cardiometabolic biomarkers: a systematic review from sham CPAP randomized controlled trials. Sleep Med Rev. 2015;21:23–38.
5. Sharabi Y, Goldstein DS, Bentho O, Saleem A, Pechnik S, Geraci MF, et al. Sympathoadrenal function in patients with paroxysmal hypertension: pseudopheochromocytoma. J Hypertens. 2007;25(11):2286–95.
6. Fogarty J, Engel C, Russo J. Hypertension and pheochromocytoma testing: the association with anxiety orders. Arch Fam Med. 1994;3:55.
7. Mann SJ. Severe paroxysmal hypertension (pseudopheochromocytoma): understanding the cause and treatment. Arch Intern Med. 1999;159(7):670–4.

# Chapter 16
# Holistic Hypercalcemia

**Irene E. Schauer**

## Case Presentation

A 54-year-old white female presented to the endocrine clinic for evaluation of hypercalcemia. She had presented to her primary care provider with a complaint of worsening constipation and nocturia. Laboratory evaluation revealed a serum calcium of 13.3 mg/dl and acute kidney injury with a serum creatinine of 1.26 mg/dl. Repeat labs were improved with serum calcium of 12.1 mg/dl and creatinine of 0.99 mg/dl. Serum PTH was low, but not fully suppressed, at 12 pg/ml. At that time she was referred to endocrinology for further evaluation.

In the endocrinology clinic, she confirmed the reported symptoms and also endorsed severe fatigue, abdominal pain, nausea, and poor appetite. She also reported increased thirst

---

I. E. Schauer (✉)
University of Colorado School of Medicine, Department of Medicine, Division of Endocrinology, Metabolism and Diabetes, Aurora, CO, USA

Rocky Mountain Regional VA Medical Center, Aurora, CO, USA
e-mail: irene.schauer@cuanschutz.edu; Irene.schauer@va.gov

© Springer Nature Switzerland AG 2019
M. T. McDermott (ed.), *Management of Patients with Pseudo-Endocrine Disorders*,
https://doi.org/10.1007/978-3-030-22720-3_16

but noted that she had been trying to limit fluid intake to minimize the need for voiding overnight. The original constipation was improved, but variably still present, with magnesium pills. She also noted that she recalled being told her calcium was borderline high in the past. ROS was otherwise positive only for headaches and some dysuria but negative for other neurological symptoms or any cardiorespiratory symptoms, bone pain, or myalgia.

Her past medical history was notable for multiple sclerosis (MS), psoriasis, and primary hypothyroidism. Medications at that time included Betaseron injections for MS and Armour Thyroid 75 mg daily. She was postmenopausal and used vaginal estrogen but no systemic hormone replacement therapy. She reported no history of smoking or other tobacco use, minimal alcohol, and a very active lifestyle with running, hiking, or weight lifting on most days. She actively limited her sun exposure and limited her dairy intake because of the popular literature regarding a possible involvement of cow's milk in the etiology of MS. Though she had taken calcium supplements in the past, she had stopped these since the diagnosis of hypercalcemia. She also denied taking a multivitamin but endorsed taking a few drops of a liquid vitamin D supplement provided by her chiropractor that was described as low dose and potentially helpful for MS symptoms.

On physical exam she was normotensive, afebrile, lean, and fit-appearing with a BMI of 20. Her exam was entirely unremarkable, notably including normal pulmonary, abdominal, musculoskeletal, neurological, and psychiatric exams.

At that time a differential diagnosis included multiple possible diagnoses for PTH-independent hypercalcemia including sarcoidosis, granulomatous disease, multiple myeloma, a PTHrp-producing tumor, and vitamin D toxicity. Milk alkali syndrome was not felt to be likely in light of her low dairy and calcium intake.

Further laboratory evaluation (Table 16.1) confirmed significant PTH-independent hypercalcemia and evidence of renal damage with a serum calcium of 13.9 mg/dl (normal

TABLE 16.1 Laboratory values

| Day from initial visit | Calcium (Nl, 8.6–10.3 mg/dl) | Albumin (Nl, 3.5–5.7 g/L) | Phosphorous (Nl, 2.5–5.0 mg/dl) | eGFR (Nl, > 60 ml/min) | 25(OH)VitD (Nl, 20–62 ng/ml) | 1,25(OH)2VitD (Nl, 19.9–79.3 pg/ml) |
|---|---|---|---|---|---|---|
| Day 0 | 13.9 | 4.6 | 2.7 | 37 | >150 | 483 |
| Day 1 | 12.7 | | | 47 | | |
| Day 2 | 12.3 | | | 45 | >150 | |
| Day 5 | 11.3 | | | 44 | | |
| Day 8 | Pamidronate infusion given | | | | | |
| Day 15 | 10.7 | 4.1 | 3.0 | 58 | | |
| Day 27 | 10.3 | | | >60 | >150 Send-out 425 | |
| Day 69 | 9.7 | | | 53 | >150 | |
| Day 130 | | | | | 148 | |

*Nl* normal, *eGFR* estimated glomerular filtration rate, *25(OH)VitD* 25 hydroxyvitamin D, *1,25(OH)2Vit D* 1,25 dihydroxyvitamin D (calcitriol) range 8.6–10.3), PTH of 5 pg/ml (normal range 12–88), and creatinine of 1.46 mg/dl corresponding to an estimated glomerular filtration rate (eGFR) of 37 ml/min. Albumin was normal, and the ionized calcium was also high at 1.76 mmol/L (normal range 0.96–1.40). Phosphorous was low normal at 2.7 mg/dl (2.5–5.0). Ultimately, PTHrp, angiotensin-converting enzyme, and SPEP were all normal. Electrolytes and bicarbonate were normal, and TSH was slightly suppressed at 0.3 mIU/L. Surprisingly, the 25-hydroxyvitamin D and 1,25-dihydroxyvitamin D levels measured >150 ng/ml (normal range 13–62) and 483 pg/ml (normal range 19.9–79.3), respectively.

The patient was called and instructed to hydrate aggressively, stop all supplements and vitamin D drops, and return for further labs. She was instructed to go the emergency department (ED) for any worsening of symptoms and informed that she would need to go to the ED if her repeat labs were not improved. She was also asked further questions about her vitamin D supplement. At that time she revealed that her chiropractor had instructed her to use one drop of the vitamin D3 liquid supplement (2000 IU/drop) daily but that she had actually been "squirting" this into her mouth daily.

Repeat serum calcium and eGFR after hydration were improved but still abnormal (Table 16.1) and remained roughly stable at these levels after a further 24 hours of aggressive oral hydration. At this time the 24-hour urine results revealed a total calcium excretion of 970 mg/day (normal 100–300) with a normal total creatinine and a volume of 6.8 liters consistent with her ongoing hydration efforts. In light of the degree of vitamin D toxicity, serum and urine calcium levels, and continued renal insufficiency with eGFR remaining in the 40s, 90 mg pamidronate IV was administered about 1 week after the initial visit. The patient noted dramatic improvement in her energy level and symptoms within a week after the infusion, though she also had some joint pain and night sweats as side effects of the infusion.

## Discussion

Vitamin D is one of the fat-soluble vitamins that has long been known to accumulate in fat tissue and has the potential for toxicity if taken at high doses. As a result, the recommended daily allowance (RDA) for vitamin D has traditionally been quite conservative with the primary goal of avoiding toxicity. During the late 1900s, for instance, Finland had gradually decreased the RDA for vitamin D in three steps from 4500 IU in 1964 to just 400 IU in 1992. However, beginning around 1990 a vast body of literature began to suggest multiple possible benefits of vitamin D supplementation. One such study demonstrated that over the time that Finland had decreased the RDA, the incidence of type 1 diabetes had steadily increased from ~18/100,000 in 1964 to 65/100,000 in 2005 [1]. Furthermore, when individual data for actual vitamin D intake from a 1966 birth cohort were analyzed, children who took the then recommended dose of 2000 IU had a relative risk (RR) of 0.22 of developing type 1 diabetes compared to those who took less [2]. During the 1990s and early 2000s, epidemiological studies demonstrated a correlation of lower vitamin D levels with increased all-cause mortality, cardiovascular mortality, type 2 diabetes prevalence, fall and fracture risk, asthma exacerbations, infection rates, adverse pregnancy outcomes, and incidence and severity of autoimmune diseases including type 1 diabetes, MS, and rheumatoid arthritis (reviewed in [3–8]). As with all epidemiological observational studies, these early studies demonstrated association but did not establish causation. However, the studies led to a general perception that more vitamin D might be a panacea for many ailments.

The epidemiological studies have since led to the performance of a large number of randomized placebo-controlled studies investigating a variety of the above outcomes. Studies varied widely in terms of the dose, frequency, duration, and type of vitamin D supplementation, inclusion of calcium supplementation, study population, and outcomes measured. Most of the studies were cost-limited and unable to include serum vitamin D level measurements in order to distinguish between repletion and supplementation or to define an optimal goal vitamin D level. Several meta-analyses and systematic reviews have attempted to combine data on specific outcomes to improve overall power [9–16].

Unfortunately, despite the large body of literature including randomized placebo-controlled studies, meta-analyses, and systematic reviews that has accumulated over the last 20 years, clear guidelines remain elusive. Results have been mixed and interpretations complicated by the variety of populations, methods, and outcomes. However, some conclusions are clear. *First*, it has become quite clear that vitamin D deficiency is a widespread issue and that existing conservative RDAs are likely inadequate. Multiple studies have found vitamin D levels <20 ng/ml in ≥50% of selected populations (for instance, 82% of African Americans [17], 69% of US Hispanics [17], 58% of Greeks [18], 49% of severely obese US children [19]). The use of sunscreens that block much of the UV wavelengths needed for vitamin D production, a general decline in time spent outdoors, and the migration of populations adapted to high sun exposure in tropical latitudes (i.e., darkly pigmented skin) to more temperate latitudes are clearly contributors. *Second*, true vitamin D deficiency is clearly implicated in fracture risk, fall risk, and autoimmunity [20], likely implicated in other inflammatory or immune-mediated processes such as prevention of infection [14, 21] and asthma exacerbations [4] and possibly implicated in other poor outcomes including increased cancer and cardiovascular mortality [3, 6, 7, 9, 12, 13, 22, 23]. *Third*, it is also clear that while enough vitamin D is important, more is not better. The issue in this case was hypercalcemia from extreme overdosing and severe vitamin D toxicity. However, many studies have now suggested that much more modest vitamin D elevations, even well within the normal range, may have negative consequences including renal damage, kidney stones, increased fall risk [21, 24–26], progression to frailty [27], and cardiovascular risk [22, 28, 29].

Many questions remain regarding the best guidelines for vitamin D supplementation. Since current data and guidelines fully support only correction of deficiency, two key questions that remain incompletely addressed are "what level constitutes deficiency?" and "at what level do risks outweigh benefits?" The 2016 US Preventive Services Task Force (USPSTF) guidelines on screening for vitamin D deficiency note that "no consensus exists on the definition of vitamin D deficiency or the optimal level of total serum 25(OH)D…" [30]. Several approaches have been taken to address the question of how low is too low. Some studies have looked at the correlation of PTH levels to 25(OH) vitamin D levels and found a strong inverse relationship at vitamin D levels <20 ng/ml (50 nmol/ml), a variable and weaker inverse relationship at levels between 20 and 30 ng/ml (50–75 nmol/ml), and a clear plateau at levels above 30 ng/ml [23, 31, 32]. Another study looked at the response of PTH and intestinal calcium transport to 8 weeks of vitamin D dosing [18]. PTH levels decreased markedly as 25 (OH) vitamin D levels increased between 8 and 15 ng/ml, less markedly from 15 to 22 ng/ml, and not significantly with an increase from 22 to 35 ng/ml. However, intestinal calcium transport continued to increase in the latter range from 45% to 65%. Taken together these studies have led to an unofficial consensus that levels <20 ng/ml are clearly deficient, while the 20–30 ng/ml range is generally considered "insufficient." Consistent with this, the reviews and meta-analyses of randomized controlled trials of vitamin D supplementation that provide vitamin D serum level data generally have found the clearest evidence of benefit in those studies where the study population was deficient or insufficient at baseline. For instance, in the Reid et al. meta-analysis [15], where vitamin D supplementation modestly improved femoral neck bone mineral density in the full analysis, the benefit was largely driven by four studies in which the baseline vitamin D level was <12 ng/ml and slightly attenuated by the one study where baseline vitamin D was >30 ng/ml.

At this point there is little or no evidence to support supplementing vitamin D to the point of increasing serum levels much above the sufficient level of 30 ng/ml (75 nmol/ml). Some studies have suggested a decrease in acute respiratory infections at higher levels but possibly at the expense of a higher fall risk [21]. Other studies have further supported an increased fall risk at vitamin D levels > ~40–50 ng/ml [24–26]. Few studies have carefully addressed optimal serum levels or doses of vitamin D for specific outcomes, but in the case of fall risk, Smith et al. broke down fall risk both by vitamin D level and by vitamin D dose [25]. They found the lowest fall risk with vitamin D levels in the 30–40 ng/ml range and vitamin D dose in the 1600–3200 IU/day range. Both higher and lower levels and doses were associated with higher fall rates. A similar U-shaped relationship was seen for progression to frailty with the optimal vitamin D level in the 20–30 ng/ml range [27]. In cardiovascular disease, a reverse J-shaped relationship has been reported for overall cardiovascular mortality with the optimal vitamin D level falling in the 20–40 ng/ml range [22], and a forward J-shaped relationship with a similar optimal range has been reported for adverse cardiac and cerebrovascular events in cardiac surgery [29]. An accumulating body of evidence supports a variety of negative cardiovascular outcomes with similarly, modestly elevated vitamin D levels (reviewed in [33]). With specific relevance to the case reported here, the existing data in MS appear to fall in line with the above results with strong support for increased incidence and disease activity in true vitamin D deficiency with levels <20 ng/ml (reviewed in [34]). However, an optimal range has not been clearly defined. Some existing evidence supports continued benefit at levels up to 37 ng/ml and a weak signal for possible further benefit at >37 ng/ml [34].

This case represents an example of non-endocrine hypercalcemia resulting from severe vitamin D overdosing and toxicity. Unfortunately, recent trends in the approach to vitamin D supplementation and popular Internet literature inflating the potential benefits of vitamin D make this an increasingly common scenario. It is important to keep vitamin D toxicity in the differential diagnosis for PTH-independent hypercalcemia and to recognize that the existing body of literature supports repletion of vitamin D deficiency but does not support supplementing to levels greater than the 30–40 ng/ml range for any indication. Furthermore, the prescribing of vitamin D repletion should always be accompanied by a discussion of the potential risks of overdose.

## References

1. Mohr SB, Garland FC, Garland CF, Gorham ED, Ricordi C. Is there a role of vitamin D deficiency in type 1 diabetes of children? Am J Prev Med. 2010;39:189–90.
2. Hypponen E, Laara E, Reunanen A, Jarvelin MR, Virtanen SM. Intake of vitamin D and risk of type 1 diabetes: a birth-cohort study. Lancet. 2001;358:1500–3.
3. Jacobs ET, Kohler LN, Kunihiro AG, Jurutka PW. Vitamin D and colorectal, breast, and prostate cancers: a review of the epidemiological evidence. J Cancer. 2016;7:232–40.
4. Kolokotroni O, Middleton N, Kouta C, Raftopoulos V, Yiallouros PK. Association of serum Vitamin D with asthma and atopy in childhood: review of epidemiological observational studies. Mini Rev Med Chem. 2015;15:881–99.
5. McCarthy EK, Kiely M. Vitamin D and muscle strength throughout the life course: a review of epidemiological and intervention studies. J Hum Nutr Diet. 2015;28:636–45.
6. Pilz S, Kienreich K, Tomaschitz A, et al. Vitamin D and cancer mortality: systematic review of prospective epidemiological studies. Anti Cancer Agents Med Chem. 2013;13:107–17.
7. Grubler MR, Marz W, Pilz S, et al. Vitamin-D concentrations, cardiovascular risk and events – a review of epidemiological evidence. Rev Endocr Metab Disord. 2017;18:259–72.
8. Smolders J, Damoiseaux J, Menheere P, Hupperts R. Vitamin D as an immune modulator in multiple sclerosis, a review. J Neuroimmunol. 2008;194:7–17.

9. Avenell A, Mak JC, O'Connell D. Vitamin D and vitamin D analogues for preventing fractures in post-menopausal women and older men. Cochrane Database Syst Rev. 2014;(4):CD000227.
10. Bischoff-Ferrari HA. Vitamin D and fracture prevention. Rheum Dis Clin N Am. 2012;38:107–13.
11. Bolland MJ, Grey A, Gamble GD, Reid IR. Vitamin D supplementation and falls: a trial sequential meta-analysis. Lancet Diabetes Endocrinol. 2014;2:573–80.
12. Bolland MJ, Grey A, Gamble GD, Reid IR. The effect of vitamin D supplementation on skeletal, vascular, or cancer outcomes: a trial sequential meta-analysis. Lancet Diabetes Endocrinol. 2014;2:307–20.
13. Ford JA, MacLennan GS, Avenell A, et al. Cardiovascular disease and vitamin D supplementation: trial analysis, systematic review, and meta-analysis. Am J Clin Nutr. 2014;100:746–55.
14. Martineau AR, Jolliffe DA, Hooper RL, et al. Vitamin D supplementation to prevent acute respiratory tract infections: systematic review and meta-analysis of individual participant data. BMJ. 2017;356:i6583.
15. Reid IR, Bolland MJ, Grey A. Effects of vitamin D supplements on bone mineral density: a systematic review and meta-analysis. Lancet. 2014;383:146–55.
16. Weaver CM, Alexander DD, Boushey CJ, et al. Calcium plus vitamin D supplementation and risk of fractures: an updated meta-analysis from the National Osteoporosis Foundation. Osteoporos Int. 2016;27:367–76.
17. Forrest KY, Stuhldreher WL. Prevalence and correlates of vitamin D deficiency in US adults. Nutr Res. 2011;31:48–54.
18. Singhellakis PN, Malandrinou F, Psarrou CJ, Danelli AM, Tsalavoutas SD, Constandellou ES. Vitamin D deficiency in white, apparently healthy, free-living adults in a temperate region. Hormones (Athens). 2011;10:131–43.
19. Turer CB, Lin H, Flores G. Prevalence of vitamin D deficiency among overweight and obese US children. Pediatrics. 2013;131:e152–61.
20. Antico A, Tampoia M, Tozzoli R, Bizzaro N. Can supplementation with vitamin D reduce the risk or modify the course of autoimmune diseases? A systematic review of the literature. Autoimmun Rev. 2012;12:127–36.
21. Ginde AA, Blatchford P, Breese K, et al. High-dose monthly vitamin D for prevention of acute respiratory infection in older

long-term care residents: a randomized clinical trial. J Am Geriatr Soc. 2017;65:496–503.
22. Durup D, Jorgensen HL, Christensen J, et al. A reverse J-shaped association between serum 25-hydroxyvitamin D and cardiovascular disease mortality: the CopD study. J Clin Endocrinol Metab. 2015;100:2339–46.
23. Lee JH, O'Keefe JH, Bell D, Hensrud DD, Holick MF. Vitamin D deficiency an important, common, and easily treatable cardiovascular risk factor? J Am Coll Cardiol. 2008;52:1949–56.
24. Sanders KM, Stuart AL, Williamson EJ, et al. Annual high-dose oral vitamin D and falls and fractures in older women: a randomized controlled trial. JAMA. 2010;303:1815–22.
25. Smith LM, Gallagher JC, Suiter C. Medium doses of daily vitamin D decrease falls and higher doses of daily vitamin D3 increase falls: a randomized clinical trial. J Steroid Biochem Mol Biol. 2017;173:317–22.
26. Bischoff-Ferrari HA, Dawson-Hughes B, Orav EJ, et al. Monthly high-dose vitamin D treatment for the prevention of functional decline: a randomized clinical trial. JAMA Intern Med. 2016;176:175–83.
27. Ensrud KE, Ewing SK, Fredman L, et al. Circulating 25-hydroxyvitamin D levels and frailty status in older women. J Clin Endocrinol Metab. 2010;95:5266–73.
28. Zittermann A, Ernst JB, Prokop S, et al. Effect of vitamin D on all-cause mortality in heart failure (EVITA): a 3-year randomized clinical trial with 4000 IU vitamin D daily. Eur Heart J. 2017;38:2279–86.
29. Zittermann A, Kuhn J, Dreier J, Knabbe C, Gummert JF, Borgermann J. Vitamin D status and the risk of major adverse cardiac and cerebrovascular events in cardiac surgery. Eur Heart J. 2013;34:1358–64.
30. USPSTF. Vitamin D deficiency screening. https://www.uspreventiveservicestaskforce.org/Page/Document/RecommendationStatementFinal/vitamin-d-deficiency-screening. 2016.
31. Atapattu N, Shaw N, Hogler W. Relationship between serum 25-hydroxyvitamin D and parathyroid hormone in the search for a biochemical definition of vitamin D deficiency in children. Pediatr Res. 2013;74:552–6.
32. Rizzoli R, Boonen S, Brandi ML, et al. Vitamin D supplementation in elderly or postmenopausal women: a 2013 update of the 2008 recommendations from the European Society for Clinical

and Economic Aspects of Osteoporosis and Osteoarthritis (ESCEO). Curr Med Res Opin. 2013;29:305–13.
33. Zittermann A. The biphasic effect of vitamin D on the musculoskeletal and cardiovascular system. Int J Endocrinol. 2017;2017:3206240.
34. Sintzel MB, Rametta M, Reder AT. Vitamin D and multiple sclerosis: a comprehensive review. Neurol Ther. 2018;7:59–85.

# Chapter 17
# Low Testosterone: Determine and Treat the Underlying Disorder

**Kenneth Tompkins and Micol S. Rothman**

## Clinical Scenario

A 54-year-old male presents to your clinic for evaluation of persistent fatigue. For over a year, he has been finding it hard to perform his regular activities. Although he sleeps 7–8 hours a night, he rarely feels rested upon waking. His wife notes that he often snores loudly while sleeping. He works a sedentary desk job and gets no regular exercise. He is obese and states that despite his best efforts with diet, he has been unable to lose weight. He notes he is under a lot of stress at his job and at home. Upon questioning, he endorses sexual issues with his wife, with decreased libido and intermittent erectile dysfunction. His issues with fatigue, failure to lose weight, and sexual dysfunction prompted him to ask you about the possibility of "low T," a condition he recently read about on an Internet site.

K. Tompkins (✉) · M. S. Rothman
University of Colorado, Department of Medicine, Division of Endocrinology, Aurora, CO, USA
e-mail: Kenneth.tompkins@ucdenver.edu

His history is otherwise notable for type 2 diabetes mellitus and "borderline hypertension." His only medication is metformin and OTC acetaminophen PRN. He takes no supplements. He drinks one to two beers a night. He denies tobacco or drug use. He has two teenage daughters. He went through puberty at the same time as his peers and had no issues with fertility. Exam reveals an obese, middle-aged male (BMI 34 kg/m$^2$). Extraocular movements are intact with normal visual fields. Neck circumference is 19 cm. Abdominal exam shows central adiposity and no visible stretch marks. GU exam reveals testes descended bilaterally, with normal size at 15 mL without palpable masses and normal consistency. Neurological exam shows normal strength without evidence of muscle wasting. Laboratory evaluation shows normal blood counts, electrolytes, kidney function, and thyroid function, and his A1c is 6.9%. In light of his complaints, a serum testosterone was also checked and returned at 224 ng/dL (normal range, 264–916).

## Discussion

Male hypogonadism, most commonly manifested by a deficiency of the sex hormone testosterone, is a frequently encountered problem in outpatient settings. One study evaluated over 2000 men, age 45 years or older, in primary care practices and found that almost 40% had a low testosterone value or were being treated with androgen therapy [1]. The symptoms of hypogonadism can include fatigue, weight gain, loss of lean muscle mass, and sexual complaints such as erectile dysfunction and decreased libido. The syndrome of "low T" has been popularized in the media and our culture; as a result, it has become common for men to approach their providers requesting an evaluation for low testosterone. The vague nature of the symptoms, the multiple etiologies of hypogonadism, the circadian variations in normal testosterone levels, and the natural decline in testosterone levels with normal aging and significant variability in testosterone labo-

Chapter 17. Low Testosterone: Determine and Treat... 217

ratory assays all contribute to unique diagnostic dilemmas and challenges when evaluating patients for suspected hypogonadism. Testosterone replacement therapy has been variably associated with increased risks of cardiovascular disease, making it crucial to make a proper diagnosis before initiating therapy. It is a common situation for providers to discover a borderline low testosterone in asymptomatic male patients. Therefore, it is key to have a framework for the proper evaluation and treatment of this condition.

Male hypogonadism is characterized by a deficiency of testosterone, impaired spermatogenesis, or both, and is usually associated with signs and symptoms. The lower limit of serum testosterone that defines hypogonadism is controversial. There is limited data on the values that are associated with clinical symptoms or sequelae of hypogonadism. A study of over 3000 men found that testosterone levels <320 ng/dl were directly correlative with sexual symptoms, including decreased morning erections, erectile dysfunction, and decreased libido [2]. Another study, utilizing a block-and-replace strategy for testosterone therapy, found that testosterone levels <200 ng/dl were associated with increased bone resorption and decreases in bone mineral density (BMD) [3].

There is a wide variety of commercially available testosterone assays, with significant variability between labs. Centers for Disease Control (CDC) validated assays use a lower limit of 264 ng/dl. In the absence of a CDC-validated assay, it may be prudent to follow the Endocrine Society guidelines, which suggest that a testosterone value <320 ng/dl may be indicative of hypogonadism [4].

Hypogonadism is classified as primary or secondary. Primary hypogonadism is due to a defect in the testicles, the organ responsible for producing testosterone and sperm. Secondary hypogonadism is due to a defect at the level of the hypothalamus or the pituitary gland. The hypothalamus-pituitary-gonadal (HPG) axis is responsible for regulating the production of testosterone and sperm within the testis. The hypothalamus synthesizes and secretes gonadotropin-releasing hormone (GnRH), which stimulates the pituitary to secrete luteinizing hormone (LH) and follicle-stimulating hormone (FSH). LH and FSH then act at the level of the testis to stimulate testosterone production and spermatogenesis, respectively. This system is tightly regulated, with each hormone feeding back on the level above it (Fig. 17.1). Disruption in either the hypothalamus, the pituitary, or the testis can lead to low testosterone.

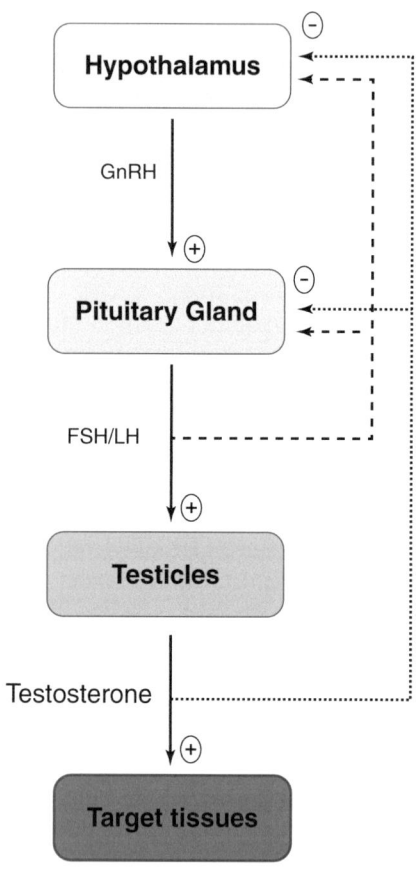

FIGURE 17.1 Hypothalamic-pituitary-gonadal axis

The differential diagnosis for hypogonadism is quite broad. Primary hypogonadism, due to testicular defects, is characterized by elevated levels of FSH and LH. This can be due to congenital disorders such as cryptorchidism, genetic conditions such as Klinefelter syndrome or acquired damage as a consequence of trauma, chemotherapy/radiation, or infections of the testes.

Secondary hypogonadism, characterized by low or inappropriately normal LH and FSH levels, is the more common type of hypogonadism. Causes of secondary hypogonadism are many and include tumors of the hypothalamus or pituitary, prolactin elevation, head trauma, iron overload syndromes, and prior pituitary surgery or radiation. Obesity, sleep disorders such as obstructive sleep apnea, depression, and excessive stress are also important and common causes of secondary hypogonadism. A number of medications, especially narcotics, marijuana, glucocorticoids, and certain body building supplements, can also cause secondary hypogonadism.

As with any evaluation, the first step in patients with suspected hypogonadism is an appropriate history and physical examination. In addition to standard symptoms associated with low testosterone, it is important to inquire about puberty and development. Late or absent puberty can signify a congenital disorder, as can a history of infertility. Loss of secondary sex characteristics, such as a decreased need to shave, can suggest more severe hypogonadism. A thorough exam including testicular palpation and measurement should be performed. Small testes, very hard or soft testes, and asymmetry of the testes can suggest a primary testicular disorder. A defect in peripheral vision suggests the presence of a pituitary mass lesion. In chronic secondary hypogonadism, with loss of the LH and FSH, the testicles may shrink in size and develop a softer consistency.

If suspicion for hypogonadism is moderate or high, measurement of serum testosterone levels is indicated. It is important to note that testosterone is a steroid hormone. As such, it is hydrophobic and only very small amounts of testosterone circulate freely in the blood. Approximately 98% of circulating testosterone is bound to circulating proteins, most importantly sex hormone-binding globulin (SHBG) [5]. Most assays measure serum total testosterone, which consists of both the free and protein-bound fractions. However, free testosterone is the only biologically active component. Low free testosterone is what causes the symptoms of hypogonadism. However, measuring free testosterone is expensive, time-consuming, and can be inaccurate depending on the assay, and thus total testosterone levels are most often used as a surrogate.

When evaluating the serum total testosterone concentration, it is important to consider that certain conditions can affect both the protein bound and free portions of testosterone. There are several common conditions that can lower the levels of SHBG, thereby lowering the concentration of protein-bound testosterone. However, the free testosterone level in these patients is often normal, and thus these men are, in fact, not hypogonadal. One of the most common conditions affecting SHBG is obesity. Several studies have shown a decline in SHBG with increasing BMI. Age also affects SHBG levels but in the opposite manner with SHBG increasing with age. A study evaluating SHBG levels in a large cohort of veterans found that the individuals most likely to have the lowest SHBG levels were young, obese men [6].

If the serum testosterone level is low, further steps need to be undertaken in the evaluation. Figure 17.2 outlines a general approach for further evaluation. Given the significant variability of testosterone levels through the day, the first step in evaluating a low testosterone level is confirming it with a repeat test. Testosterone has diurnal and circadian variation and can also be affected by glucose and food intake. Therefore, a low testosterone should prompt a fasting repeat test in the AM, when testosterone levels are naturally highest, to confirm [4].

If the serum total testosterone level is unequivocally low (<150 ng/dl), there is likely a true pathologic cause of the

Chapter 17. Low Testosterone: Determine and Treat... 221

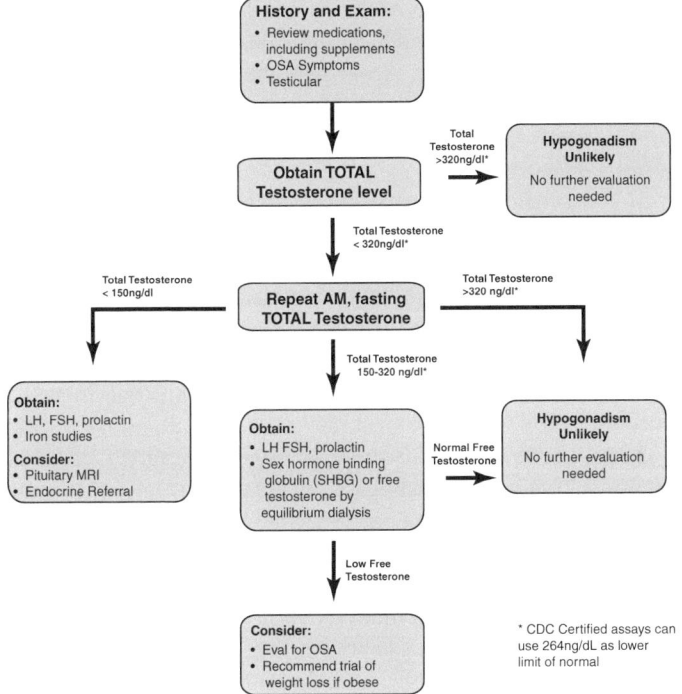

FIGURE 17.2 Approach to a patient with low testosterone

hypogonadism, and the workup below should ensue. If the level is low normal or mildly low (>150 ng/dl), this could be related to low SHBG or other etiologies. In this scenario it is reasonable to check an SHBG level. Online calculators can be used to give an accurate estimate of the free testosterone concentration based on the patient's total testosterone, SHBG, and albumin levels. If the free testosterone level is normal, then this is likely a binding protein issue, and this can be evaluated separately. Alternatively, if free testosterone is low, this points toward a pathologic cause of hypogonadism.

Free testosterone levels by equilibrium dialysis can also be checked. This is different than the standard free testosterone platform assays that are routinely available; these assays generally use an immunoprecipitation-based approach and are notoriously unreliable. Free testosterone by equilibrium dialysis is a more reliable test but is more time-consuming, cumbersome, and expensive than the other assays. As such, it is not routinely used.

If the serum total testosterone level is frankly low on at least two occasions, or if estimations of the free testosterone concentration suggest that it is low, a workup for the cause is warranted. It is important to initiate this workup before beginning any treatment for two reasons. First, testosterone supplementation will artificially suppress the HPG axis, making it difficult to interpret laboratory testing going forward. Second, many of the conditions known to cause low serum testosterone levels are reversible. Ideally, whenever possible, the underlying cause should be treated to allow normal endogenous testosterone production to return rather than artificially supplementing it with exogenous testosterone.

Once a low serum testosterone level is confirmed, the next step is to order measurement of serum FSH and LH. In the setting of primary hypogonadism, the FSH and LH are elevated. In this circumstance, the hypothalamus and pituitary are functioning normally, and therefore without the inhibitory feedback effect of testosterone, FSH and LH appropriately rise. If the workup is suggestive of primary hypogonadism, the evaluation should then focus on finding a defect in the testicles themselves. A directed history exploring trauma or prior treatments such as chemotherapy or radiation is important. A dedicated physical exam should assess for undescended testes or any asymmetry. A history of infertility along with very small testes should prompt one to think about Klinefelter syndrome and consider ordering a karyotype.

In secondary hypogonadism, which is more common than primary, the FSH and LH are generally low or inappropriately normal, usually in the single digits. It is appropriate to order a serum prolactin level and iron studies in all patients with secondary hypogonadism to rule out hyperprolactinemia and hemochromatosis. If the testosterone level is significantly low

(<150 ng/dl), this can suggest pituitary dysfunction. In this case, evaluating all the pituitary hormones and considering dedicated imaging, such as a pituitary MRI, may be warranted [4].

Obesity-related complications are among the most common causes of HPG axis dysfunction. Obesity can lower total testosterone levels by lowering SHBG levels, but it can also lead to mild lowering of the free testosterone itself. Weight reduction has been shown to improve testosterone levels back to normal levels in obese men [7]. Thus, when faced with an obese male without clear a cause of hypogonadism, the treatment plan should focus on strategies to reduce weight rather than replace testosterone. In most cases, it is perfectly reasonable to withhold replacement therapy during evaluation and while trialing other treatment options before initiating replacement therapy.

Hypogonadism is a common and complex disorder. Given its prevalence and prominence in modern culture, a groundwork for the appropriate workup and treatment of hypogonadism is important for most providers to understand, especially in the primary care and endocrine settings. The diagnosis of hypogonadism should be made based on, as discussed above, a history of compatible symptoms, a good physical examination, distinctly low serum testosterone levels, and an evaluation for the cause of low testosterone, if present.

It cannot be emphasized enough that male hypogonadism is often due to other medical conditions or medications that cause suppression of the male reproductive axis and is not due to organic failure of the HPG axis. Often these conditions are far more serious than the low serum testosterone levels that they cause. "Low T" is therefore often an indication of much more serious underlying health issues. Therefore, to maximize benefit and minimize harm to patients, it is important, whenever possible, to identify and treat reversible causes of low testosterone prior to starting testosterone therapy. Obesity, sleep apnea, and depression should be identified and treated; efforts should be made to remove offending medications, especially opiates and glucocorticoids. These measures will often normalize serum testosterone levels and sexual function. Treating prolactin elevations will also usually return testosterone levels to normal. Resection of pituitary adenomas commonly restores normal gonadal function postoperatively. In many patients, strategies focusing on eliminating the primary cause can lead to restoration of testosterone levels, without having to expose patients to the risks of testosterone therapy.

Replacement should only be initiated once true hypogonadism is confirmed. Testosterone therapy can be administered in multiple ways, including transdermal gels, transdermal patches, axillary gels, trans-buccal patches, intramuscular injections, and injections of pellets. When testosterone replacement therapy is undertaken, patients should be informed that this medication will likely suppress their own reproductive axis, resulting in further impairment of testosterone production and often significant reductions in sperm production resulting in infertility. Once initiated, appropriate serum testosterone targets should be set and strictly adhered to. An appropriate target is to maintain the serum testosterone level in the middle of the normal range for males during transdermal therapy or midway between intramuscular injections.

Excessive testosterone levels should be carefully avoided. It is not unusual, however, for some practitioners to prescribe higher doses with hopes or promises of improved benefits from high normal or frankly elevated serum testosterone levels. We have seen numerous patients who have received testosterone pellet injections (which are advertised aggressively on Internet websites) and who subsequently had moderate to highly elevated serum testosterone levels as well as high hematocrits and elevated prostate-specific antigen (PSA) levels. Though the data are somewhat mixed, some studies have shown an association of testosterone replacement therapy with higher risks of cardiovascular disease [8, 9]. In addition, conditions such as untreated obstructive sleep apnea may be worsened by testosterone replacement therapy [10]. No clinical evidence supports the notion that high normal or frankly elevated serum testosterone levels provide any type of symptomatic or health benefit compared to physiologic levels and, indeed, supraphysiologic testosterone levels are those that are most likely to result in significant side effects and complications. There is no published evidence currently to support either the efficacy or safety of this practice. We consider this type of therapy to be dangerous and unethical and discourage our patients from engaging in this type of therapeutic strategy.

## *Back to the Patient*

This patient has multiple potential causes for having low serum testosterone levels. He is obese. He probably has sleep apnea based on his loud snoring. He is also under a great deal of stress. These are all issues that can be approached with lifestyle measures or medical therapy. His provider should discuss all of these matters with him and inform him of the serious impact his obesity, sleep apnea, and stressful life are having on his body; his low serum testosterone is just one example of this. He should be further advised that starting testosterone replacement therapy is only a Band-Aid masking the underlying problem. We have found that explaining the causes of low testosterone to men in a professional and caring manner is well accepted. Most men are happy to know that there is no significant permanent pathology within their reproductive tract and that their low testosterone levels can be improved by lifestyle measures that will allow them to avoid a lifetime of dependency on testosterone replacement therapy.

# References

1. Mulligan T, Frick MF, Zuraw QC, Stemhagen A, McWhiter C. Prevalence of hypogonadism in males aged at least 45 years: the HIM study. Int J Clin Pract. 2006;60(7):762–9.

2. F W, Tajar A, Beynon J, (the EMAS Group), et al. Identification of late onset hypogonadism in middle-aged and elderly men. N Engl J Med. 2010;363:123–35.
3. Finkelstein J, Lee H, Leder B, et al. Gonadal steroid-dependent effects on bone turnover and bone mineral density in men. J Clin Invest. 2016;126(3):1114–25.
4. Bhasin S, Brito J, Cunningham G, et al. Testosterone therapy in men with hypogonadism: an Endocrine Society clinical practice guideline. J Clin Endocrinol Metab. 2018;103(5):1715–44.
5. Dunn J, Nisula B, Robboard A. Transport of steroid hormones: binding of 21 endogenous steroids to both testosterone-binding globulin and corticosteroid-binding globulin in human plasma. J Clin Endocrinol Metab. 1981;53(1):58–68.
6. Cooper L, Page S, Amory J, Anawalt B, Matsumoto A. The association of obesity with sex hormone-binding globulin is stronger than the association with ageing – implications for the interpretation of total testosterone measurements. Clin Endocrinol. 2015;83:828–33.
7. Camacho EM, Huhtaniemi IT, O'Neill TW, (the EMAS Group), et al. Age-associated changes in hypothalamic–pituitary–testicular function in middle-aged and older men are modified by weight change and lifestyle factors: longitudinal results from the European Male Ageing Study. Eur J Endocrinol. 2013;168:445–55.
8. Basaria S, Coviello A, Travison T, et al. Adverse events associated with testosterone administration. N Engl J Med. 2010;363(2):109–22.
9. Budoff M, Ellenberg SS, Lewis CE, et al. Testosterone treatment and coronary artery plaque volume in older men with low testosterone. JAMA. 2017;317(7):708–16.
10. Hoyos C, Killick R, Yee B, Grunstein R, Liu PY. Effects of testosterone therapy on sleep and breathing in obese men with severe obstructive sleep apnoea: a randomized placebo-controlled trial. Clin Endocrinol. 2012;77(4):599–607.

# Chapter 18
# Inappropriate Use of Mifepristone to Treat Diabetes Mellitus

**Eveline Waring and Beatrice Hull**

Like most good stories in medicine, this one begins with a patient.

"Mrs. Smith" had been seen by another endocrinologist 6 months prior but had subsequently been referred to our practice for another opinion. Like most second opinions, it became clear very quickly that this was a complicated case.

This 62-year-old female had multiple medical problems including but not limited to diabetes, morbid obesity, trichotillomania, irritable bowel syndrome, depression/anxiety/PTSD, gout, untreated sleep apnea, coronary artery disease, recurrent upper respiratory infections requiring intermittent courses of glucocorticoids, and chronic pain requiring frequent "injections." Her pertinent surgical history was a laminectomy at an unknown level, cholecystectomy, and appendectomy. She was married, did not use tobacco or alcohol, had two daughters, and was retired from clerical work. She was allergic to codeine and Percocet, both of which caused itching. Her family history was notable for hypertension, obesity, diabetes, and hypothyroidism throughout.

Six months prior to our appointment, Mrs. Smith was informed by her previous endocrinologist that she had an elevated cortisol level and was immediately placed on mifepristone (Korlym) for treatment of Cushing's syndrome. She was on Korlym for 3 weeks but stopped it after developing a rash, generalized weakness, and "feeling awful." She did not have labs at the time of discontinuing Korlym and therefore did not know the status of her potassium at that time. After stopping Korlym, her symptoms resolved within 1 week.

In keeping with her complicated medical history, she was on multiple medications at the time of her first appointment in our practice: valproic acid, brexipiprazole, allopurinol, amitriptyline, levothyroxine, pregabalin, pantoprazole, lubiprostone, rosuvastatin, metformin, empagliflozin, and dulaglutide.

Mrs. Smith was accompanied by her husband at her initial consultation. Their questions were why she had been placed on treatment for Cushing's syndrome, what was Cushing's syndrome, and did she indeed have it?

On physical exam, Mrs. Smith was anxious, tearful, and morbidly obese. Her blood pressure was 125/84 mmHg with a pulse of 82 and a BMI of 44 kg/m$^2$. She had male pattern baldness, a buffalo hump, thin skin with ecchymoses on extensor surfaces, central adiposity, and plethoric facies. She did not have abdominal striae, and hirsutism was not noted.

Her accompanying medical records noted an incidental right-sided adrenal nodule of 1.6 cm, described as benign per radiological parameters. Her laboratory records were extensive and showed fluctuating glucose control with a hemoglobin A1C of 8%. Her potassium and renal function were normal. There was no complete blood count with her initial labs. Her 24-h urine cortisol was 12 mcg/24 h (normal, 0–50 mcg/24 h). After 1 mg overnight dexamethasone suppression test, her morning cortisol was 1.5 mcg/dl (with a dexamethasone level of 170 ng/dL) and ACTH of 3.0 pg/ml (normal, 7.2–63.3 pg/ml). Plasma metanephrine was 30 pg/ml (normal,

0–62 pg/ml) with a mildly elevated normetanephrine of 147 pg/ml (normal, 0–145 pg/ml), DHEA-S was 25.9 mcg/dl (normal, 29.4–220.5 mcg/dl), plasma aldosterone 30 ng/dl, plasma renin activity 11.78 ng/ml/h, insulin level of 44.1 uIU/ml (normal, 2.6–24.9 uIU/ml), TSH 6.3 mU/L (normal, 0.45–4.5 mU/L), TPO antibodies 126 IU/ml (normal, 0–34 IU/ml), and free T4 0.53 ng/dl (normal, 0.58–1.64 ng/dl).

Further history was obtained. The patient noted that she had not gained weight in years and had maintained the exact same shape since her last pregnancy 30 years prior. Interestingly, she added that her entire family favored one another in appearance and showed a photo to solidify her claim. She admitted to problems with depression and knew that she was a "stress eater" and preferred "comfort foods" of potatoes and pasta to the foods recommended to her previously for her diabetes. As to her male pattern baldness, she confessed that she pulled her hair out as part of her PTSD from childhood trauma. She was having a difficult time finding a regimen that addressed her depression/anxiety adequately and was constantly adjusting her psychiatric medications accordingly. She had had multiple courses of oral glucocorticoids in the preceding few years and countless injections in her lumbar spine, hips, and knees for pain.

This is a particularly difficult patient, with multiple comorbidities and a striking appearance consistent with Cushing's syndrome. That said, there were significant confounding variables that were not necessarily taken into account before the diagnosis of Cushing's was applied to this patient. As we know from a preceding chapter in this book, pseudo-Cushing's can be caused by depression, obesity, alcoholism, and poorly controlled diabetes. In this particular patient, all of the above apply with the exception of alcoholism. Further, the patient had been treated with exogenous steroids on multiple occasions over the previous several years prior to her arrival in our office.

We were curious about the diagnosis of Cushing's syndrome for this patient and, subsequently, about her treatment with mifepristone, so we did some digging into the literature.

Mifepristone, a glucocorticoid and progesterone receptor antagonist, is marketed as Korlym and is approved by FDA to control hyperglycemia occurring secondary to hypercortisolism in patients with endogenous Cushing's syndrome who have diabetes mellitus type 2 or glucose intolerance and who have failed surgery or who are not surgical candidates.

As you see from our example, the indication for mifepristone use was arrived at in reverse: the patient presented with difficult-to-control metabolic syndrome (obesity, hypertension, diabetes, depression), and then the search for hypercortisolemia was undertaken, culminating in the patient being placed on mifepristone.

In order to know if mifepristone can and *should* be used in our reference patient, three questions need to be answered: (1) How prevalent is autonomous cortisol secretion? (2) How should the diagnosis of autonomous cortisol secretion be made? (3) Has the appropriate risk-benefit analysis been done comparing mifepristone with other treatment options?

Autonomous cortisol secretion is a state of altered hypothalamic-pituitary-adrenal axis cortisol secretion without classic features of overt cortisol excess. It is reportedly present in 5–30% in patients with adrenal incidentalomas [1]. Because adrenal masses are common in the general population (4–7%), the prevalence of autonomous cortisol secretion in adults in general population is estimated to be 0.2–2% [1].

The majority of studies evaluating the diagnostic approach to autonomous cortisol secretion have been done in patients with adrenal incidentalomas. The overnight 1 mg dexamethasone suppression test (1 mg DST), 24-h urinary free cortisol (UFC), midnight salivary cortisol (MSC), and ACTH measurement have all been studied as diagnostic tests for this condition with very variable results in sensitivity and specificity [1]. Subsequently, the definition of autonomous cortisol secretion varies, and there is no one reliable test to diagnose this condition, leading physicians to utilize multiple available tests to try to make an accurate diagnosis [1], but it also creates the situation where the interpretation of tests results can to be interpreted "loosely" depending on physician personal bias and experience.

In their practice guidelines for the management of adrenal incidentalomas published in 2016, the European Society of Endocrinology advises use of 1 mg DST as a screening test with a level below 1.8 mcg/dl excluding autonomous cortisol secretion, the level >3 mcg/dl confirming it, and the level between 1.9 and 2.9 mcg/dl requiring additional testing [2].

Meta-analyses of 14 studies published in 2017 showed that among 2827 type 2 diabetic patients, the pooled prevalence of hypercortisolism and Cushing's syndrome was 3.4% (95% CI, 1.5–5.9) and 1.4% (95% CI, 0.4–2.9), respectively [2]. Screening tests used to diagnose hypercortisolism varied considerably among studies (1 mg DST with variable cutoffs and MSC being most commonly used) [3]. Fifty-two percent of patients with hypercortisolism had adrenal tumors [3]. Some, but not all, studies suggested that poor glycemic control was associated with the increased prevalence of hypercortisolism [4].

It is logical to think that autonomous cortisol secretion can be associated with metabolic disorders (diabetes, hypertension, obesity) and cardiovascular disease, just as overt Cushing's syndrome can. To date, studies evaluating possible health implications of hypercortisolism have yielded variable results confounded by disease definition and sample populations. Hypertension and impaired glucose metabolism are more prevalent in patients with hypercortisolism; however, the prevalence range for type 2 diabetes is quite wide (5–69%) [4]. Several studies show that patients with adrenal adenomas and hypercortisolism have an increased risk to develop cardiovascular disease and increased mortality attributable to cardiovascular disease and infectious complications [5].

Studies that evaluate treatment options in patients with autonomous cortisol production are few. Most evaluate patients with autonomous cortisol secretion and adrenal adenomas comparing conservative management with adrenalectomy.

Good-quality studies are lacking and available studies suffer from retrospective study designs, small sample sizes, variable diagnostic criteria for hypercortisolism and comorbidities, and variable follow-up times. In a meta-analysis of 26 such studies published in 2016, low-to-moderate quality evidence suggested that adrenalectomy in patients with autonomous cortisol secretion and adrenal adenoma shows improvement in cardiovascular risk factors and improvement in hypertension (RR 11, 95% CI, 4.3–27.8) and diabetes mellitus type 2 (RR 3.9, 95% CI, 1.5–9.9), but not dyslipidemia or obesity when compared with conservative management [6]. Aggressive medical management of comorbidities has never been compared to adrenalectomy. No studies have been done to evaluate management outcomes in patients with hypercortisolemia without adrenal adenomas or in patients with subclinical Cushing's syndrome and pituitary adenomas.

Mifepristone was studied in patients with Cushing's syndrome who had type 2 diabetes mellitus, glucose intolerance, and hypertension [7]. These study end points were used as surrogate markers of antiglucocorticoid effect of mifepristone: glycemic control improved in 60% of patients, diastolic blood pressure improved in 38%, and 87% of patients reported improvement in signs and symptoms and overall wellbeing [7]. Side effects were common: fatigue (48%), nausea (48%), headache (44%), hypokalemia (34%), arthralgia (30%), vomiting (26%), edema (26%), and endometrial thickening in women (20%) [7].

There is only one published study assessing the use of mifepristone in patients with autonomous cortisol secretion and adrenal incidentalomas treating six subjects with mifepristone for 4 weeks [8]. These patients did not have abnormal glucose metabolism at baseline. Treatment with mifepristone showed a decrease in insulin resistance indices in five out of six patients [8]. One subject withdrew from the study due to fatigue, and hypokalemia was found in two subjects [8].

To date, there are no studies evaluating mifepristone efficacy in patients with hypercortisolemia without an adrenal adenoma. There are also no long-term outcome and safety studies comparing mifepristone with aggressive management of comorbidities.

In summary, autonomous cortisol secretion is quite prevalent, especially in high-risk populations such as poorly controlled diabetic and hypertensive patients with adrenal incidentalomas, but the diagnosis of this condition is difficult to establish properly owing to the lack of a single best test. Good-quality, long-term studies evaluating different treatment options (aggressive management of comorbidities versus adrenalectomy versus management of hypercortisolemia) are lacking. Appropriate studies evaluating the efficacy and safety of mifepristone in patients with autonomous cortisol secretion with or without adrenal adenomas are insufficient. In our opinion, it is important to examine the current state of evidence when considering prescribing medication with the potential for myriad side effects and an exorbitant price tag (up to $240,400 for 1 year). It would therefore seem advisable to exercise patience and await larger clinical trial data.

# References

1. Chiodini I. Diagnosis and treatment of subclinical hypercortisolism. J Clin Endocrinol Metab. 2011;96(5):1223–35.
2. Fassnacht M, et al. Management of adrenal incidentalomas: European Society of endocrinology clinical practice guideline in collaboration with the European network for the study of adrenal tumors. Eur J Endocrinol. 2016;175:G1–G34.
3. Steffensen C, et al. Prevalence of hypercortisolism in type 2 diabetes patients: a systemic review and meta-analysis. Eur J Endocrinol. 2016;175(6):R247–53.
4. Cansu GB, et al. Which type 2 diabetes mellitus patients should be screened for subclinical Cushing's syndrome? Hormones (Athens). 2017;16(1):22–32.
5. Di Dalmazi G, et al. Subclinical hypercortisolism: a state, a syndrome, or a disease? Eur J Endocrinol. 2015;173:M61–71.
6. Bancos I, et al. Improvement of cardiovascular risk factors after adrenalectomy in patients with adrenal tumors and subclinical

Cushing's syndrome: a systemic review and meta-analysis. Eur J Endocrinol. 2016;175(6):R283–95.
7. Fieseriu M, et al. Mifepristone, a glucocorticoid receptor antagonist, produces clinical and metabolic benefits in patients with Cushing's syndrome. J Clin Endocrinol Metab. 2012;97(6):239–49.
8. Debono M, et al. Mifepristone reduces insulin resistance in patient volunteers with adrenal incidentaloma that secrete low levels of cortisol: a pilot study. PLoS One. 2013;8(4):e60984.

# Chapter 19
## Insulin-like Growth Factor-1 Deficiency

**Thomas Ittoop and S. Sethu K. Reddy**

## Introduction

Insulin-like growth factor-1 is a peptide hormone primarily synthesized in the liver and is an essential component of an individual's growth [1]. Secretion of GH from the pituitary gland stimulates the hepatic production of IGF-1 and its release into circulation. IGF-1 lengthens bones by its action at the epiphyses (it is estimated that 2/3 of all bone growth is directly due to the effects of IGF-1). Other IGF-1 effects include modulating cellular growth, proliferation, differentiation, and survival against apoptosis. The effects of IGF-1 are mediated through the IGF-1 receptor (IGF-1R) and its signaling pathway. The IGF-1R is structurally and functionally similar to the insulin receptor. Thus, IGF-1 can bind to insulin

T. Ittoop · S. S. K. Reddy (✉)
Central Michigan University College of Medicine,
Mt. Pleasant, MI, USA
e-mail: sethu.reddy@cmich.edu

receptors but at a much lower affinity than insulin. It is also known that insulin can bind to the IGF-1R but at a lower affinity than IGF-1. Unlike insulin, however, there are several IGF-1-binding proteins (IGF-BP) that help to increase the circulating half-life and delivery of IGF to tissues, modulating IGF-1 interactions with IGF-1R by holding on to or releasing IGF-1, ultimately regulating the bioavailability of IGF-1.

Over the last 20 years, the IGF-1 system has been recognized as far more complex than a simple GH-IGF-1-bone axis [2]. IGF-1 has paracrine and autocrine functions as well as classic endocrine actions, and the IGF-1 + IGF-BP + IGF-1R system interacts with other growth factors, cytokines, lipoproteins, reactive oxygen species, and hemodynamic forces. In addition, there is cross talk between the IGF system and other growth factors and integrin receptors. There is accumulating evidence of a role for IGF-1 in multiple vascular pathologies, including atherosclerosis, hypertension, restenosis, angiogenesis, and diabetic vascular disease [3].

The IGF-BP family (at least six members) serves as transporter proteins and as storage pools for IGF-1. The expression of IGF-BPs is tissue- and developmental stage-specific and the concentrations of IGF-BPs in different body compartments are different. The functions of IGF-BPs are regulated by phosphorylation, proteolysis, polymerization, and cell or matrix association of the IGF-BP. All six IGF-BPs are known to inhibit IGF-1 action, but IGF-BP-1, IGF-BP-3, and IGF-BP-5 have also been shown to stimulate IGF-1 action.

The acid-labile subunit (ALS) functions to maintain the balance of the circulating IGF/IGF-BPs in the system; ALS is critical to the maintenance of a large reservoir of IGFs by extending their half-life from 10 min (free forms) to 30–90 min in binary complexes (early periods of human life) and later to more than 12 hours, when bound into tertiary complexes. ALS deficiency can lead to low IGF-1 levels and cause primary IGF-1 deficiency and thus qualify for IGF-1 therapy. The measurement of IGF-1 levels is challenging with at least six commercially available assays. The measurement of IGF-

BPs, in particular IGF-BP3, is also critical. IGF-1 levels rise incrementally from infancy to adulthood and then slowly fall after age 30.

A deficiency of IGF-1 should be considered in patients, specifically children, who present with short stature or delayed onset of puberty [4]. IGF-1 deficiency presents similar to growth hormone deficiency (GHD) and involves the following clinical features: severe growth failure after birth, delayed bone maturation and puberty, prominent forehead, small face, shallow orbits, blue sclera, and delayed dental eruption. It also includes an increased tendency to develop low blood glucose levels, walking and motor development delays, and a tendency for excess fat deposition around the trunk. Long-term IGF-1 deficiency in adults is thought to causally relate to neurodegeneration and dementia and is associated with coronary artery disease.

The causes of IGF-1 deficiency can be classified into two main types: primary and secondary. Primary IGF-1 deficiency refers to IGF-1 impairment but with normal GH secretion. Secondary IGF-1 deficiency refers to IGF-1 impairment due to some dysregulation in GH secretion. IGF-1 impairment can be attributed to different molecular aspects of both primary and secondary deficiency, as seen in Table 19.1. It is important to note that IGF-1 is activated downstream of GH and that any pathological reduction in GH will ultimately result in reduced IGF-1 as well, as seen in any case of secondary IGF-1 deficiency. Until primary vs secondary IGF-1 deficiency is determined, causes of GH reduction should be under careful consideration. This chapter, however, will put an emphasis on primary IGF-1 deficiency.

## Diagnosis of IGF-1 Deficiency

Suspicion of a growth deficiency should arise when tracking a patient's height, weight, and growth velocity. If a patient's progress is concerning for short stature, then an X-ray of the hand and wrist can be obtained to determine the level of

TABLE 19.1 Molecular causes of IGF-1 deficiency

| Classification of IGF deficiency | Pathogenesis |
|---|---|
| *Primary IGF-1 deficiency*: | IGF-1 impairment, normal growth hormone (GH) secretion |
| Dysfunction in GH action | Anti-GH antibodies Excess GH binding proteins GH receptor (GHR) dysfunction: GHR antibodies, GHR gene defects JAK-STAT secondary messenger system dysfunction |
| Defects in IGF-1 production | IGF-1 gene mutation/deletion Disruption of IGF-1 cofactors |
| Dysfunction in IGF-1 action | Lack of IGF-1-binding proteins (IGF-BP) Excess binding proteins Deficiency of acid-labile subunit (ALS) IGF-1 receptor (IGF-R) dysfunction: antibodies to IGF-R or gene mutation |
| *Secondary IGF-1 deficiency*: | IGF-1 impairment due to dysregulation in GH secretion |
| GH production defect | Somatopause |
| GH-releasing hormone (GHRH) defect/GHRH receptor defect | Receptor/genetic defect of GHRH receptor |

skeletal growth plate maturation, along with a measurement of serum IGF-1 levels [5]. At this time, measurement of IGF-BP-3, or the binding protein for IGF-1, can be ordered as well, as these levels can affect the bioavailability of IGF-1. If the IGF-1 levels are low, then a GH stimulation test can be administered to differentiate between primary and secondary IGF-1 deficiency. Failure of IGF-1 to rise after GH stimula-

Chapter 19. Insulin-like Growth Factor-1 Deficiency    239

tion indicates a primary IGF-1 deficiency. If IGF-1 rises after the stimulation test, then further evaluation of GH deficiency and secondary causes must be considered.

## Clinical Causes of IGF-1 Deficiency

There are multiple factors that can contribute to the molecular changes shown in Table 19.1 that result in primary IGF-1 deficiency. When diagnosing a patient with IGF-1 deficiency, it is important to look into correlating diseases, nutrition, and genetics to understand the root of the deficiency, for all of these can contribute to a reduction in IGF-1.

## Associated Diseases

Different underlying conditions can lead to a deficiency in IGF-1. A prime example is liver disease. Since the liver is the main site of IGF-1 synthesis, patients with cirrhosis can present with an IGF-1 deficiency [6]. The liver is not the only site of IGF-1 synthesis. Studies have shown that local (paracrine) IGF-1 can have overlapping effects with liver IGF-1, but it cannot replace liver-derived IGF-1 for the major phenotypic functions [7]. Thus, a lack of IGF-1 production from a cirrhotic liver can manifest as a clinical phenotype of IGF-1 deficiency. Recent evaluation has found that IGF-1, when studied in 64 hospitalized patients with cirrhosis over a 2-year period, is not regulated by nutrition. Patients with IGF-1 Z-scores < median values (−2.5) showed lower long-term survival rates compared with patients with IGF-1 Z-scores > −2.5 ($P < 0.01$). IGF-1 Z-scores were not different in patients with or without signs of energy malnutrition, as defined by values of midarm muscle circumference (MAMC) and/or triceps skinfold (TSF) <5th percentile. These data indicate that serum IGF-1 is not related to energy malnutrition in cirrhotic patients, while it appears to be a good predictor of survival and an early marker of liver dysfunction.

Hypothyroidism can also lead to reduced IGF-1 levels. One study reported that removing l-thyroxine from patients who underwent a thyroidectomy decreased levels of both IGF-1 and IGF-BP [8].

IGF-1 deficiency is associated with chronic kidney disease as well, specifically through GH resistance [9]. One of the major mechanisms that contributes to this correlation is the reduced levels of free IGF-1 circulating through the body. This is caused by an increased level of IGF-1-binding proteins (IGF-BPs) due to decreased renal excretion caused by chronic kidney disease. As a result, more IGF-1 is bound to IGF-BPs, and IGF-1 is not free to fulfill its physiological purpose, causing a functional primary IGF-1 deficiency. Other mechanisms seen in chronic kidney disease include an impaired secondary messenger system, specifically in JAK/STAT signaling, from the GH receptor and an overall reduced concentration of GH receptors.

Laron syndrome [10] is characterized by the inability to utilize GH. As an autosomal recessive disorder, it is a form of primary IGF-1 deficiency that results from a deletion or mutation in the GH receptor gene. Because the defect is in the GH receptor, serum GH levels are elevated. Although Laron syndrome is an extremely rare disease [around 350 people have been diagnosed in the world [11]], it is an important congenital model used for IGF-1 deficiency research and reference. Individuals with Laron syndrome exhibit the classic characteristics expected of an inability to produce IGF-1, including growth defects/dwarfism, obesity, and delayed puberty. Interestingly, those with Laron syndrome have been shown to be protected from cancer development, likely as a result of the IGF-1 deficiency [12], highlighting the involvement of IGF-1 in certain cancers. Nevertheless, an understanding of the molecular basis of Laron syndrome and its clinical manifestations is important for the thorough understanding of primary IGF-1 deficiency.

Reduced IGF-1 is also seen in malabsorption diseases, including cystic fibrosis, inflammatory bowel disease, and celiac disease. It is also a characteristic of diseases with significant energy requirements, such as cardiac disease (those involving cyanosis or congestive heart failure) and HIV infections [13]. These diseases are categorized together because of their relation to nutrition, caloric deficits, and specific mineral deficiencies, which is the next point of discussion.

## Nutrition

Nutritional disturbances should be a key differential in analyzing an IGF-1 deficiency. There are many aspects of nutrition that contribute to this deficiency. For example, obesity has been shown to lead to insulin/IGF-1 resistance. One study even linked this obesity-related insulin/IGF-1 resistance to an exacerbation of neurodegeneration in disorders such as Alzheimer's disease, Parkinson's disease, and Huntington's chorea [14]. More often, however, forms of undernutrition are the source of IGF-1 deficiency.

GH resistance can result from undernutrition via the GH receptor signaling pathway. During fasting, fibroblast growth factor 21 (FGF21) is produced in adipocytes. FGF21 subsequently decreases phosphorylation of signal transducer and activator of transcription 5 (STAT5) [15]. Phosphorylation of STAT5 is an important step in the secondary messenger cascade of the GH receptor that leads to IGF-1 production. Studies have also shown that restriction of calorie intake and protein intake both result in reduced levels of IGF-1 [16]. It is important to determine if a patient with decreased IGF-1 levels is ingesting enough calories and protein to match the amount of energy he or she expends. Calorie and protein deficiencies can be especially prevalent in areas with lack of access or education to enough healthy food needed to maintain IGF-1 levels. There are a multitude of other reasons why a patient might not be receiving enough calories in their diet, including fear of obesity and side effects of medication. Therefore, a thorough history is needed to determine the underlying cause of such nutritional deficiency. Although low IGF-1 levels in preclinical models are associated with vitamin B6 [17], magnesium [18], and zinc [19] deficiencies, their physiological importance in man remains unclear. Iodine deficiency has also been correlated with reduced IGF-1 levels, but iodine supplements should not be administered, given the risk of hypothyroidism and an additional reduction in IGF-1 [20].

## Low IGF-1 Levels in Adults

IGF-1 deficiency may be considered by some to be a GH insensitivity or GH resistance syndrome. However, while IGF-1 excess is usually related to GH excess, IGF-1 deficiency may not necessarily be due to GH deficiency. Thus, an adult syndrome similar to the Laron syndrome is unlikely. Most patients with severe IGF-1 deficiency have normal concentrations of GH. This primary form of severe IGF-1 deficiency (with normal or high GH levels) is differentiated from secondary forms of IGF-1 deficiency, such as in malnutrition or liver disease.

For adults with newly discovered IGF-1 deficiency, one must conduct formal endocrine testing for reduced GH secretion prior to initiating GH therapy. At present, a low IGF-1 itself does not support access to GH therapy.

## Potential Clinical Implications of Low IGF-1 Levels

Low IGF-1 levels are associated with impaired glucose intolerance [21] and type 2 diabetes [22]. Low IGF-1 levels may also be related to hepatic insulin resistance and impaired beta cell function [23]. However, it is not clear whether these associations are related to underlying impairments in cell function because portal insulin is an important promoter of hepatic IGF-1 synthesis [7]. Thus, evaluation of healthy adults will be useful in delineating the physiological roles of IGF-1.

Though more evidence is needed to prove causality, there is some suggestion that low IGF-1 levels may be associated with more rapidly progressive vascular dementia, Alzheimer's dementia [24], and Parkinson's disease [25], increased risk of ischemic stroke, and a lower risk of some cancers [26, 27]. Future delineation of these associations will no doubt depend upon clarification of the endocrine (systemic) vs. paracrine (local) effects of IGF-1; it is possible that circulating levels of IGF-1 do not reflect local tissue-specific IGF-1 regulation [14].

IGF-1 and its signaling pathway play a primary role in normal growth and aging. Recent studies suggest that IGF-1 is essential for neurogenesis in the adult brain, and thus, the reduction of IGF-1 with aging may contribute to age-related cognitive decline [28].

Initially, low IGF-1 levels may serve as biomarkers of prognostic significance [29] in certain disorders such as liver disease [30], nonalcoholic steatohepatitits (NASH) [31], and overall nutrition, including obesity [32].

## *IGF-1 and Longevity [33]*

In vivo studies of preclinical models have established that a downregulated GH/IGF-1 system may be associated with increased longevity. Data in humans has been more controversial. The rationale for this concept arises from caloric restriction-associated increased life span and nutritional status-associated IGF-1 biology [34]. There are conflicting results from a variety of centenarian cohorts [35], from higher levels of IGF-1/IGF-BP3 levels to low IGF-1 levels being associated with longevity [36].

## Treatment Guidelines for IGF-1 [37]

Increlex (mecasermin) contains recombinant DNA-engineered human IGF-1 (rhIGF-1). rhIGF-1 is approved in Europe and the USA for the treatment of growth failure in children with severe primary IGF-1 deficiency as it stimulates linear growth. Patients with severe primary IGF-1 deficiency (primary IGFD) fail to produce adequate levels of IGF-1, due to disruption of GH stimulated IGF-1 release.

Increlex (rhIGF-1) is specifically indicated for the long-term treatment of growth failure in pediatric patients with primary IGFD or with GH gene deletion who have developed neutralizing antibodies to GH. It is not indicated to treat secondary IGFD resulting from GH deficiency, malnutrition, hypothyroidism, or other causes; it is not a substitute for GH therapy.

For children with GH resistance and IGF-1 deficiency, the FDA has approved IGF-1 as a therapeutic agent for severe forms of IGF-1 deficiency. A combination of IGF-1 with IGF-BP-3 (IGF-1/BP-3 complex) has also been approved by the FDA but is not currently in use due to legal issues. For primary IGF-1 deficiency, the following three criteria must be met prior to use of rhIGF-1: basal IGF-1 and height should be three standard deviations (SD) or below for age and sex; stimulated GH should be normal or elevated [GH peak level greater than 10 ng/ml or basal (unstimulated) serum GH level greater than 5 ng/ml] [38]. Of note, the growth response in these children tends to be less than the response seen by GH-deficient children treated with GH.

Increlex is supplied as a sterile, aqueous, clear, and colorless solution intended for subcutaneous injection. Dosing should be titrated on a per-patient basis: the recommended initial dose is 40–80 mcg/kg twice daily. The dose can be increased in 40 mcg/kg/dose increments if well tolerated for 1 week, to a maximum dose of 120 mcg/kg twice daily.

The authors are not aware of any initiatives to seek approval of IGF-1 therapy for adult IGF-1 deficiency.

## Summary and Clinical Tips

1. IGF-1 biology is far more complex than the original concept of GH-stimulated hepatic release of IGF-1 to result in systemic effects of growth and development. IGF-binding proteins play a key role in IGF-action as well as cross talk between IGF-1 receptor activation and a multitude of other second messenger systems.
2. IGF-1 deficiency is usually the result of conditions other than pure GH deficiency. Thus low IGF-1 levels by themselves have to be investigated further. Treating the underlying cause will usually result in improvement in the IGF-1 deficiency.
3. There is early human data that IGF-1 levels may be a marker of healthy aging but also of progression of liver disease, CNS-degenerative conditions, atherosclerosis, and many other disorders.
4. Future studies are needed to delineate the differential effects of endocrine IGF-1 vs. paracrine IGF-1 and abnormalities in IGF-1 action cross talk, to truly understand the effects of IGF-1 in humans.

# References

1. Frysak Z, Schovanek J, Iacobone M, Karasek D. Insulin-like Growth Factors in a clinical setting: review of IGF-I. Biomed Pap Med Fac Univ Palacky Olomouc Czech Repub. 2015;159(3):347–51.
2. Gallagher EJ, LeRoith D. World leaders describe the latest in IGF research. J Mol Endocrinol. 2018;61(1):E1–3.
3. Higashi Y, Gautam S, Delafontaine P, Sukhanov S. IGF-1 and cardiovascular disease. Growth Hormon IGF Res. 2019;45:6.
4. Backeljauw P. Insulin-like growth factor 1 deficiency [Brochure]. Author. 2008. Retrieved from http://hgfound.org/wp-content/uploads/2015/02/Insulin-Like-Growth-Factor-I-Deficiency.pdf.
5. Ranke MB. Growth hormone deficiency: diagnostic principles and practice. In: Ranke MB, Mullis P-E, editors. Diagnostics of

endocrine function in children and adolescents. 4th ed. Basel: Karger; 2011. p. 102–37.
6. de la Garza RG, Morales-Garza LA, Martin-Estal I, Castilla-Cortazar I. Insulin-like growth factor-1 deficiency and cirrhosis establishment. J Clin Med Res. 2017;9(4):233–47.
7. Ohlsson C, Mohan S, Sjögren K, Tivesten A, Isgaard J, Isaksson O, Jansson JO, et al. The role of liver-derived insulin-like growth factor-I. Endocr Rev. 2009;30(5):494–535.
8. Angervo M. Thyroxine withdrawal is accompanied by decreased circulating levels of insulin-like growth factor-binding protein-1 in thyroidectomized patients. J Clin Endocrinol Metab. 1993;76(5):1199–201. https://doi.org/10.1210/jc.76.5.1199.
9. Mahesh S, Kaskel F. Growth hormone axis in chronic kidney disease. Pediatr Nephrol (Berlin, Germany). 2007;23(1):41–8.
10. Laron Z, Kauli R, Lapkina L, Werner H. IGF-1 deficiency, longevity and cancer protection of patients with Laron syndrome. Mutat Res Rev Mutat Res. 2017;772:123–33. https://doi.org/10.1016/j.mrrev.2016.08.002.
11. Laron syndrome – Genetics Home Reference – NIH. n.d. Retrieved from https://ghr.nlm.nih.gov/condition/laron-syndrome#statistics.
12. Shevah O, Laron Z. Patients with congenital deficiency of IGF-1 seem protected from the development of malignancies: a preliminary report. Growth Hormon IGF Res. 2007;17(1):54–7. https://doi.org/10.1016/j.ghir.2006.10.007.
13. Hawkes CP, Grimberg A. Insulin-like growth factor-I is a marker for the nutritional state. Pediatr Endocrinol Rev: PER. 2015;13(2):499–511.
14. Spielman LJ, Little JP, Klegeris A. Inflammation and insulin/IGF-1 resistance as the possible link between obesity and neurodegeneration. J Neuroimmunol. 2014;273(1):8–21.
15. Guasti L, Silvennoinen S, Bulstrode NW, Ferretti P, Sankilampi U, Dunkel L. Elevated FGF21 leads to attenuated postnatal linear growth in preterm infants through GH resistance in chondrocytes. J Clin Endocrinol Metabol. 2014;99(11):E2198. https://doi.org/10.1210/jc.2014-1566.
16. Smith WJ. Effects of caloric or protein restriction on insulin-like growth factor- I (IGF-1) and IGF-binding proteins in children and adults. J Clin Endocrinol Metab. 1995;80(2):443–9. https://doi.org/10.1210/jc.80.2.443.

17. Rao KJ, Mohan P. Plasma somatomedin activity, growth-hormone and insulin levels in vitamin B6 deficient rats. Horm Metab Res. 1982;14(11):580–2. https://doi.org/10.1055/s-2007-1019086.
18. Dørup I, Flyvbjerg A, Everts ME, Clausen T. Role of insulin-like growth factor-1 and growth hormone in growth inhibition induced by magnesium and zinc deficiencies. Br J Nutr. 1991;66(03):505. https://doi.org/10.1079/bjn19910051.
19. Cesur Y, Yordam N, Doğan M. Serum insulin-like growth factor-I and insulin-like growth factor binding protein-3 levels in children with zinc deficiency and the Effect of zinc supplementation on these parameters. J Pediatr Endocrinol Metab. 2009;22(12):1137–44. https://doi.org/10.1515/jpem.2009.22.12.1137.
20. Safarinejad MR, Shafiei N, Safarinejad S. Relationship of insulin-like growth factor (IGF) binding protein-3 (IGFBP-3) gene polymorphism with the susceptibility to development of prostate cancer and influence on serum levels of IGF-1, and IGFBP-3. Growth Hormon IGF Res. 2011;21(3):146–54. https://doi.org/10.1016/j.ghir.2011.03.008.
21. Sesti G, Sciacqua A, Cardellini M, Marini MA, Maio R, Vatrano M, Succurro E, Lauro R, Federici M, Perticone F. Plasma concentration of IGF-I is independently associated with insulin sensitivity in subjects with different degrees of glucose tolerance. Diabetes Care. 2005;28(1):120–5.
22. Friedrich N, Thuesen B, Jørgensen T, Juul A, Spielhagen C, Wallaschofksi H, Linneberg A. The association between IGF-I and insulin resistance: a general population study in Danish adults. Diabetes Care. 2012;35(4):768–73.
23. Thankamony A, Capalbo D, Marcovecchio ML, Sleigh A, Jørgensen SW, Hill NR, Mooslehner K, et al. Low circulating levels of IGF-1 in healthy adults are associated with reduced-beta cell function, increased intramyocellular lipid, and enhanced fat utilization during fasting. J Clin Endocrinol Metab. 2014;99:2198–207.
24. Westwood AJ, Beiser A, DeCarli C, Harris TB, Chen TC, He XM, et al. Insulin-like growth factor-1 and risk of Alzheimer dementia and brain atrophy. Neurology. 2014;82(18):1613–9.
25. Picillo M, Pivonello R, Santangelo G, Pivonello C, Savastano R, Auriemma R, Amboni M, et al. Serum IGF-1 is associated

with cognitive functions in early, drug-naïve Parkinson's disease. PLoS One. 2017;12(10):e0186508.
26. Anisimov VN, Bartke A. The key role of growth hormone–insulin–IGF-1 signaling in aging and cancer. Crit Rev Oncol Hematol. 2013;87(3):201–23.
27. Levine ME, Suarez JA, Brandhorst S, Balasubramanian P, Cheng CW, Madia F, et al. Low protein intake is associated with a major reduction in IGF-1, cancer, and overall mortality in the 65 and younger but not older population. Cell Metab. 2014;19(3):407–17.
28. Frater J, Lie D, Bartlett P, McGrath JJ. Insulin-like growth factor 1 (IGF-1) as a marker of cognitive decline in normal ageing: a review. Ageing Res Rev. 2018;42:14–27.
29. Carlzon D, Svensson J, Petzold M, Karlsson MK, Ljunggren Ö, Tivesten Å, et al. Both low and high serum IGF-1 levels associate with increased risk of cardiovascular events in elderly men. J Clin Endocrinol Metabol. 2014;99(11):E2308–16.
30. Caregaro L, Alberino F, Amodio P, Merkel C, Angeli P, Plebani M, Bolognesi M, Gatta A. Nutritional and prognostic significance of insulin-like growth factor 1 in patients with liver cirrhosis. Nutrition. 1997;13(3):v–190.
31. Dichtel LE, Corey KE, Misdraji J, Bredella MA, Schorr M, Osganian SA, Young BJ, Sung JC, Miller KK. The association between IGF-1 levels and the histologic severity of nonalcoholic fatty liver disease. Clin Transl Gastroenterol. 2017;8(1):e217.
32. Thankamony A, Capalbo D, Marcovecchio ML, Sleigh A, Jørgensen SW, Hill NR, et al. Low circulating levels of IGF-1 in healthy adults are associated with reduced β-cell function, increased intramyocellular lipid, and enhanced fat utilization during fasting. J Clin Endocrinol Metab. 2014;99(6):2198–207.
33. Milman S, Atzmon G, Huffman DM, Wan J, Crandall JP, Cohen P, Barzilai N. Low insulin-like growth factor-1 level predicts survival in humans with exceptional longevity. Aging Cell. 2014;13(4):769–71.
34. Junnila RK, List EO, Berryman DE, Murrey JW, Kopchick JJ. The GH/IGF-1 axis in ageing and longevity. Nat Rev Endocrinol. 2013;9(6):366–76.
35. Vitale G, Barbieri M, Kamenetskaya M, Paolisso G. GH/IGF-I/insulin system in centenarians. Mech Ageing Dev. 2017;165:107–14. https://doi.org/10.1016/j.mad.2016.12.001.
36. Vitale G, Pellegrino G, Vollery M, Hofland LJ. ROLE of IGF-1 system in the modulation of longevity: controversies and new

insights from a centenarians' perspective. Front Endocrinol. 2019;10:27. https://doi.org/10.3389/fendo.2019.00027.
37. Moore B, Whitehead A, Davies K. Short stature, growth hormone deficiency, and primary IGF-1 deficiency. In: Advanced practice in endocrinology nursing. Cham: Springer; 2019. p. 13–37.
38. Chernausek SD, Backeljauw PF, Frane J, Kuntze J, Underwood LE. Long-term treatment with recombinant insulin-like growth factor (IGF)-I in children with severe IGF-I deficiency due to growth hormone insensitivity. J Clin Endocrinol Metab. 2007;92:902–10.
39. Le Roith D. Seminars in medicine of the Beth Israel Deaconess Medical Center. Insulin-like growth factors. N Engl J Med. 1997;336:633–40.

# Chapter 20
# Non-thyroidal Hypothyroidism

James V. Hennessey

The Case: A 71-year-old Caucasian woman seeks consultation for a 3-month history of tiredness and feeling depressed. The first question to be answered is how likely is it that she is hypothyroid based on this clinical presentation? Over 20 years ago, a series of observations were made in regard to the association of symptoms of hypothyroidism and the presence of biochemically documentable disease. Canaris et al. reported in 1997 that when considering the frequency with which symptoms consistent with the presence of hypothyroidism were reported, the biochemical confirmation of a hypothyroid state was variable [1]. When considering subjects with no symptoms of hypothyroidism, about 40% of euthyroid subjects fit this profile as did just over 35% of those with documented subclinical hypothyroidism (SCHypo) and about 28% of patients with overt hypothyroidism (OHypo). Those complaining of one or two

J. V. Hennessey (✉)
Harvard Medical School, Beth Israel Deaconess Medical Center, Boston, MA, USA
e-mail: jhenness@bidmc.harvard.edu

symptoms of hypothyroidism were nearly equally distributed across the spectrum of euthyroidism to overt hypothyroidism, but when four or more symptoms were present, overtly hypothyroid subjects were present in statistically significantly higher rates (about ¼) when compared to those with SCHypo (about 22%) and the euthyroid group where nearly 18% complained of symptoms consistent with the presence of hypothyroidism [1]. Clearly the ability of a clinician to accurately identify those with biochemical hypothyroidism based on the presence of symptoms is poor. In another report in 2000, the same authors examined the frequency with which specific symptoms were reported in subjects with OHypo and biochemically euthyroid controls without thyroid disease [2]. The most commonly reported symptom, dry skin, was noted by fewer than 30% of those with OHypo, while 25% of euthyroid controls had the same complaint. Because of the large number of subjects participating in this study, this difference was statistically significant, but again a seasoned clinician immediately recognizes that the specificity of this finding is lacking. These authors performed similar analysis of 14 symptoms consistent with hypothyroidism and found similar overlapping but statistically significant differences in 12 parameters. Although the authors concluded that the symptoms of hypothyroidism are noted more frequently in those with OHypo, the high prevalence of the same complaints among euthyroid individuals [2], who according to guidelines would not be candidates for thyroid hormone replacement [3], again provides a clear clinical caveat for the use of symptoms to make clinical decisions regarding thyroid hormone replacement. More recently, Carle et al. have looked at this issue using a different set of complaints that were found to be associated with hypothyroidism [4]. These authors analyzed the likelihood of finding biochemical hypothyroidism based on symptoms among subjects stratified by gender and age. The number of symptoms reported by patients with OHypo vs. euthyroid controls without thyroid disease was significantly higher in younger subject, but the frequencies were far more similar in those over 60 and completely overlapping in those over 70 years of age [4]. Among the younger subjects (less than 50 years of age), those with three or fewer symptoms were unlikely to be hypothyroid, while in those over 60, the presence of one symptom predicted the absence of hypothyroidism [4]. While the likelihood of finding hypothyroidism did significantly increase as the number of symptoms rose above 4 in the younger group (<50 years), there was no significant predictive value of symptoms seen in the older subjects when 2–8+ symptoms were present [4]. Lastly, when stratified by age and gender, receiver operator curve analysis indicated that symptoms performed best for men under 50 and far worse for women over 60 years of age [4]. So to try to answer the first question posed, this patient is unlikely to be hypothyroid based on this clinical presentation.

But the patient is in her primary care MD's office expecting that her complaints will be addressed, so what does one do after a complete history and physical exam? Is there an indication for measuring thyroid function tests (TFTs) in a patient with this presentation? Of course, so who are the patients who are most frequently assessed with thyroid function testing in the primary care setting? Bould et al. systematically reviewed the thyroid function test ordering patterns of primary care practitioners in Bristol, England [5]. These authors reviewed the thyroid function test results associated with the indications for test ordering in 325 subjects who met all inclusion criteria of this prospective study. The thyroid function assessments had been ordered at the clinical discretion of the primary care physician. Those with tests ordered were invited to participate in this study which involved the completion of three questionnaires assessing psychiatric distress (GHQ-12), likelihood of depression (PHQ-9), and thyroid symptomatology (TSQ). The results of thyroid function testing on the 325 subjects, 78% of whom were women with a mean age of

45.7 years, were then correlated with the symptom scores of the 3 assessment tools. Overall, only 6.2% of the population had a TSH greater than 4.0 which the authors designated as potential SCHypo [5]. Further breakdown of the thyroid function documented in this group of clinically eligible patients indicated that only 4% had a single TSH over 4.5 and no subjects with OHypo were reported. The mean TSQ score was 15.7 (1–32); when I took the TSQ, I scored a 6 and I learned that there are few if any standardized expected score ranges in euthyroid individuals. Overall psychiatric stress levels were high with 54.2% of the population indicating caseness on the GHQ-12 and 55.1% reflecting possible depression on the PHQ-9 scale [5]. None of these scales predicted the elevation of TSH which would have indicated a potential thyroid etiology of the symptoms [5]. Comparison of the TSQ-12 scores of the individuals in the Bould study to the control subjects, administered the same questionnaire by Saravanan et al., indicated that TSQ scores were worse in Bould's report (TSQ = 16) versus a TSQ of 12 in Saravanan's controls and 13 in those treated with LT4 for well-documented hypothyroidism [6]. Likewise the GHQ-12 rating of caseness (about 54%) was much higher [5] than the controls and LT4-treated subjects in the Saravanan report (25–35%), so the context of these ratings is limited. A TSH greater than 4.0 mIu/mL was not correlated with any of the quality of life (QOL) measures [5] further limiting the utility of factoring in patient-reported symptoms in clinical decision-making. Bould's report documents that those referred for thyroid function testing in the course of primary care practice (PCP) have high rates of psychological stress. There is a low correlation of symptoms and abnormal TFTs. Identification of mild TSH elevations often results in the initiation of LT4 Rx which assumes the symptoms are actually due to hypothyroidism. As a diagnostic label will be professionally affixed to the patient, the search for alternative explanations of symptoms usually ends. If LT4 is initiated in a patient without significant thyroid dysfunction, the therapy is likely to fail to cure what should be considered *non*-thyroid symptoms [7] resulting in patient dissatisfaction and confusion. The authors of the Bould study specifically requested that PCPs keep psychological morbidity in mind and avoid prematurely labeling subjects as hypothyroid [5].

Who actually gets treated with LT4 in PCP offices? After appropriate exclusions, a study of 52,298 subjects receiving LT4 prescriptions over a 9-year period was assessed through the United Kingdom Clinical Practice Research Datalink [8]. The authors considered TSH and FT4 values obtained pre-LT4, and again after 5 years of LT4 therapy, correlations with demographic and concomitant diagnosis information were initiated and investigated. The TSH value available at the time of L-thyroxine initiation was less than 4.0 mIu/L (euthyroid) in about 6%; TSH was between 4.0 and 10.0 in 55.1% and greater than 10 in 38.8% [8]. The authors report a concerning trend of a decreasing TSH threshold for initiation of LT4 in successive years; this is mainly accounted for by an increase in the number of prescriptions written for TSH between 4.0 and 10.0 mIu/L, while prescriptions issued to subjects with TSH greater than 10.0 declined and LT4 offered to those with TSH less than 4.0 remained essentially unchanged over time [8]. This data is of concern as euthyroid subjects are apparently being offered a treatment that is unlikely to be of clinical benefit [7] and more patients are receiving treatment for degrees of hypothyroidism demonstrated to be unresponsive from a symptomatic perspective [9]. The sum of this data further documents the need to verify the presence of hypothyroidism prior to initiating or altering thyroid hormone replacement in patients with symptoms consistent with hypothyroidism.

Back to the case, recall that this 71-year-old woman sought consultation for a 3-month history of tiredness and feeling depressed. Her past medical history is as follows: a gradual 60 lb. weight gain following birth of her third child at age 36 along with decreased physical activity and plantar fasciitis when her TSH was documented to be 1.4 mIu/L and further a diagnosis of hypertension at age 45 (TSH 1.8) which had been treated with propranolol for the past 27 years. Next a diagnosis of hypercholesterolemia was made at age 49 when her TSH was documented to be 2.0. She reports being treated since then with simvastatin initially and now atorvastatin. At age 62 she was given a diagnosis of depression and had her TSH was documented to be 3.3 mIU/mL. She has been treated with SSRIs since that diagnosis. Relevant evaluation at age 70 includes thyroid function tests ordered by her PCP 12 months prior (age 70 years). TSH 4.6 mIU/mL (0.4–4.12 mIU/mL) at 16:30.

Again the question: is this patient hypothyroid and should she be treated now to relieve her symptoms? If we assume that SCHypo is potentially the basis of the patient's current symptoms and recognize that there was no indication that hypothyroidism played a role in the etiology of her other medical problems, a review of the incidence, the prediction of persistently elevated TSH, and if a single elevated TSH actually predicts progression to overt hypothyroidism are appropriate.

In a study of 3594 (non-LT4 using) subjects, ≥65 years of age, 85% ($n$ = 3057) were euthyroid at baseline and 2.7% became SCHypo by a 2-year follow-up. A total of 12.8% ($n$ = 459) met criteria for SCHypo at the baseline visit. Of the 369 completing a 2-year follow-up evaluation, 56% remained SCHypo, 35% reverted to euthyroidism, 2% progressed to overt hypothyroidism, and 7% had been started on LT4 [10]. At 4 years of follow-up among subjects with SCHypo at the 2-year follow-up, 58% remained SCHypo and 8% reverted to normal, 2% progressed to overt hypothyroidism, and 11% were on LT4. The bottom line here is that one set of TFTs with an elevated TSH consistent with SCHypo misclassifies more than 40% of the elderly. Clinical diagnosis requires more than one set of TFTs to establish SCHypo. In this observational study, TSH values greater than 10 increased the risk of persistent SCHypo and OHypo and the eventual clinical initiation of LT4 treatment [10].

Returning to the patient once again, relevant information at age 71 included thyroid function tests by her PCP 12 months prior (age 70) with a TSH 4.6 mIU/mL (0.4–4.12 mIU/mL) at 16:30 and a TSH of 5.3 mIU/mL 1 month later at 08:00. The FT4 1.5 ng/ml (0.8–1.7) and a TT3 81 ng/dL (80–200) were noted to be "low normal" in the PCP's note. Do these findings identify an individual with clinically relevant hypothyroidism that is likely to benefit from thyroid hormone replacement? To answer that question, we would need to consider what an upper normal cutoff for TSH is. Although in the past we have received recommendations suggesting a TSH >2.0 was too high, this was based on risk of developing overt hypothyroidism in the 20-year follow-up of a community-based thyroid health study [11]. Another recommendation was a statistically derived suggestion of 2.5 mU/L [12]. A more practical answer to this question may lie in analyzing TSH distribution patterns stratified by age in thyroid disease-free populations. One such study of the NHANES III population indicates that across all ages an upper limit cutoff of normal individuals falls at 4.12 mU/L [13]. When broken out by age groups however, a different pattern appears. For example, for those 20–29 years of age, the upper limit of normal (97.5%) appears to be 3.56 mIU/L, and only 2.4% of this normal population would be expected to have a TSH greater than 4.5 mIu/mL (the limit expected of the assay used in this analysis) [14]. Meanwhile, for those 70–79 years, the 97.5% was observed to be 5.9 mIU/L and fully 9.9% of this disease-free group would be expected to have a TSH greater than 4.5. Likely most telling is the observation that in those over 80 years, the upper normal cutoff would be 7.49 mIU/L and 12.0% of this presumably thyroid disease-free subpopulation would have a TSH over 4.5 [14]. Reproducible evidence of increasing TSH normal cutoffs with increasing age are found in several publications [15–17] with the 97.5%ile of TSH values being expected to be as high as 7.96 in those over 90 [18]. Other factors that may impact upon the upper limit of TSH may include gender with women demonstrating higher levels than men and variation by time of blood draw showing peak TSH values overnight and nadir results in the afternoon [15]. TSH varies by season in colder latitudes where not only is there an enhanced conversion of T4 to T3 in the winter months [19], but also higher TSH results are seen in the winter-spring season in both euthyroid and SCHypo subjects [20] and those treated with LT4 [21, 22]. Although the upper limit of TSH varies from study to study, a fairly clear increase in the expected upper normal TSH is observed in several studies, but at this time, it is unusual for clinical laboratories to stratify expected TSH results by age or by these other factors, and most clinical results are reported using a fixed upper normal of about 4–4.5 mIu/mL. Given this, it is likely safe to say that, as one set of TFTs with an elevated TSH consistent with SCHypo misclassifies more than 40% of the elderly, we should require at the very least that TSH elevations be persistent to establish the diagnosis of SCHypo. Finally as reproducible TSH values greater than 10 increase risk of persistent SCHypo and progression to OHypo, the initiation of LT4 therapy should be primarily focused on those meeting these criteria [3, 10].

Returning to the case, remember the evaluation at age 71 reviewed the thyroid function tests done by the primary care physician (PCP) 12 months prior to referral were a TSH of 4.6 mIU/mL (0.4–4.12 mIU/mL) at 16:30, and a repeat TSH of 5.6 mIU/mL was noted 1 month later when drawn at 08:00. Her FT4 was 1.5 ng/ml (0.8–1.7) and a TT3 of 81 ng/dL (80–200) which the PCP noted to be "low normal." Anti-thyroid antibodies were not done. The PCP started LT4 therapy for subclinical hypothyroidism at 50 mcg/day and this resulted in a follow-up TSH of 2.1 within 8 weeks. Based upon the discussion above, this patient does meet one of the recommended criteria for therapy [3], but more recent published data may require a reconsideration of this indication for a trial of LT4 in subjects with TSH greater than the upper limit of local laboratory normal and less than 10 mIU/mL [3].

Does thyroid hormone therapy have an impact on symptoms in SCHypo? Does age impact LT4 response? In a study of 27 children with SCHypo, a questionnaire of 16 items typical of hypothyroidism was administered and showed significantly more symptoms in those with SCHypo in 3 of the 16 parameters versus controls [23]. Each of these subjects had been classified as SCHypo based on a TSH greater than 4.94 mIU/mL on two separate occasions, and all had FT4 within the normal range. Treatment with LT4 was titrated to a normal TSH. After 6 months of euthyroidism, the 16-item questionnaire was readministered, some improvement was noted in most symptoms, but this was statistically significant in only 2 of the 16 [23]. The results of a large study of LT4 impact on SCHypo on older adults with SCHypo were recently published [24]. The *T*hyroid Hormone *R*eplacement for *U*ntreated older adults with *S*ubclinical hypothyroidism – a randomized placebo controlled *T*rial (TRUST) study reported on 737 appropriately qualified adults ≥65 years (mean age, 74.4 years) with persistent (X 2) elevations in TSH > 4.6 ranging up to 19.99 mIU/L. The mean TSH at baseline was 6.40 indicating that few had TSH levels either greater than their age expected upper normal or 10 mIU/L. The follow-up TSH levels declined to 5.48 in the *placebo-treated* group by 1 year indicating a normalization of TSH in a substantial number of subjects without any treatment. TSH was significantly lower (3.63 mIu/L) in the *LT4*-treated group by the end of the first year of follow-up. At baseline and after LT4 therapy, the primary outcome measure was the *Thy*roid-Related Quality-of-Life *P*atient-*R*eported *O*utcome (ThyPRO) with focus on the hypothyroid symptoms score (four items) and the tiredness score (seven items). A planned secondary quality-of-life outcome was measured by generic health-related QOL assessments along with anthropometric parameters. Subjects were randomized 1:1 to either LT4 or matching placebo at a dose of 50 mcg daily to start, and blinded dose adjustments were made to normalize TSH [24]. ThyPRO outcomes indicated that very few symptoms were present at baseline with a score of 0 or *NO* symptoms on the hypothyroid scale found in (27%) of participants and (8.7%) scored 0 in the tiredness scale. After 1 year F/U, comparing the LT4-treated versus placebo groups, there was no significant difference in symptoms [24]. Among the multiple secondary outcome measures, most demonstrated no significant effect of LT4 therapy except for one: the EQ-5D descriptive rating was worse at 12 months in those treated with LT4 but paradoxically was rated as better than placebo during prolonged follow-up. Within the confines of this trial, the safety of LT4 therapy was reassuring, but the clinical impact of treating older individuals' symptoms with slight elevations of TSH was not evident.

So where does this leave our patient? At the first endocrine visit, we are faced with a 72-year-old woman with persistent tiredness and depression, sleeping poorly who cannot lose weight. She has discovered online that "LT4 does not work for most patients with hypothyroidism" and asked her PCP for additional laboratory testing and the addition of LT3, a switch to a natural thyroid hormone extract (THExtract), or to refer her to an "expert" who will accomplish these tasks for the patient. On physical exam you find that her pulse is 109 and seems irregularly irregular. Her BMI is 35.9 kg/m2 and the current LT4 dose is 175 mcg/day. The PCP's most recent laboratory assessment shows a TSH < 0.01, FT4 1.9, TT3 175, and rT3 28 (10–24 ng/dL). The patient suggests that she would like three grains of thyroid extract. You ask yourself, how can these symptoms persist with these circulating thyroid hormone levels?

Is there a correlation between circulating T3 and rT3 and are these symptoms consistent with hypothyroidism? Phrased in a different way, is the lack of endogenous T3 production and subsequent inadequate T3 levels the basis of poor QOL? In a study of 143 patients (69.2% women, mean age 50.2 yrs.) who had undergone total thyroidectomy and 131-I ablation for differentiated thyroid cancer, at least 1 year prior to study inclusion, LT4 suppressive therapy as clinically appropriate was administered to avoid frank thyrotoxicosis [25]. The investigators assessed QOL with the RAND-36, thyroid-specific QOL with the ThyPRO instrument, and fatigue with a Multidimensional Fatigue Inventory (MFI). The results of these QOL measures were correlated with circulating TFTs. Unique to this study population but similar to our patient, median TSH was 0.042 mU/L (ref 0.4–4.3), median FT4 25.6 pmol/l (ref 11–25), and median TT3 1.93 nmol/l (ref 1.4–2.5), while the median rT3 was 0.53 nmol/l (ref 0.22–0.54). Based upon these assessments, athyreotic subjects with thyroid cancer on LT4 scored lower than Dutch reference for QOL, but none of the TFTs were associated with their QOL. Determinates of QOL showed a negative association with the total number of drugs used and a positive association time since diagnosis, but there was no association with either RAND-36 or ThyPRO and curation, BMI, or the presence of hypoparathyroidism [25]. Associations with general fatigue, physical fatigue, reduced motivation, and reduced physical activity as measured by the MFI were positive only for the number of drugs used. The authors concluded that higher than normal but not thyrotoxic circulating FT4 and TT3 (remained within the normal range) were not associated with QOL and those with the lowest TT3 levels did not differ when compared to the higher levels. There was no relationship between TFTs and complaints of fatigue or impaired QOL [25]. A study gleaned from the Swedish Cancer Registry study involved 279 (79% response rate) subjects with DTC (diagnosed 1995–1998), who completed a SF-36 14–17 years after their initial diagnosis. Although only 19 (7%) reported a recurrence of their DTC, 239/279 (85%) reported at least 1 thyroid-related symptom such as fatigue (77%), sleep disorder (59%), irritability(57%), and lower stress resistance (56%), being the most frequently reported. The presence of any thyroid-related symptoms or surgery/131-I symptoms resulted in lower health-related QOL [26]. Further insights into the relationship of fatigue and physical activity in hypothyroid subjects treated with thyroid hormone are evident in a similar survey of 205 (63.1% response rate) DTC survivors, ¾ of whom were women, with a mean age of 52.5 years, 6.8 years out from their initial diagnosis. These individuals were surveyed and their outpatient records were reviewed [27]. The subjects completed a Brief Fatigue Inventory (BFI) as well as an International Physical Activity Questionnaire (IPAQ-7). Based on these responses, moderate-to-severe fatigue was reported by 41.4%. Women did not report worse fatigue than in men, but individuals who were unemployed or unable to work had higher levels of fatigue ($p < 0.001$). Increased physical activity was associated with lower levels of fatigue ($p = 0.002$) [27], and as seen in the Massolt study, biochemical variables and ATA risk staging were *not* associated with complaints of fatigue [27]. Indeed it has been noted that simply the awareness of having a chronic disease results in diminished QOL in patients with hypothyroidism treated with LT4 [28].

Complaints of fatigue and lower QOL in those with various forms of hypothyroidism on LT4 have been documented for some time. In 2002 Saravanan reported on 597 LT4-treated hypothyroid patients (T4-P), 397 of whom were said to have a "normal" TSH (0.1–6.0 mU/L) in the previous 12 months, and compared their QOL to 551 non-hypothyroid controls [6]. Both groups were subjected to the *G*eneral *H*ealth *Q*uestionnaire-12 (GHQ-12) and the *T*hyroid *S*ymptom *Q*uestionnaire-12 (TSQ-12). A GHQ-12 score greater than 3 (maximum score 36) was considered caseness, and 25.6% of the normal euthyroid controls (mean score 11.39) were designated as cases. This control frequency was compared to the 34.4% of those with a normal TSH on LT4 (mean score 12.11) designated as cases; of course this resulted in a statistically significant difference

($p < 0.05$). TSQ scores were also slightly but significantly higher in the LT4-treated subjects [6]. Side-by-side comparisons in bar graph data show substantial overlap in the mean scores and designated caseness rates of both the GHQ-12 and TSQ-12 results making an objective clinical identification of those suffering from truly inadequate LT4 treatment problematic as there was obviously no way to blind results to the LT4 treatment and the inherent bias of known chronic disease. A subsequent publication from the same group on an expanded cohort of 697 LT4-treated hypothyroid patients with TSH values in a more narrow "normal" range (0.3–4.0 mIu/mL) showed a correlation with the GHQ-12 score with FT4 and the log TSH but not FT3, rT3, rT3/FT4, rT3/FT3, nor TPO antibody positivity. TSQ-12 was found to correlate with FT4, log TSH, FT3/FT4, rT3/FT4, but not FT3, rT3, FT3/rT3, nor TPO. An additional assessment of depression with the Hospital Anxiety and Depression Scale (HADS) found no correlation with any thyroid function parameter [29]. Treatment with LT4 for hypothyroidism does demonstrate a significant positive impact on QOL as documented in 10 of the 11 parameters evaluated by Nygaard et al. [30]. These investigators also found no correlation between individual TFTs and QOL measures [30] further bringing into question our patient's request for additional thyroid function testing.

Does baseline T3 predict LT4/LT3 (combination therapy as requested by the patient) success rates? In a study of 37 subjects on LT4 with persistent hypothyroid symptoms, all with normal TFTs and no comorbidities who were treated openly with LT4/LT3 (in a 17/1 ratio as per ETA [31] recommendations), each subject had TSH, FT4, TT3, and FT3I measured at baseline, 3 months, 6 months, and 12 months [32]. After adding in the LT3, the subjects were to self-classify as a responder or nonresponder. By 3 months, 70% reported feeling better and 30% reported no improvement in their symptoms, by 12 months 65% reported being better, and by now 35% did not feel improved compared to LT4 alone. Obviously this result does not objectively tell us much other than how patients will feel when trying something new that they believe in, but the fact that the thyroid function results were unknown at the time LT4/LT3 was initiated is of interest in determining the utility of checking TFTs to predict this subjective response. Neither age, BMI, baseline TSH, TT3, nor FT3 index predicted the patient-reported response to the addition of the LT3 [32]. So it would appear that our patient's request for more thyroid function testing would be unlikely to provide any useful information which would help her clinician to manage her symptoms.

A summary of the above information should in a narrow sense have us thinking that patient selection and expectations for the utility of thyroid hormone intervention go a long way in providing symptomatic relief of hypothyroid symptoms to those with actual hypothyroidism. A series of assumptions have been made in this case which have "thyroidised" this patient's symptoms and associated these symptoms with thyroid function test results that likely do not provide conclusive evidence of a thyroid etiology of her clinical presentation. A decision to initiate LT4 therapy has been made which advances us along the road to thyroid predation, creating a vision seen through a thyroid tunnel and cementing this diagnosis in the patient's mind. These circumstances are far more acceptable to the patient and apparently more easily treatable than other, more likely explanations of her complaints. She is losing her faith in the primary diagnoser and prescriber of her LT4 and has driven this otherwise objective practitioner to advance the dose of the thyroid hormone replacement to toxic levels associated with not only cardiac [8, 33–36] but also skeletal [33, 37, 38] risk for the patient. Her frustration in seeking relief from her symptoms has driven her to the Internet where she has "discovered" that she is not being managed as the experts on several non-endocrine-based websites suggest, and she pressures her PCP to request more extensive testing, which we have learned is unlikely to provide any helpful information for management of her "thyroid condition." It would appear that her PCP has succumbed to her pressure for further testing but has thankfully drawn the line and will not add LT3 or thyroid hormone extract to an already iatrogenically thyrotoxic patient.

Back to the patient one more time, at the initial visit, the endocrinologist assembles all of the relevant data and recognizes that the TSH elevations that triggered the assumption that this patient's symptoms were thyroid related are essentially within the expected range for a woman of this age. That in fact she might not be hypothyroid at all and therefore would not be expected to respond to thyroid hormone intervention [7] is perhaps not the primary message to convey to this Internet-inspired patient at the first encounter. The fact however must not be lost as it must be recognized that we are most likely involved with a case of non-thyroid-related "hypothyroidism," and the optimal end goal would be to effectively remedy this situation. At the first visit, the fact that the patient was already thyrotoxic on the LT4 is excuse enough to avoid adding LT3 or substituting extract at this visit, and a plan to decrease the current LT4 dosage to "safe" levels to avoid potential cardiac and skeletal issues was the first step. Plans for follow-up after sufficient time to allow equilibrium on the lower dose, to obtain further TFTs at that time, and to include anti-thyroid antibodies to assess the risk of potentially "real" thyroid disease underlying the initial findings are put in motion. Three months later the TSH is still suppressed, anti-thyroid antibodies are negative, and further dose reductions are planned as the patient is sleeping better now although several of her symptoms persist. The PCP is alerted to the fact that the symptoms may be *non*-thyroidal. A differential diagnosis of non-thyroidal considerations for her symptoms is offered (Table 20.1). And the endocrinologist lives happily ever after.

TABLE 20.1 Alternative physical etiologies for the nonspecific symptoms considered consistent with hypothyroidism

| Endocrine/ autoimmune | Nutritional | Lifestyle |
|---|---|---|
| Diabetes mellitus | Vitamin B12 deficient | Stressful life events |
| Adrenal insufficiency | Folate deficiency | Poor sleep pattern |
| Hypopituitarism | Vitamin D deficiency | Work exhaustion |
| Celiac disease | Iron deficiency | Alcohol excess |
| Pernicious anemia | *Metabolic* | *Others* |
| *Hematologic* | Obesity | Obstructive sleep apnea |
| Anemia | Hypercalcemia | Viral syndromes |
| Multiple myeloma | Electrolyte abnormality | Post-viral syndromes |
| *End-organ damage* | *Drugs* | Chronic fatigue syndrome |
| Chronic kidney disease | Beta-blockers | Carbon monoxide poisoning |
| Chronic liver disease | Statins | Depression/anxiety |
| Congestive heart failure | Opiates | Polymyalgia rheumatic |
|  |  | Fibromyalgia |

Modified from Okosieme et al. [39]

# References

1. Canaris GJ, Steiner JF, Ridgway EC. Do traditional symptoms of hypothyroidism correlate with biochemical disease? J Gen Intern Med. 1997;12(9):544–50.
2. Canaris GJ, Manowitz NR, Mayor GH, Ridgway EC. The Colorado thyroid disease prevalence study. Arch Intern Med. 2000;160(4):526–34.

3. Garber JR, Cobin RH, Gharib H, Hennessey JV, Klein I, Mechanick JI, Pessah-Pollack R, Singer PA, Woeber KA. Clinical practice guidelines for hypothyroidism in adults: cosponsored by the American Association of Clinical Endocrinologists and the American Thyroid Association. Thyroid. 2012;22(12):1200–35. https://doi.org/10.1089/thy.2012.0205.
4. Carle A, Pedersen IB, Knudsen N, Perrild H, Ovesen L, Andersen S, Laurberg P. Hypothyroid symptoms fail to predict thyroid insufficiency in old people: a population-based case-control study. Am J Med. 2016;129(10):1082–92. https://doi.org/10.1016/j.amjmed.2016.06.013.
5. Bould H, Panicker V, Kessler D, Durant C, Lewis G, Dayan C, Evans J. Investigation of thyroid dysfunction is more likely in patients with high psychological morbidity. Fam Pract. 2012;29(2):163–7. https://doi.org/10.1093/fampra/cmr059.
6. Saravanan P, Chau W-F, Roberts N, Vedhara K, Greenwood R, Dayan CM. Psychological well-being in patients on "adequate" doses of L-thyroxine: results of a large, controlled community-based questionaire study. Clin Endocrinol. 2002;57:577–85.
7. Pollock MA, Sturrock A, Marshall K, Davidson KM, Kelly CJG, McMahon AD, McLaren EH. Thyroxine treatment in patients with symptoms of hypothyroidism but thyroid function tests within the reference range: randomized double blind placebo controlled crossover trial. Br Med J. 2001;323(20 October):891–5.
8. Taylor PN, Iqbal A, Minassian C, Sayers A, Draman MS, Greenwood R, Hamilton W, Okosieme O, Panicker V, Thomas SL, Dayan C. Falling threshold for treatment of borderline elevated thyrotropin levels-balancing benefits and risks: evidence from a large community-based study. JAMA Intern Med. 2014;174(1):32–9. https://doi.org/10.1001/jamainternmed.2013.11312.
9. Stott DJ, Rodondi N, Kearney PM, Ford I, Westendorp RGJ, Mooijaart SP, Sattar N, Aubert CE, Aujesky D, Bauer DC, Baumgartner C, Blum MR, Browne JP, Byrne S, Collet TH, Dekkers OM, den Elzen WPJ, Du Puy RS, Ellis G, Feller M, Floriani C, Hendry K, Hurley C, Jukema JW, Kean S, Kelly M, Krebs D, Langhorne P, McCarthy G, McCarthy V, McConnachie A, McDade M, Messow M, O'Flynn A, O'Riordan D, Poortvliet RKE, Quinn TJ, Russell A, Sinnott C, Smit JWA, Van Dorland HA, Walsh KA, Walsh EK, Watt T, Wilson R, Gussekloo J. Thyroid hormone therapy for older adults with subclinical hypothyroidism. N Engl J Med. 2017;376(26):2534–44. https://doi.org/10.1056/NEJMoa1603825.

10. Somwaru LL, Rariy CM, Arnold AM, Cappola AR. The natural history of subclinical hypothyroidism in the elderly: the cardiovascular health study. J Clin Endocrinol Metab. 2012;97(6):1962–9. https://doi.org/10.1210/jc.2011-3047.
11. Vanderpump MPJ, Tunbridge WMG, French JM, Appleton D, Bates D, Clark F, Grimley Evans J, Hasan DM, Rodgers H, Tunbridge F, Young ET. The incidence of thyroid disorders in the community: a twenty-year follow-up of the Whickham Survey. Clin Endocrinol. 1995;43:55–68.
12. Baloch Z, Carayon P, Conte-Devolx B, Demers LM, Feldt-Rasmussen U, Henry JF, LiVosli VA, Niccoli-Sire P, John R, Ruf J, Smyth PP, Spencer CA, Stockigt JR. Laboratory medicine practice guidelines. Laboratory support for the diagnosis and monitoring of thyroid disease. Thyroid. 2003;13(1):3–126. https://doi.org/10.1089/105072503321086962.
13. Hollowell JG, Staehling NW, Flanders WD, Hannon WH, Gunter EW, Spencer CA. Serum TSH, T4, and thyroid antibodies in the United States population(1988 to 1994): National Health and Nutrition Survey (NHANES III). J Clin Endocrinol Metab. 2002;87:489–99.
14. Surks MI, Hollowell JG. Age-specific distribution of serum thyrotropin and antithyroid antibodies in the US population: implications for the prevalence of subclinical hypothyroidism. J Clin Endocrinol Metab. 2007). doi:jc.2007-1499 [pii];92(12):4575–82. https://doi.org/10.1210/jc.2007-1499.
15. Ehrenkranz J, Bach PR, Snow GL, Schneider A, Lee JL, Ilstrup S, Bennett ST, Benvenga S. Circadian and circannual rhythms in thyroid hormones: determining the TSH and free T4 reference intervals based upon time of day, age, and sex. Thyroid. 2015;25(8):954–61. https://doi.org/10.1089/thy.2014.0589.
16. Bremner AP, Feddema P, Leedman PJ, Brown SJ, Beilby JP, Lim EM, Wilson SG, O'Leary PC, Walsh JP. Age-related changes in thyroid function: a longitudinal study of a community-based cohort. J Clin Endocrinol Metab. 2012;97(5):1554–62. https://doi.org/10.1210/jc.2011-3020.
17. Fontes R, Coeli CR, Aguiar F, Vaisman M. Reference interval of thyroid stimulating hormone and free thyroxine in a reference population over 60 years old and in very old subjects (over 80 years): comparison to young subjects. Thyroid Res. 2013;6(1):13. https://doi.org/10.1186/1756-6614-6-13. 1756-6614-6-13 [pii].
18. Waring AC, Arnold AM, Newman AB, Buzkova P, Hirsch C, Cappola AR. Longitudinal changes in thyroid function in the

oldest old and survival: the cardiovascular health study all-stars study. J Clin Endocrinol Metab. 2012;97(11):3944–50. https://doi.org/10.1210/jc.2012-2481.
19. Konno N. Comparison between the thyrotropin response to thyrotropin-releasing hormone in summer and that in winter in normal subjects. Endocrinol Jpn. 1978;25(6):635–9.
20. Kim TH, Kim KW, Ahn HY, Choi HS, Won H, Choi Y, Cho SW, Moon JH, Yi KH, Park DJ, Park KS, Jang HC, Kim SY, Park YJ. Effect of seasonal changes on the transition between subclinical hypothyroid and euthyroid status. J Clin Endocrinol Metab. 2013;98(8):3420–9. https://doi.org/10.1210/jc.2013-1607.jc.2013-1607 [pii].
21. Konno N, Morikawa K. Seasonal variation of serum thyrotropin concentration and thyrotropin response to thyrotropin-releasing hormone in patients with primary hypothyroidism on constant replacement dosage of thyroxine. J Clin Endocrinol Metab. 1982;54(6):1118–24. https://doi.org/10.1210/jcem-54-6-1118.
22. Gullo D, Latina A, Frasca F, Squatrito S, Belfiore A, Vigneri R. Seasonal variations in TSH serum levels in athyreotic patients under L-thyroxine replacement monotherapy. Clin Endocrinol. 2017;87(2):207–15. https://doi.org/10.1111/cen.13351.
23. Catli G, Anik A, Unver Tuhan H, Bober E, Abaci A. The effect of L-thyroxine treatment on hypothyroid symptom scores and lipid profile in children with subclinical hypothyroidism. J Clin Res Pediatr Endocrinol. 2014;6(4):238–44. https://doi.org/10.4274/Jcrpe.1594.
24. Stott DJ, Rodondi N, Bauer DC. Thyroid hormone therapy for older adults with subclinical hypothyroidism. N Engl J Med. 2017;377(14):e20. https://doi.org/10.1056/NEJMc1709989.
25. Massolt ET, van der Windt M, Korevaar TI, Kam BL, Burger JW, Franssen GJ, Lehmphul I, Kohrle J, Visser WE, Peeters RP. Thyroid hormone and its metabolites in relation to quality of life in patients treated for differentiated thyroid Cancer. Clin Endocrinol. 2016;85:781. https://doi.org/10.1111/cen.13101.
26. Hedman C, Djarv T, Strang P, Lundgren CI. Effect of thyroid-related symptoms on long-term quality of life in patients with differentiated thyroid carcinoma: a population-based study in Sweden. Thyroid. 2017;27(8):1034–42. https://doi.org/10.1089/thy.2016.0604.
27. Alhashemi A, Jones JM, Goldstein DP, Mina DS, Thabane L, Sabiston CM, Chang EK, Brierley JD, Sawka AM. An exploratory study of fatigue and physical activity in Canadian

thyroid cancer patients. Thyroid. 2017;27(9):1156–63. https://doi.org/10.1089/thy.2016.0541. 10.1089/thy.2016.0541 [pii]
28. Ladenson PW. Psychological wellbeing in patients. Clin Endocrinol. 2002;57(5):575–6. doi:1682 [pii]
29. Saravanan P, Visser TJ, Dayan CM. Psychological well-being correlates with free thyroxine but not free 3,5,3′-triiodothyronine levels in patients on thyroid hormone replacement. J Clin Endocrinol Metab. 2006;91(9):3389–93. jc.2006-0414 [pii] 10.1210/jc.2006-0414.
30. Nygaard B, Jensen EW, Kvetny J, Jarlov A, Faber J. Effect of combination therapy with thyroxine (T4) and 3,5,3′-triiodothyronine versus T4 monotherapy in patients with hypothyroidism, a double-blind, randomised cross-over study. Eur J Endocrinol. 2009;161(6):895–902. https://doi.org/10.1530/EJE-09-0542. EJE-09-0542 [pii].
31. Wiersinga WM, Duntas L, Fadeyev V, Nygaard B, Vanderpump MP. 2012 ETA guidelines: the use of L-T4 + L-T3 in the treatment of hypothyroidism. Eur Thyroid J. 2012;1(2):55–71. https://doi.org/10.1159/000339444. etj-0001-0055 [pii].
32. Medici BB, la Cour JL, Michaelsson LF, Faber JO, Nygaard B. Neither baseline nor changes in serum triiodothyronine during levothyroxine/Liothyronine combination therapy predict a positive response to this treatment modality in hypothyroid patients with persistent symptoms. Eur Thyroid J. 2017;6(2):89–93. https://doi.org/10.1159/000454878. etj-0006-0089 [pii].
33. Flynn RW, Bonellie SR, Jung RT, MacDonald TM, Morris AD, Leese GP. Serum thyroid-stimulating hormone concentration and morbidity from cardiovascular disease and fractures in patients on long-term thyroxine therapy. J Clin Endocrinol Metab. 2010;95(1):186–93. https://doi.org/10.1210/jc.2009-1625. jc.2009-1625 [pii].
34. Mammen JS, McGready J, Oxman R, Chia CW, Ladenson PW, Simonsick EM. Thyroid hormone therapy and risk of thyrotoxicosis in community-resident older adults: findings from the Baltimore longitudinal study of aging. Thyroid. 2015;25(9):979–86. https://doi.org/10.1089/thy.2015.0180.
35. Sawin CT, Geller A, Wolf PA, Belanger AJ, Baker E, Bacharach P, Wilson PWF, Benjamin EJ, D'Agostino RB. Low serum thyrotropin concentrations as a risk factor for atrial fibrillation in older persons. N Engl J Med. 1994;331:1249–52.

36. Cappola AR, Fried LP, Arnold AM, Danese MD, Kuller LH, Burke GL, Tracey RP, Ladenson PW. Thyroid status, cardiovascular risk, and mortality in older adults. JAMA. 2006;295(9):1033–41.
37. Bauer DC, Ettinger B, Nevitt MC, Stone KL. Group, S.o.O.F.R.: risk for fracture in women with low levels of thyroid-stimulating hormone. Ann Intern Med. 2001;134(7):561–8.
38. Blum MR, Bauer DC, Collet TH, Fink HA, Cappola AR, da Costa BR, Wirth CD, Peeters RP, Asvold BO, den Elzen WP, Luben RN, Imaizumi M, Bremner AP, Gogakos A, Eastell R, Kearney PM, Strotmeyer ES, Wallace ER, Hoff M, Ceresini G, Rivadeneira F, Uitterlinden AG, Stott DJ, Westendorp RG, Khaw KT, Langhammer A, Ferrucci L, Gussekloo J, Williams GR, Walsh JP, Juni P, Aujesky D, Rodondi N. Subclinical thyroid dysfunction and fracture risk: a meta-analysis. JAMA. 2015;313(20):2055–65. https://doi.org/10.1001/jama.2015.5161.
39. Okosieme O, Gilbert J, Abraham P, Boelaert K, Dayan C, Gurnell M, Leese G, McCabe C, Perros P, Smith V, Williams G, Vanderpump M. Management of primary hypothyroidism: statement by the British Thyroid Association Executive Committee. Clin Endocrinol. 2016;84(6):799–808. https://doi.org/10.1111/cen.12824.

# Chapter 21
# Wilson's Syndrome (Low T3 Syndrome)

Catherine J. Tang and Jeffrey R. Garber

## Case Description

A 48-year-old woman with asthma and hypertension presents with fatigue and insomnia. She reports that her energy level has gradually declined since the birth of her first child 10 years ago but has gotten progressively worse in the last year. She is having more trouble focusing than before, and although she is still working full time, she struggles to get through her day. In addition, she has difficulty falling and staying asleep. She goes to bed around 11 PM to midnight

C. J. Tang (✉)
Division of Endocrinology, Diabetes, and Metabolism, Harvard Medical School, Beth Israel Deaconess Medical Center,
Boston, MA, USA
e-mail: ctang@bidmc.harvard.edu

J. R. Garber
Division of Endocrinology, Diabetes, and Metabolism, Harvard Medical School, Beth Israel Deaconess Medical Center,
Boston, MA, USA

Atrius Health, Boston, MA, USA

© Springer Nature Switzerland AG 2019
M. T. McDermott (ed.), *Management of Patients with Pseudo-Endocrine Disorders*,
https://doi.org/10.1007/978-3-030-22720-3_21

and wakes up at 6 AM. She snores but denies choking or gasping for air at night. She does not feel refreshed in the morning and occasionally feels sleepy during the day. She was evaluated by her primary care physician who found no abnormalities on her physical examination or laboratory tests, including a normal complete blood count, electrolytes, and serum thyroid-stimulating hormone (TSH).

A co-worker has recommended the patient to look into "Wilson's syndrome." Upon reading about it on the Internet, she believes that many of her symptoms overlap with what is described for Wilson's syndrome. She is here now to be evaluated for Wilson's syndrome and for its treatment.

Review of systems is positive for weight gain of 10 pounds in the last 5 years, increased hair loss, dry skin, intermittent nausea, and occasional dizziness. All other review of systems is otherwise reviewed and negative. A thorough physical examination is unremarkable.

# "Wilson's Syndrome" (Also Known as "Low T3 Syndrome")

E. Denis Wilson MD first coined "Wilson's syndrome" or "Wilson's temperature syndrome" after himself in 1990 to describe a constellation of common and nonspecific symptoms including, but not limited to, fatigue, chilliness, constipation, weight gain, dry skin, swelling, joint pains, hair loss, brittle nails, insomnia, depression, and anxiety. The diagnosis is made by any combination of these symptoms, normal thyroid hormone levels in the bloodstream, and oral temperatures consistently averaging below 98.2 °F.

Dr. Wilson postulated that these common symptoms, which also often overlap with those of hypothyroidism, are due to low levels of circulating triiodothyronine (T3). Thus, the hallmark of "Wilson's syndrome" is T3 levels that are below the reference range. Hence, this has also been called the "low T3 syndrome." He suggested that under severe stress, the body converts less thyroxine (T4) to T3, hypothetically resulting in lower T3 levels despite normal serum TSH levels. In turn, the low T3 levels slow down metabolism and lower the body temperature, which manifests as various symptoms as previously mentioned. As such, Dr. Wilson started treating his patients with thyroid hormones (both T3 and T4) despite their normal serum thyroid function tests (TFTs), and the symptoms reportedly all resolved upon treatment. On Dr. Wilson's website, he describes several successful anecdotes, including his wife, who had benefited from this treatment strategy [1]. Moreover, Dr. Wilson advocates treatment with herbal supplements and co-founded an herbal supplement company with a naturopathic practitioner to provide these herbs [1]. It is worthwhile to note that Dr. Wilson is no longer a practicing physician, as his Florida license had been suspended since the 1990s and he was ordered by the Florida Board of Medicine to undergo psychological testing [2].

# Molecular Action of Thyroid Hormone

## Intracellular Regulation of Thyroid Hormone

The thyroid gland is a vital endocrine organ in the human body. It produces thyroxine (T4), a prohormone, and its active form triiodothyronine (T3). Thyroid hormone (TH) acts on nearly every tissue in the body and regulates essential metabolic pathways, including energy balance, thermogenesis, normal growth, and development [3–5]. Under normal physiologic conditions, the vast majority of TH produced by the thyroid gland is T4, which is then converted to the more potent T3 in peripheral tissues in a highly regulated process, mediated by tissue-specific deiodinase enzymes and transmembrane transporters [3]. Type I deiodinase (D1) is primarily expressed in the liver and kidney, whereas type II deiodinase (D2) is mainly found in the pituitary, hypothalamus, white adipose tissue, brown adipose tissue, and skeletal muscle. D1 and D2 are both expressed in the thyroid. Whereas D1 and D2 convert T4 to T3, type III deiodinase

(D3) converts T4 and T3 to reverse T3 (RT3) and diiodothyronine (T2), respectively; RT3 and D2 are inactive forms of T3. D3 is highly expressed in the placenta, vascular tissue, and skin [4]. D3 is activated by hypoxia, and its expression in the placenta may protect the fetus from maternal hyperthyroidism [4, 6].

Animal knockout models have demonstrated that D1 is not essential for TH action [7]. In humans, D2 is the primary generator of serum and intracellular T3; the activity of D2 is increased by low levels of T4 and adrenergic activation [4]. Polymorphisms in the D2 gene have been linked with type 2 diabetes and obesity [8]. Additionally, one study has shown that hypothyroid patients with a specific D2 gene polymorphism (Thr92Ala) experienced improvement in symptoms when they were treated with combined T4/T3 therapy as compared to T4 monotherapy to achieve normal TSH levels [9].

In addition to deiodinase enzymes, intracellular levels of T3 are also regulated by cell surface transporters including monocarboxylate and organic ion transporter families [3, 4]. Notably, mutations in the monocarboxylate transporter 8 (MCT8) gene cause a severe neurological disorder called Allan-Herndon-Dudley syndrome. The MCT8 gene is encoded on the X-chromosome and is highly expressed in the brain and hypothalamus. Affected males have severe neurological abnormalities, including developmental delay, low IQ, dystonia, and progression to quadriplegia [4, 10].

## *Mechanism of Thyroid Hormone Action*

There are four thyroid hormone receptor (TR) isoforms, TRα1, TRα2, TRβ1, and TRβ2, which are alternatively spliced products of *TRA* and *TRB* genes, respectively. Only three of these are biologically active: TRα1, TRβ1, and TRβ2. In contrast, TRα2 lacks a T3-binding domain, rendering it unable to bind T3; its role is, therefore, not well understood [4]. The TRα1 and TRα2 genes are located on chromosome 17, and the

TRβ1 and TRβ2 genes are located on chromosome 3. They share a similar molecular structure, with an N-terminal activation domain, a DNA-binding domain, and a C-terminal ligand-binding domain. Like the deiodinase enzymes, TRs are also tissue-specific. TRα1 is primarily expressed in the heart, bone, and small intestines. TRβ1 is highly expressed in the liver, kidney, and inner ear. TRβ2 is preferentially expressed in the brain, hypothalamus, pituitary, and retina [3–5, 11]. The functional role of each TR isoform appears to be dictated by its tissue-specific expression as shown by multiple mouse models where individual receptor isoforms have been knocked out [4, 11, 12].

The primary mechanism of TH action is via gene transcription. The TR and the retinoid X receptor (RXR) form heterodimers that bind to thyroid hormone response elements (TRE) in the promoter regions of target genes. In the absence of T3, TR binds to corepressor proteins that silence target gene expression. Upon ligand (T3) binding, corepressors dissociate from TR, and coactivator proteins are recruited in order to activate gene transcription [3–5, 12]. In more recent years, there has been increasing recognition that TH also exerts nongenomic actions, such as altering the phosphorylation of protein kinases and interacting with integrin receptors that activate downstream pathways [4]. In addition, T3 exerts several nongenomic actions on the cardiovascular system, including reducing systemic vascular resistance and modulating the cardiac myocyte membrane ion channels [13].

The actions of the various TR isoforms depend on their structure and their tissue of expression. This has been extensively studied in animal models with various isoform mutations and is underscored by the clinical syndrome of resistance to thyroid hormone (RTH syndromes). Refetoff et al. reported the first case of RTH, now known as RTH β, in 1967 [14]; the case was eventually shown to be due to a mutation in the ligand-binding domain of TRβ such that the receptor had reduced T3-binding affinity and the binding of T3 did not promote the dissociation of transcriptional corepressors [4]. Biochemical studies in TRH patients often show a normal serum TSH level but with elevated serum T3 and T4 levels. Patients may present with a goiter but are generally euthyroid, except for having tachycardia and sometimes delayed bone age. These symptoms are due to the unopposed action of TH on predominantly TRα-expressing tissues, including the heart and bone [4]. More recently, Bochukova et al. reported the first case of RTH α in 2012; the affected 6-year-old girl presented with developmental delay, short stature, delayed tooth eruption, and severe constipation and was found to have a mutation in the TRα gene [15]. Biochemical studies in the few reported cases have demonstrated normal serum TSH levels, low or low-normal T4 levels, and high or high-normal T3 concentrations. TSH remains normal because regulation of the hypothalamic-pituitary axis is mediated by TRβ, which remains functional. Therefore the TH feedback is normal, and there is no compensatory increase in T3 and T4, consistent with the phenotype of hypothyroidism [4, 15].

## Use of T3 in Hypothyroidism

There are many causes of low serum T3 levels, but there has not been conclusive evidence that T3 therapy is indicated in most of them (Table 21.1). As mentioned in the earlier section, there is evidence that hypothyroid patients with a specific D2 gene polymorphism (Thr92Ala) experienced improved symptoms when they were treated with combined T4 and T3 therapy as compared to T4 monotherapy to achieve normal TSH levels, suggesting that this polymorphism may cause a defect in peripheral or brain T4 to T3 conversion [9]. Another study of 140 thyroidectomized patients on levothyroxine (LT4) monotherapy found that those with the Thr92Ala D2 polymorphism had significantly reduced serum free T3 (FT3) levels as compared to those without the polymorphism (whose FT3 levels were similar to pre-surgery levels) [16]. Similarly, in vivo studies in muscle cells and pituitary cells have demonstrated that mutant D2 is less efficient in converting T4 to T3 [16]. Note that these

TABLE 21.1 Causes of relatively low serum T3 levels and the role of T3 therapy

| Condition | TSH | T4 | T3 | Clinical presentation | Role of T3 Rx |
|---|---|---|---|---|---|
| Levothyroxine treatment for hypothyroidism | Normal | Normal or ↑ | Normal or ↓ | Most patients show symptom improvement, but a small percentage may have ongoing hypothyroid symptoms despite normal TSH level | Generally not indicated due to lack of conclusive data [20] |
| Sick euthyroid syndrome | Normal or ↓ | Normal or ↓ | ↓ Mildly, moderately, or severely (depending on the severity of the illness) | Most patients have an acute or chronic non-thyroidal illness Commonly seen in hospitalized patients Usually transient Lower T3 is potentially protective during illnesses. | Neither T4 or T3 has shown to be helpful and may even be harmful [38] |

(continued)

Table 21.1 (continued)

| Condition | TSH | T4 | T3 | Clinical presentation | Role of T3 Rx |
|---|---|---|---|---|---|
| Thyroid binding globulin (TBG) deficiency | Normal | ↓ Or normal | ↓ Or normal | Causes of TBG deficiency include familial (X-linked), hyperandrogenism (anabolic steroid abuse), glucocorticoid excess, malnutrition, nephrotic syndrome, and drug-induced Patients are generally euthyroid, and the free T4 and free T3 levels are normal | Not indicated |
| D2 gene polymorphism | Normal | Normal (if hypothyroid and treated with T4 therapy) | Normal or ↓ (if hypothyroid and treated with T4 therapy) | Most commonly reported D2 polymorphism is Thr92Ala. Note that euthyroid patients with D2 polymorphisms have normal serum T4 and T3 levels | May benefit from combined T4 and T3 therapy [9] but not applicable in the clinical setting yet. No commercial testing is available |

| | | | | |
|---|---|---|---|---|
| RTH α | Normal | ↓ Or normal | ↑ Or normal | Very rare, mostly case reports. Intellectual disability, developmental delay, short stature, delayed tooth eruption, constipation, bradycardia, anemia, abnormal bone development | In children, T4 therapy may improve bone development, growth, and intellectual ability In adults, T4 therapy can improve constipation |
| RTH β | ↑ Or normal | ↑ Or normal | ↑ Or normal | Incidence is 1 in 40,000. Can be euthyroid or have a goiter, tachycardia, hyperactivity, delayed bone age, and intellectual disability. | Triiodothyroacetic acid (Triac), a T3 analog, is used in some cases to lower TSH and TH levels. It works by having a higher affinity for TRβ than for TRα Cardiac symptoms can be treated with a beta-blocker |

Abbreviations: *T4* thyroxine, *T3* triiodothyronine

studies were done in hypothyroid patients with the Thr92Ala polymorphism. In contrast, euthyroid patients with D2 gene polymorphisms have similar thyroid hormone levels as other euthyroid patients without the polymorphism [17].

Furthermore, a clinical study of 1811 Italian athyreotic patients on LT4 monotherapy reported that 7.2% had significantly higher free T4 (FT4) levels and 15.2% had significantly lower FT3 levels as compared to matched euthyroid controls who were not thyroidectomized [18]. A limitation of this study was that the athyreotic patients all had a history of thyroid cancer and it is not clear how the physiology may differ from patients without this history. Peterson et al. confirmed these findings in a cross-sectional study of the US National Health and Nutrition Examination Survey (NHANES) data. Here they found that patients whose serum TSH levels were normal on LT4 therapy had 15–20% lower serum total and free T3/T4 ratios as compared to matched controls, raising the question of whether many LT4 treated patients with normal TSH levels are truly euthyroid [19]. They also found that in patients on LT4 therapy, lower T3 levels were associated with older age and lower calorie consumption (<1000 calories per day), possibly because of reduced muscle mass with older age (D2 is expressed in skeletal muscle) and reduced levels of insulin (which stimulates T3 production) [19].

Despite the molecular evidence of the effects of D2 polymorphisms on intracellular T3 levels, there is insufficient data on the clinical application of this information [20]. First, there is no commercially available assay to detect D2 polymorphisms. In addition, there is no clear evidence that D2 gene polymorphisms are associated with negative clinical outcomes [21] or with alterations of circulating thyroid hormone levels [9]. Nonetheless, larger and well-powered studies are still needed to investigate the role of D2-Thr92Ala in regulating thyroid parameters and clinical consequences. Moreover, in their review of 13 randomized-controlled trials and 4 systemic reviews or meta-analyses, the American Thyroid Association (ATA) concluded that there is no consistent evidence that combination T4 and T3 therapy is superior to T4 alone in patients with primary hypothyroidism either as the initial therapy or in those who continue to feel unwell on T4 monotherapy [20]. Importantly, there is no long-term data on the efficacy or safety of liothyronine (LT3) as monotherapy and its use are hampered by the peaks and troughs after its administration owing to its short half-life [20].

A key component of "Wilson's syndrome" is a low body temperature. However, studies have shown that our body temperatures actually fluctuate throughout the day, dispelling the notion that 98.6 °F is the only "normal" body temperature [22]. Moreover, while lower T3 levels have been associated with acute or chronic illnesses, including psychiatric disorders, no research has definitively shown that T3 therapy can improve or restore wellness. It is worthwhile to mention that TH has been used as an adjunct treatment for psychiatric disorders, including depression and bipolar disorder, since there is some evidence that it may hasten the rate of treatment response and improve the quality of the response in patients with clinical or subclinical hypothyroidism [23]. The evidence for patients with hypothyroid symptoms but normal TFTs is less clear [23].

Furthermore, the reported success of T3 treatment for "Wilson's syndrome" is entirely anecdotal and has never been submitted to rigorous research or published in peer-reviewed journals. In addition, Dr. Wilson advocates using herbal supplements, which are not FDA-regulated, and their ingredients cannot be verified. In fact, because the intracellular conversion of T4 to T3 is tightly regulated, giving excessive T3 may actually cause harm, including symptoms of thyrotoxicosis such as palpitations, worsening anxiety, night sweats, transaminitis, and heart failure, due to significant peaks after its administration.

In summary, "Wilson's syndrome" is not an evidence-based diagnosis and is not accepted by the medical community. In its public health statement, the ATA strongly refuted the notion of "Wilson's syndrome" due to its lack of scientific evidence and its contradiction of our current knowledge of

TH synthesis, metabolism, and action [24]. The Mayo Clinic similarly refutes the existence of this diagnosis [25]. LT4 monotherapy remains the first-line treatment for primary hypothyroidism. There is no conclusive evidence that combination therapy with LT4 and LT3 is superior to LT4 alone, and there is no long-term data on the safety of LT3 monotherapy.

## Evaluation and Management of this Case

Nonspecific complaints are common in the endocrinology practice, and sometimes patients may present with multiple nonspecific complaints that appear to be unrelated. The patients have often struggled with these symptoms for quite some time (generally months and years) before seeking medical attention and come to the endocrinology office after a normal evaluation by their primary care providers and occasionally other specialists. While it can be confusing at times to find a common thread among the many complaints, it is crucial not to dismiss them as these patients frequently are already frustrated with not getting the answers they were hoping for from the previous providers. The key is to listen carefully, show empathy, and complete an evaluation that is appropriate to the level and severity of their complaints. This case demonstrates the key components of this type of evaluation.

However, these symptoms are real and can cause significant suffering and functional disability in affected people. While many of these symptoms overlap with those of hypothyroidism, they are also commonly found in the general population. One study reported that 60% of participants with normal serum TSH levels had at least one hypothyroid symptom and 15% had four or more hypothyroid symptoms. In contrast, 70% of participants with elevated TSH levels had at least one hypothyroid symptom, and 25% had four or more hypothyroid symptoms [26]. Indeed, none of the individual hypothyroid symptoms were sensitive in patients with elevated TSH levels, with the highest sensitivity of 28% for drier skin and the lowest sensitivity of 3% for deeper voice [26].

In this case, checking a serum TSH level is indicated. Unless there is a suspicion for a pituitary etiology of the patient's symptoms, generally a TSH alone is sufficient, without the need for additional thyroid function tests such as T4 and T3 levels. Generally, checking a T3 level is not helpful in making a diagnosis of hypothyroidism as T3 levels can be decreased during or following an acute illness or with comorbid conditions including aging. In addition, the T3 immunoassays are less accurate in the lower end of the assay range [27]. Furthermore, no studies have shown that patients with normal TSH values and relatively low T3 levels have negative consequences [28]. If her TSH is elevated, then therapy should be considered. According to the current ATA guidelines [20], LT4 is the preferred therapy for hypothyroidism because it mimics the body's physiologic way of providing thyroid hormone to the cells (provision of T4 as a prohormone allowing tissues specific conversion of T4 to T3, as discussed in detail in a prior section). Although the use of LT3 is not recommended for routine use in treating primary hypothyroidism, as was previously discussed, it may be considered in selected patients as an adjunct to LT4 [9, 29]. However, it is important to note that several systemic reviews and meta-analyses concluded that LT4/LT3 combination therapy is not superior to LT4 monotherapy [30–33]. Clinical judgment must be exercised with prudence; physicians should discuss its' controversial use with the patients, including its' risks, and if both agree to proceed with combination LT4/LT3, caution must be taken to avoid excessive T3 treatment.

In addition, one may also check an 8 AM serum cortisol to screen for adrenal insufficiency if the suspicion is moderate to high. This patient has significant fatigue with some GI symptoms (nausea), so it may be reasonable to assess for other etiologies such as irritable bowel syndrome, gastroesophageal reflux disease, and celiac disease. In the presence of vomiting, dizziness, weight loss, and muscle weakness, adrenal insufficiency should also be assessed.

If these initial tests are normal, we should consider non-endocrine causes for her symptoms. For instance, she exhibits some symptoms associated with sleep apnea, including not feeling refreshed in the morning and daytime sleepiness. Sleep apnea is a common but underdiagnosed disorder that can cause fatigue, and thus a sleep study is indicated in this case [34]. If she proves to have comorbid conditions such as the gastrointestinal or other disorders noted above, their management should be optimized first. Furthermore, the timing of her fatigue coincides with the birth of her first child, and it may be worth exploring the psychosocial aspects of her life, including her mental health, social support, work, and personal life. This is best done with her primary care physician and mental health providers, particularly if she seems overwhelmed, anxious, or depressed. Finally, although this case did not provide enough information on her reproductive history, she may be approaching menopause and having its associated symptoms, so it is worth obtaining additional history.

If the evaluation is unremarkable, provide reassurance to the patient, and always show empathy. Often the symptoms are multifactorial and do not require medical intervention. It is reasonable to discuss alternative approaches that other patients have found helpful, including cognitive behavioral therapy, exercise, acupuncture, and tai chi [35–37]. The support that we demonstrate to these patients can go a long way.

# References

1. Wilson ED. Wilson's temperature syndrome. 2018. https://www.quackwatch.org/04ConsumerEducation/News/wilson.html.
2. Barrett S. Government actions against Richard A. Marschall, N.D. 2018. https://www.quackwatch.org/04ConsumerEducation/News/wilson.html.
3. Astapova I. Role of co-regulators in metabolic and transcriptional actions of thyroid hormone. J Mol Endocrinol. 2016;56(3):73–97.

4. Mullur R, Liu YY, Brent GA. Thyroid hormone regulation of metabolism. Physiol Rev. 2014;94(2):355–82.
5. Ramadoss P, Abraham BJ, Tsai L, Zhou Y, Costa-e-Sousa RH, Ye F, et al. Novel mechanism of positive versus negative regulation by thyroid hormone receptor beta1 (TRbeta1) identified by genome-wide profiling of binding sites in mouse liver. J Biol Chem. 2014;289(3):1313–28.
6. Simonides WS, Mulcahey MA, Redout EM, Muller A, Zuidwijk MJ, Visser TJ, et al. Hypoxia-inducible factor induces local thyroid hormone inactivation during hypoxic-ischemic disease in rats. J Clin Invest. 2008;118(3):975–83.
7. Schneider MJ, Fiering SN, Thai B, Wu SY, St Germain E, Parlow AF, et al. Targeted disruption of the type 1 selenodeiodinase gene (Dio1) results in marked changes in thyroid hormone economy in mice. Endocrinology. 2006;147(1):580–9.
8. Estivalet AA, Leiria LB, Dora JM, Rheinheimer J, Boucas AP, Maia AL, et al. D2 Thr92Ala and PPARgamma2 Pro12Ala polymorphisms interact in the modulation of insulin resistance in type 2 diabetic patients. Obesity (Silver Spring). 2011;19(4):825–32.
9. Panicker V, Saravanan P, Vaidya B, Evans J, Hattersley AT, Frayling TM, et al. Common variation in the DIO2 gene predicts baseline psychological well-being and response to combination thyroxine plus triiodothyronine therapy in hypothyroid patients. J Clin Endocrinol Metab. 2009;94(5):1623–9.
10. Hollenberg AN. The endocrine society centennial: the thyroid leads the way. Endocrinology. 2016;157(1):1–3.
11. Mendoza A, Astapova I, Shimizu H, Gallop MR, Al-Sowaimel L, MacGowan SMD, et al. NCoR1-independent mechanism plays a role in the action of the unliganded thyroid hormone receptor. Proc Natl Acad Sci U S A. 2017;114(40):E8458–E67.
12. Mendoza A, Hollenberg AN. New insights into thyroid hormone action. Pharmacol Ther. 2017;173:135–45.
13. Klein I, Danzi S. Thyroid disease and the heart. Curr Probl Cardiol. 2016;41(2):65–92.
14. Refetoff S, DeWind LT, DeGroot LJ. Familial syndrome combining deaf-mutism, stuppled epiphyses, goiter and abnormally high PBI: possible target organ refractoriness to thyroid hormone. J Clin Endocrinol Metab. 1967;27(2):279–94.
15. Bochukova E, Schoenmakers N, Agostini M, Schoenmakers E, Rajanayagam O, Keogh JM, et al. A mutation in the thyroid hormone receptor alpha gene. N Engl J Med. 2012;366(3):243–9.

16. Castagna MG, Dentice M, Cantara S, Ambrosio R, Maino F, Porcelli T, et al. DIO2 Thr92Ala reduces deiodinase-2 activity and serum-T3 levels in thyroid-deficient patients. J Clin Endocrinol Metab. 2017;102(5):1623–30.
17. Butler PW, Smith SM, Linderman JD, Brychta RJ, Alberobello AT, Dubaz OM, et al. The Thr92Ala 5′ type 2 deiodinase gene polymorphism is associated with a delayed triiodothyronine secretion in response to the thyrotropin-releasing hormone-stimulation test: a pharmacogenomic study. Thyroid. 2010;20(12):1407–12.
18. Gullo D, Latina A, Frasca F, Le Moli R, Pellegriti G, Vigneri R. Levothyroxine monotherapy cannot guarantee euthyroidism in all athyreotic patients. PLoS One. 2011;6(8):e22552.
19. Peterson SJ, McAninch EA, Bianco AC. Is a normal TSH synonymous with "Euthyroidism" in levothyroxine monotherapy? J Clin Endocrinol Metab. 2016;101(12):4964–73.
20. Jonklaas J, Bianco AC, Bauer AJ, Burman KD, Cappola AR, Celi FS, et al. Guidelines for the treatment of hypothyroidism: prepared by the american thyroid association task force on thyroid hormone replacement. Thyroid. 2014;24(12):1670–751.
21. Wouters HJ, van Loon HC, van der Klauw MM, Elderson MF, Slagter SN, Kobold AM, et al. No effect of the Thr92Ala polymorphism of deiodinase-2 on thyroid hormone parameters, health-related quality of life, and cognitive functioning in a large population-based cohort study. Thyroid. 2017;27(2):147–55.
22. Mackowiak PA, Wasserman SS, Levine MM. A critical appraisal of 98.6 degrees F, the upper limit of the normal body temperature, and other legacies of Carl Reinhold August Wunderlich. JAMA. 1992;268(12):1578–80.
23. Kalra S, Balhara YP. Euthyroid depression: the role of thyroid hormone. Recent Pat Endocr Metab Immune Drug Discov. 2014;8(1):38–41.
24. American Thyroid Association Statement on "Wilson's Syndrome". 2005. https://www.thyroid.org/american-thyroid-association-statement-on-wilsons-syndrome/.
25. Nippoldt T. Is Wilson's syndrome a legitimate ailment? 2018. https://www.mayoclinic.org/diseases-conditions/hypothyroidism/expert-answers/wilsons-syndrome/faq-20058414.
26. Canaris GJ, Manowitz NR, Mayor G, Ridgway EC. The Colorado thyroid disease prevalence study. Arch Intern Med. 2000;160(4):526–34.

27. Soukhova N, Soldin OP, Soldin SJ. Isotope dilution tandem mass spectrometric method for T4/T3. Clin Chim Acta. 2004;343(1–2):185–90.
28. Jonklaas J, Bianco AC, Bauer AJ, Burman KD, Cappola AR, Celi FS, et al. Guidelines for the treatment of hypothyroidism: prepared by the american thyroid association task force on thyroid hormone replacement. Thyroid. 2014;24(12):1701.
29. Kim BW, Bianco AC. For some, L-thyroxine replacement might not be enough: a genetic rationale. J Clin Endocrinol Metab. 2009;94(5):1521–3.
30. Escobar-Morreale HF, Botella-Carretero JI, Escobar del Rey F, Morreale de Escobar G. REVIEW: treatment of hypothyroidism with combinations of levothyroxine plus liothyronine. J Clin Endocrinol Metab. 2005;90(8):4946–54.
31. Grozinsky-Glasberg S, Fraser A, Nahshoni E, Weizman A, Leibovici L. Thyroxine-triiodothyronine combination therapy versus thyroxine monotherapy for clinical hypothyroidism: meta-analysis of randomized controlled trials. J Clin Endocrinol Metab. 2006;91(7):2592–9.
32. Joffe RT, Brimacombe M, Levitt AJ, Stagnaro-Green A. Treatment of clinical hypothyroidism with thyroxine and triiodothyronine: a literature review and metaanalysis. Psychosomatics. 2007;48(5):379–84.
33. Ma C, Xie J, Huang X, Wang G, Wang Y, Wang X, et al. Thyroxine alone or thyroxine plus triiodothyronine replacement therapy for hypothyroidism. Nucl Med Commun. 2009;30(8):586–93.
34. Motamedi KK, McClary AC, Amedee RG. Obstructive sleep apnea: a growing problem. Ochsner J. 2009;9(3):149–53.
35. Wang C, Schmid CH, Fielding RA, Harvey WF, Reid KF, Price LL, et al. Effect of tai chi versus aerobic exercise for fibromyalgia: comparative effectiveness randomized controlled trial. BMJ. 2018;360:k851.
36. Deare JC, Zheng Z, Xue CC, Liu JP, Shang J, Scott SW, et al. Acupuncture for treating fibromyalgia. Cochrane Database Syst Rev. 2013;5:CD007070.
37. Voet N, Bleijenberg G, Hendriks J, de Groot I, Padberg G, van Engelen B, et al. Both aerobic exercise and cognitive-behavioral therapy reduce chronic fatigue in FSHD: an RCT. Neurology. 2014;83(21):1914–22.
38. Utiger RD. Altered thyroid function in nonthyroidal illness and surgery. To treat or not to treat? N Engl J Med. 1995;333(23):1562–3.

# Chapter 22
# Reverse T3 Dilemma

**Katarzyna Piotrowska and Mark Lupo**

## Abbreviations

DI   Deiodinase
ICU  Intensive care unit
NTI  Nonthyroidal illness
rT3  Reverse T3
TSH  Thyroid-stimulating hormone

**Case** 48-year-old female present for evaluation of abnormal thyroid function tests and.

symptoms of hypothyroidism. She has a history of fibromyalgia, chronic fatigue, anxiety,

---

K. Piotrowska (✉)
Thyroid and Endocrine Center of Florida, Sarasota, FL, USA
e-mail: kpiotrowska@thyroidflorida.com

M. Lupo
Thyroid and Endocrine Center of Florida, Florida State University, College of Medicine, Sarasota, FL, USA

© Springer Nature Switzerland AG 2019
M. T. McDermott (ed.), *Management of Patients with Pseudo-Endocrine Disorders*,
https://doi.org/10.1007/978-3-030-22720-3_22

insomnia, and inability to lose weight. No family history of thyroid dysfunction. She is taking over-the-counter biotin, turmeric, and coenzyme Q10.

She did research online and came to the conclusion that all her symptoms are consistent with hypothyroidism. First, she sought help with her primary care physician and was told that her labs were normal. Based on her online resources and as well as a book she purchased, she was convinced that she was one of many patients who have hypothyroidism even with normal labs. She also learned from her research that her doctors may not know about this disorder; therefore she further sought answers.

She visited a practitioner who ran thyroid function tests which showed a TSH, free T4 in normal range, low normal total T3, and reverse T3 which was mildly elevated.

He diagnosed her with "reverse T3 syndrome" and started 20mcg of T3 as well as an adrenal support supplement which was sold in the practitioner's office. Since this approach was not covered by insurance, she was not able to continue the treatment plan due to cost and therefore presented to our office. She does note that she did not feel better with the T3 treatment; in fact she was experiencing heart palpitations intermittently.

Physical exam showed a female with BMI of 28. Vital signs normal. Physical exam was unremarkable; specifically, her thyroid gland was not enlarged and no nodules were palpable.

**Approach to the Patient**

In the recent years, the reverse T3 syndrome has received quite a bit of attention, with patients convinced that mainstream medicine is ignoring their symptoms and that there is a secret cure to their ailments, citing that physicians treating patients according to traditional medicine either do not understand or do not want to treat their thyroid disorder.

Before seeing the patient, it is important to remember that each patient visiting our office has symptoms that prompted them to visit us. The suffering is real for the patient, and the approach should be an empathetic, patient-centric exploration into potential causes.

The first step is to listen to the patient's story, the symptoms they are experiencing, and the struggle they went through to get to the point where they are now. The next step is to acknowledge that the patient's symptoms are real and that you are there for them to evaluate possible reasons for the symptoms including a thorough evaluation for thyroid dysfunction.

It is important to be aware of the information and theories being proposed by other providers in order to be able to clearly address the patient's questions. Additionally, it is important to discuss the research or, more often, the lack of research to support certain tests and therapies that the patient is requesting in addition to pointing out the potential harm of some of the treatments.

## Explaining Reverse T3 to Patients

There is indeed quite a bit of hype on reverse T3. An April 2018 PubMed literature search for any article (with human subjects) with reverse T3 in the title revealed nothing since 2010. Does this represent a knowledge gap or a case closed?

### *Thyroid Hormone Physiology*

Thyroxine (T4) is a prohormone produced solely in the thyroid gland that is converted to the active hormone, triiodothyronine (T3), which binds to cellular thyroid hormone receptors in order to exert a metabolic action. Deiodinase enzymes predominately in the liver, kidney, muscle and pituitary are responsible for this conversion as well as the conversion of T4 to an inactive hormone, rT3 (see Fig. 22.1).

Reverse T3 syndrome proponents suggest that elevated rT3 causes hypothyroidism in two ways: 1) rT3 potently blocks the action of T3 by competing with binding to the

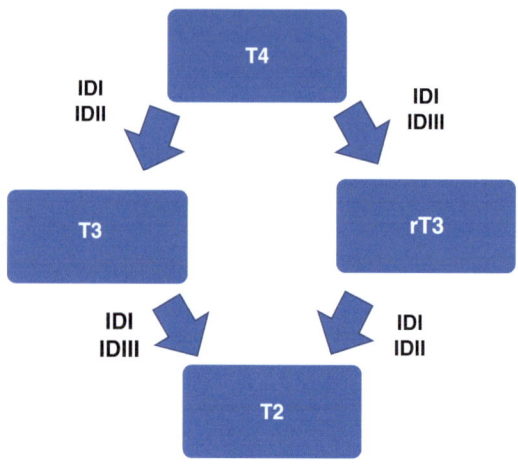

FIGURE 22.1 Thyroid hormone deiodination pathways

thyroid hormone receptor and 2) rT3 blocks the conversion of T4 to T3. There is evidence to show that the affinity of T3 for the cellular thyroid binding receptor is more than 100 times greater than that of rT3 [1], undermining the proposal that rT3 potently antagonizes T3 action. To understand the physiologic reason that rT3 inhibits the conversion of T4 to T3, we need to review the clinical scenario in which the measurement of rT3 may be useful.

## Nonthyroidal Illness

In acutely ill, hospitalized patients, thyroid function should not be assessed unless there is a high suspicion for underlying thyroid disease. Acutely ill patients may have low T4 and T3 as well as low TSH, but not because of thyroid disease; this is referred to as nonthyroidal illness. The finding of an elevated rT3 can help confirm that the abnormal thyroid labs are due to another illness.

80% of T3 is produced by 5′-monodeiodinase (D1 and D2); this reaction decreases in response to illness [2], while the D3 activity increases causing conversion of T4 to rT3. With decrease in activity of D1 and D2, the clearance of rT3 also decreases, causing a further elevation in rT3 levels (see Fig. 22.1).

When the body is under stress, this protective conversion of T4 to rT3 helps to prevent catabolism [3]. The observation that rT3 itself further inhibits T4 to T3 conversion is part of this self-protective mechanism during acute illness.

Studies with thyroid hormone replacement have been done in patients with NTI during fasting [4, 5], critical illness [6, 7] and coronary artery bypass patients [5, 8–12]. These have not shown evidence of clinical benefit.

## Reverse T3 Syndrome

Some alternative medicine websites discussing reverse T3 syndrome propose that in the past NTI was only pertinent to sick patients in the ICU/hospital but now is seen in ambulatory patients and should be addressed by treating patients with T3 to "flush out" the rT3. Often these websites cite a quantifiable goal: free T3 to rT3 ratio of >0.2 to be utilized in the titration of T3 treatment. The body alters thyroid hormone levels during stress for a reason – the best way to "fix" the situation is to address the underlying cause. It is misinformed to make physiology into a syndrome.

It is an important educational point for the patient that we currently do not have data supporting T3 supplementation for improved well-being and health outcomes in patients with elevated rT3. On the contrary, we do have evidence and data that unnecessary treatment with T3 supplementation increases risk of arrhythmia, stroke and bone loss.

Most proponents of the rT3 syndrome advocate (and sell) supplements such as selenium, zinc and thyroid support formulations. There is no data to support that low selenium has a primary role in rT3 elevation in these patients. Some hypothesized that selenium deficiency may be responsible for reverse T3 syndrome, but there is insufficient evidence to support this [13].

It is reassuring to note that many of the recommendations from practitioners adhering to the reverse T3 syndrome revolve around addressing the underlying cause(s) – commonly citing insulin resistance, inflammation, food/chemical sensitivities, gut imbalances, and abnormal cortisol levels. These may be pertinent but as addressed in other chapters of this book have their own inherent uncertainties and potential for the selling of supplements and products the patient may not need or that may cause harm. We can all agree, however, that it is essential to help the patient address good sleep habits, stress management, exercise, and a healthy diet.

## *Identifying the Cause of Elevated rT3*

After reviewing the physiology of rT3 production, our patient became more open into exploring other causes of her symptoms and recognized that "hypothyroid" symptoms are very nonspecific and often are due to other conditions. For such patients who come in with prior testing showing high rT3, this is a good opportunity to highlight the importance of getting to the source cause of abnormality (see Table 22.1).

It is our duty to try to help the patient. While part of this includes understanding why the elevated rT3 does not mean they have a thyroid condition, our obligation is to assist in the evaluation of their symptoms and attempt to guide them down the correct path. In addition to confirming if the patient is up to date with yearly physical and preventive screenings, testing should include complete blood counts, comprehensive metabolic panel, screening for depression/anxiety, and evaluation for sleep apnea.

Identify the potential stresses in the patient's life and determine coping mechanisms. This may include increased exercise and/or referral to counseling to explore relationship and job dynamics, for example. In all cases, emphasizing the importance of introducing regular daily physical activity, as

**Table 22.1** Causes of increase in RT3

| |
|---|
| Severe illness |
| Fasting/starvation |
| Obstructive sleep apnea |
| Trauma |
| Malignancies |
| Stress |
| Psychiatric illness |
| Heart failure/myocardial infraction |
| Liver cirrhosis |
| Diabetic ketoacidosis |
| Inflammatory diseases (via cytokines) |
| HIV infection |
| Heat/burns |
| Hypoxia, ischemia (5 up-to-date ref) |

well as good sleep and dietary habits (including the avoidance of excess alcohol), is critical.

Diet is a prolonged discussion that would require a chapter (or book) in itself. Most of us will attempt the discussion but may require help from a nutritionist/dietitian. Since as noted above fasting and starvation will increase reverse T3, a well-balanced diet with an appropriate amount of calories is recommended.

If there are chronic underlying comorbidities, discuss that reverse T3 may be continuously elevated unless the underlying disorder is resolved, reinforcing that there is no indication for treatment with T3.

We all face time restrictions in our offices, but if the above issues are not addressed, the patient will continue to struggle and continue to seek answers. This may require several visits and referrals to other health-care providers.

## Conclusion

Reverse T3 syndrome can seem like a convenient way to explain many nonspecific symptoms that are increasingly common in our patients. However, the "syndrome" exploits normal physiology in place to protect the body during times of illness and stress. There is no compelling evidence to support the argument that an elevated rT3 means the patient is hypothyroid in the absence of other thyroid function abnormalities. Treatment with T3 is not likely to help the symptoms and may cause harm. The focus should be on educating the patient and together charting a course to determine the underlying cause of the symptoms.

## References

1. Schuster L, Schwartz H, Oppenheimer J. Nuclear receptors for 3,5,3'- triiodothyronine in human liver and kidney: characterization, quantitation and similarities to rat receptors. J Clin Endocrinol Metab. 1979;48(4):627–32.
2. Davidson MB, Chopra IJ. Effect of carbohydrate and noncarbohydrate sources of calories on plasma 3,5,3'-triiodothyronine concentrations in man. J Clin Endocrinol Metab. 1979;48:577.
3. Utiger RD. Altered thyroid function in nonthyroidal illness and surgery. To treat or not to treat? N Engl J Med. 1995;333:1562.
4. Vignati L, Finley RJ, Hagg S, Aoki TT. Protein conservation during prolonged fast: a function of triiodothyronine levels. Trans Assoc Am Phys. 1978;91:169.
5. Gardner DF, Kaplan MM, Stanley CA, Utiger RD. Effect of tri-iodothyronine replacement on the metabolic and pituitary responses to starvation. N Engl J Med. 1979;300:579.
6. Becker RA, Vaughan GM, Ziegler MG, et al. Hypermetabolic low triiodothyronine syndrome of burn injury. Crit Care Med. 1982;10:870.
7. Brent GA, Hershman JM. Thyroxine therapy in patients with severe nonthyroidal illnesses and low serum thyroxine concentration. J Clin Endocrinol Metab. 1986;63(1)
8. Broderick TJ, Wechsler AS. Triiodothyronine in cardiac surgery. Thyroid. 1997;7:133.

9. Novitzky D, Fontanet H, Snyder M, et al. Impact of triiodothyronine on the survival of high-risk patients undergoing open heart surgery. Cardiology. 1996;87:509.
10. Klemperer JD, Klein I, Gomez M, et al. Thyroid hormone treatment after coronary-artery bypass surgery. N Engl J Med. 1995;333:1522.
11. Kaptein EM, Sanchez A, Beale E, Chan LS. Clinical review: thyroid hormone therapy for postoperative nonthyroidal illnesses: a systematic review and synthesis. J Clin Endocrinol Metab. 2010;95:4526.
12. Choi YS, Shim JK, Song JW, et al. Efficacy of perioperative oral triiodothyronine replacement therapy in patients undergoing off-pump coronary artery bypass grafting. J Cardiothorac Vasc Anesth. 2013;27:1218.
13. Gärtner R. Selenium and thyroid hormone axis in critical ill states: an overview of conflicting view points. J Trace Elem Med Biol. 2009;23(2):71–4.

# Chapter 23
## Persistent Hypothyroid Symptoms Despite Adequate Thyroid Hormone Replacement

**Michael T. McDermott**

## Case 1

A 42-year-old man is referred for persistent symptoms despite levothyroxine therapy. Hypothyroidism was diagnosed 6 months ago. He still experiences fatigue, mild depression, and difficulty losing weight. He says that his TSH does not reflect his true thyroid status and requests further thyroid testing and medication adjustment.

PMH: Hypothyroidism    Meds: Levothyroxine 150 mcg/day

PE: BP 122/84   P 76   Ht 6′1″   Wt 203 lb.

General Exam: Normal   Thyroid: Enlarged, granular

Lab:   TSH 1.6 mU/l (nl, 0.45–4.5)

Free T4 1.4 ng/dl (nl, 0.8–1.8)

You say: "It's not your thyroid."

He says: "But what else could it be?"

---

M. T. McDermott (✉)
University of Colorado Hospital, Aurora, CO, USA
e-mail: michael.mcdermott@cuanschutz.edu

## Case 2

A 35-year-old woman was diagnosed with hypothyroidism 6 months ago. She is still experiencing fatigue, mild depression, and difficulty losing weight. She has done an extensive Internet search. She requests T3 therapy.

---

PMH: Hypothyroidism   Meds: Levothyroxine 125 mcg/day

PE: BP 122/84   P 80   Ht 5′6″   Wt 172 lb.

General Exam: Normal   Thyroid: Mildly enlarged, firm

Lab:   TSH 1.2 mU/l (nl, 0.45–4.5)

Free T4 1.3 ng/dl (nl, 0.8–1.8)

---

## Discussion

Hypothyroidism is a state of deficient thyroid hormone action throughout the body [1, 2]. Hypothyroidism is most often caused by primary thyroid gland failure but can also be caused by hypothalamic or pituitary disease; conditions that promote excessive peripheral thyroid hormone consumption/metabolism; and disorders of cellular transmembrane thyroid hormone transport, intracellular thyroid hormone metabolism, and thyroid hormone receptor binding (Table 23.1). Certainly additional causes of tissue thyroid hormone deficiency will be identified in the future.

Since most tissues in the body are dependent on thyroid hormone for normal function, symptoms due to thyroid hormone deficiency usually increase in number and severity with increasing magnitude of the total body thyroid hormone deficit; for uncertain reasons, however, symptoms may be minimal or absent in some patients with biochemically overt disease and can be numerous in patients with only mild disease. The most common clinical features of thyroid hormone deficiency are fatigue, dry skin, cold intolerance, puffy eyelids, and weight gain [2–5]. However, these and other features of hypothyroidism are mostly nonspecific; similar symptoms

TABLE 23.1 Classification and etiology of hypothyroidism

**Primary hypothyroidism**

*Chronic lymphocytic thyroiditis (Hashimoto's thyroiditis)*
*Iatrogenic hypothyroidism*
 Thyroidectomy
 Radiation damage
  Radioiodine (I-131) ablation
  Radiation therapy for non-thyroid cancer
 Medications
  Lithium
  Amiodarone
  Alpha interferon
  Tyrosine kinase inhibitors
  Antituberculosis drugs (second line)
  Checkpoint inhibitors (ipilimumab, nivolumab)
  Thalidomide and pomalidomide (used to treat multiple myeloma)
*Transient thyroiditis*
 Postpartum thyroiditis
 Silent (painless) thyroiditis
 Subacute (De Quervain's) thyroiditis
 Palpation thyroiditis (e.g., after parathyroidectomy)
*Iodine disorders*
 Iodine excess (severe)
 Iodine deficiency (severe)
*Infiltrative disease*
 Sarcoidosis
 Malignancy (lymphoma, metastatic non-thyroid cancer)
*Congenital hypothyroidism*
 Genetic disorders of thyroid development
 Genetic disorders of thyroid hormone synthesis

**Central hypothyroidism**

*Hypothalamic-pituitary disorders*
 Tumors
 Surgical removal
 Radiation therapy
 Trauma (traumatic brain injury)
 Hemorrhage/infarction (apoplexy, Sheehan's syndrome)
 Infiltrative disorders (sarcoidosis, TB, hemochromatosis, histiocytosis X)
 Medications (dopamine, opioids, glucocorticoids, somatostatin analogs, metyrapone, bexarotene)

(continued)

Table 23.1 (continued)

**Peripheral hypothyroidism**

Consumptive hypothyroidism [deiodinase 3 (D3) expressing tumors]
Thyroid hormone resistance syndromes (TRβ, TRα, MCT8, SECISBP2 mutations)

Adapted from Ref. [1]
*TRβ* thyroid hormone receptor beta, *TRα* thyroid hormone receptor alpha, *MCT8* monocarboxylate transporter 8, *SECISBP2* selenocysteine insertion sequence-binding protein 2 (SECISBP2)

may also occur with numerous other conditions unrelated to the thyroid system [4, 5].

Oral levothyroxine (LT4) is the recommended medication of choice for hypothyroid patients because of its proven efficacy, long-term experience with its benefits, favorable side effect profile, good gastrointestinal absorption, ease of administration, long serum half-life, and low cost [1, 2, 6–8]. Thyroxine (T4) itself is not well absorbed from the gastrointestinal tract, but absorption is enhanced significantly by replacing one hydrogen ion with a sodium to produce synthetic LT4. The molecular structures of T4 and LT4 are identical aside from this sodium substitution (Fig. 23.1); T4 and LT4 are therefore considered bioidentical [9]. LT4 is rapidly absorbed in the duodenum and has a serum half-life of 5–7 days; a steady state is reached approximately 5–6 weeks after initiation of LT4 or a change in the LT4 dose. Oral liquid LT4 preparations have been reported to have better and less variable absorption compared to LT4 tablets in hypothyroid patients, including those with issues that interfere with absorption such as gastrointestinal diseases and the concomitant use of proton pump inhibitor medications [10–12].

Synthetic liothyronine (LT3) preparations are similarly identical to the triiodothyronine (T3) produced by the human thyroid gland. Desiccated thyroid extract (DTE) preparations are made by drying and powdering animal thyroid glands, most commonly porcine thyroid glands. DTE products consist of about 80% T4 and 20% T3 (approximately a 4:1 ratio of T4 to T3). The T4 to T3 ratio may vary somewhat

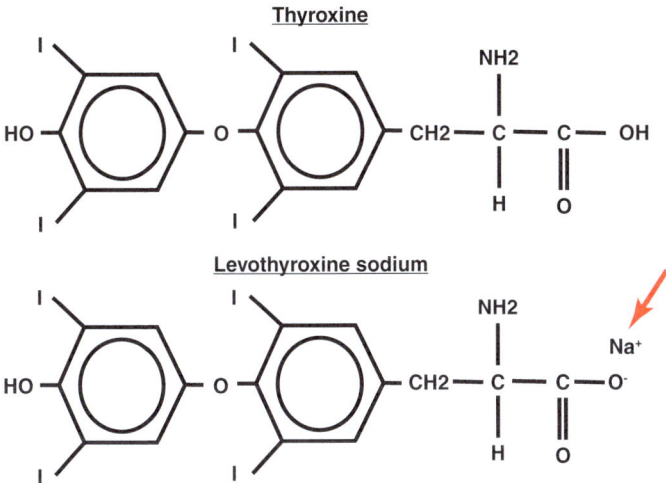

Figure. 23.1 Molecular structures of thyroxine and levothyroxine sodium (Ref. [2])

in DTE products, depending on the brand and manufacturing process [9].

The majority of patients with overt hypothyroidism who are treated with adequate doses of LT4 experience rapid resolution of their hypothyroid symptoms [1, 2, 13–15]. One exception to this may be body weight. Since weight gain is often a feature of hypothyroidism, it would be anticipated that LT4 therapy in hypothyroid patients would result in weight loss. It is somewhat surprising, therefore, that published research has not verified this [16], although randomized controlled trials have not been performed. Nonetheless, observational studies have reported minimal or no weight loss after the institution of thyroid hormone therapy for hypothyroidism; weight loss that did occur in two studies was attributed mainly to the resolution of edema or loss of lean mass [16].

Despite the well-documented efficacy of LT4 and extensive clinical experience with its use, some patients continue to experience symptoms consistent with thyroid hormone deficiency despite taking adequate LT4 replacement therapy that maintains serum TSH levels within the reference range [1, 2, 9, 13–15, 17–21]. The American Thyroid Association (ATA) conducted a mail survey of 12,000 hypothyroid patients who were receiving thyroid hormone replacement therapy (95% female); among the survey respondents, 60% were treated with LT4 alone, 25% were receiving combination LT4 and LT3, and 10% were taking DTE or a compounded thyroid hormone preparation. The mean satisfaction score with therapy among respondents was 5 (visual analog scale, 1–10). Dissatisfaction was most commonly due to persistent fatigue/ low energy (75%), body weight issues (70%), memory problems (55%), mood problems (45%), and other issues (35%). The respondents' mean satisfaction score with their physician was 5–6, and the score for their belief that their physician was knowledgeable was also 5–6 (visual analog scale, 1–10). Furthermore, 10–45% of the respondents had changed physicians 1–4 times and 10% had changed physicians 5–10 times because of persistent symptoms and thyroid management issues [21].

Hypothyroid patients taking LT4 replacement in doses sufficient to maintain serum TSH levels within the population reference range have been reported to have persistently low resting energy expenditure (REE) [22, 23]. Additionally, LT4-treated patients have higher free T4 levels, lower free T3 levels, and lower free T3/T4 ratios compared to euthyroid individuals with similar serum TSH levels [24, 25]. LT4-treated hypothyroid subjects in the NHANES cohort had higher body weights than controls despite reporting higher levels of exercise and similar caloric intakes; they also used antidepressant medications more often [25]. In light of this data, some investigators and clinicians now question whether traditional LT4 therapy is truly physiological and is the most appropriate therapy for all patients [14, 25].

Interestingly, one study presented data suggesting that chronic lymphocytic thyroiditis (Hashimoto's thyroiditis) may possibly cause symptoms that are not related to and are independent of serum thyroid hormone levels [26]. Patients with Hashimoto' thyroiditis are also known to develop other autoimmune conditions more frequently [27, 28], adding further complexity to symptom evaluation and management. Hypoparathyroidism, either overt or subtle, may also coexist in patients with postsurgical or post-ablative hypothyroidism and could be an additional source of symptoms if not adequately managed [29]. Symptoms in these patients may also not be thyroid-related or endocrine-related at all [2, 8]. Potential causes of persistent symptoms suggestive of thyroid hormone deficiency in adequately treated hypothyroid patients are shown in Table 23.2 [8]. Table 23.3 lists other autoimmune disorders that occur more commonly in patients with Hashimoto' s thyroiditis [27, 28].

Persistent symptoms continue to frustrate some hypothyroid patients who appear to be adequately treated with thyroid hormone replacement therapy managed carefully by experienced clinicians. These unfortunate patients have posed major challenges for the devoted clinicians who share their frustrations and sincerely strive to relieve their symptoms and restore their optimal quality of life. Improving their patients' quality of life is the main reason most physicians have dedicated their talents, energy, and careers to the patients who honor them by entrusting their health care to them.

Satisfactory outcomes for persistently symptomatic patients require a skillful and compassionate approach by the physician. Attentively listening to the patient's symptoms and ongoing concerns, without interruption, will help set the stage for progress. It is often useful then to explain briefly to the patient, in understandable language, pertinent aspects of thyroid physiology and how and why we order and interpret the tests we use. We should emphasize that our current tests are highly accurate and that we have extensive experience with their interpretation. However, an acknowledgment that everything is not known about thyroid function and that there could be conditions, yet to be identified, for which we currently do not have diagnostic tests, can be helpful. It is also vitally important for the patient to understand that symptoms that are frequently attributed to hypothyroidism are nonspecific and could be due to other conditions unrelated to the thyroid system [2, 8]. Accordingly, one should consider offering additional testing, if not done already, for other endocrine-related and metabolic conditions, such as diabetes mellitus, calcium abnormalities, adrenal disorders,

TABLE 23.2 Possible causes of persistent symptoms in patients treated for hypothyroidism

*Inadequate levothyroxine dose*
*Lifestyle measures suboptimal*
  Unhealthy diet
  Lack of exercise
  Inadequate sleep
  Excess stress
*Coexisting disease*
  Chronic Fatigue Syndrome
  Fibromyalgia
  Sleep Apnea
  Climacteric Syndrome
  Iron Deficiency
  Vitamin D Deficiency
  Vitamin B12 Deficiency
  Other Autoimmune Disease
  Other Medical Illness
    Kidney, Liver, Heart, Lung, Blood
    Viral and Post-viral Syndromes
*Deiodinase 2 polymorphisms*
  Thr92Ala Polymorphism
*Other subtle disorder of thyroid regulation or action*
*Psychiatric illness (depression especially)*
*Substance abuse*

Adapted from Ref. [8]

TABLE 23.3 Autoimmune diseases that occur with increased frequency in patients with chronic lymphocytic thyroiditis (495 subjects)

| **Autoimmune condition** | **Women (%)** | **Men (%)** |
|---|---|---|
| Rheumatoid arthritis | 4.7 | 1.5 |
| Vitamin B12 deficiency | 4.5 | 0 |
| Adrenal insufficiency | 1.2 | 3 |
| Celiac disease | 1.2 | 0 |
| Multiple sclerosis | 0.7 | 1.5 |
| Inflammatory bowel disease | 0.7 | 1.5 |
| Systemic lupus erythematosus | 0.7 | 0 |

Adapted from Ref. [27]

hypogonadism, celiac disease, vitamin D deficiency, vitamin B12 deficiency, sleep apnea, and depression. Alternatively, the endocrine-specific provider can explain that additional general medical testing may be more efficiently done by their primary care provider [2].

In addition to the available clinical data (history, physical examination, laboratory results, and individual patient concerns), the discerning clinician should consider multiple possibilities that may cause or contribute to persistent symptoms in their hypothyroid patients. The current thyroid hormone dose may be adequate but not optimal; the thyroid regimen may not be physiological for that individual patient; the patient may possibly have a hypothalamic or pituitary disorder, rendering the serum TSH an unreliable test. As educated and trained thyroid experts, endocrinologists must also consider that there could be a subtle, or possibly not yet identifiable, genetic, epigenetic, or other acquired disorder somewhere within the thyroid hormone regulatory or response system for which tests are not readily accessible or not yet available.

Management advice to improve patients' overall well-being should include lifestyle measures, emphasizing a well-balanced diet, regular exercise, adequate sleep, and stress reduction. Treatment of other endocrine and metabolic disorders uncovered during the evaluation should be discussed or implemented. Contributing non-endocrine medical and psychiatric conditions can be discussed but are often more appropriately managed by primary care providers or other specialists.

Some endocrinologists and primary care providers will also consider a trial of combination LT4/LT3 or DTE therapy. Combination LT4/LT3 therapy has been evaluated compared to LT4 treatment alone in multiple published randomized controlled trials since the first report in 1999. Some studies reported improvement in symptoms and a preference among study subjects for combination LT4/LT3 therapy. However, the majority of the investigations reported no subjective or objective benefits from combination therapy [1, 2]. The studies were mostly small and of short duration and did not specifically evaluate patients who had persistent symptoms on LT4 monotherapy, leaving investigators unconvinced of combination therapy efficacy but uncertain about whether adequate studies had been done [1, 2].

The largest and longest study consisted of over 600 hypothyroid subjects who were randomized to combination LT4/LT3 therapy or LT4 alone and were followed for 1 year. Consistent with most of the other trials, benefits from combination LT4/LT3 therapy compared to LT4 therapy were not demonstrated. Subsequently, this group reported genotyping over 500 of their original subjects and identified a polymorphism of the deiodinase 2 (D2) enzyme, Thr92Ala, in 16% of the cohort. The subset of subjects with this D2 polymorphism had more symptoms at baseline and showed statistically significant symptom improvement on combination LT4/LT3 therapy (30); the authors postulated that this relatively common D2 variation might be causally related to poorer psychological well-being and a better response to combination LT4/LT3 therapy [30]. In contrast, a previous study reported that the D2 Thr92Ala polymorphism was not associated with impaired well-being or neurocognitive functioning or with a subject preference for combined LT4/LT3 treatment [31].

The clinical consequences of the Thr92Ala polymorphism on D2 function are not entirely clear. Investigators have suggested that D2 activity might be reduced, causing decreased T4 to T3 conversion in the brain under hypothyroid conditions. The D2 enzyme is normally ubiquitinated causing subsequent proteolytic D2 degradation when T4 concentrations are high, whereas D2 degradation is prevented by de-ubiquitination when the prevailing T4 supply is low. However, the Thr92Ala substitution is located in the D2 instability loop, which is closely linked to ubiquitination, and may somehow impair D2 rescue under hypothyroid conditions, resulting in greater dependence on circulating T3 levels to maintain an adequate T3 supply to the brain. The D2 Thr92Ala polymorphism and a D2 Ala92Ala polymorphism have more recently been shown to be associated with reduced serum T3 levels and reduced intracellular T3 concentrations in thyroidectomized patients replaced with LT4 alone [32]. Clinical genetic testing to determine in advance who may and who may not benefit from this therapy (pharmacogenetics) is not currently available.

When combination LT4/LT3 therapy is utilized, it is suggested that an LT4 to LT3 ratio of approximately 14:1 to 10:1 be administered to mirror the human physiological T4 to T3 secretion ratio of 14:1. Because LT3 has a much shorter half-life than LT4, some clinicians administer LT3 in twice-daily divided doses approximately 8–12 hours apart. Many, but not all, clinicians recommend that patients on combination LT4/LT3 therapy have serum TSH levels measured in the morning before taking either LT4 or LT3 because of the abrupt rise in serum T3 levels that occurs in the first few hours after LT3 is ingested. Serum TSH levels in these patients, as with those on LT4 monotherapy, should be maintained within the reference range to avoid the toxicities and complications of chronic thyroid hormone excess [2].

The use of DTE is a much older approach to combination T4/T3 therapy. Currently available DTE products are made from porcine thyroid glands; patients who avoid pork products for religious or other reasons should be made aware of the source of DTE preparations. Some websites and individuals promote DTE as being "natural" thyroid hormone replacement because the DTE hormones are not synthetic. However, porcine thyroid glands and physiology are not the same as their human counterparts. Human thyroid glands normally secrete a T4/T3 molar ratio of approximately 14:1, while porcine thyroid glands contain a T4/T3 ratio of about 4:1. Therefore desiccated porcine thyroid glands contain much higher T3 concentrations than human thyroid glands. Taken orally, these DTE products produce an abrupt rise in serum T3 levels, often transiently into the suprapsysiological range. Potentially, this transient T3 excess could cause short-term harm or the long-term complications known to occur with thyroid hormone excess [9].

DTE therapy was evaluated in a short-term randomized controlled trial that included 70 LT4-treated hypothyroid patients who received 16 weeks of treatment with either DTE or continued LT4. TSH levels were similar in both groups, but DTE-treated patients had lower serum free T4 levels and higher total T3 levels during the treatment period. Symptoms during the trial did not differ between the groups, but the DTE-treated group lost a small amount of weight; 48.6% of subjects expressed a preference for DTE, while 18.6% preferred LT4. There were no adverse events reported in either group [33]. A 2017 mail survey study of physicians who were frequent thyroid hormone prescribers was conducted by members of ATA, the American Association of Clinical Endocrinologists (AACE), and the Endocrine Society; the surveyed physicians reported a high incidence of adverse events in patients taking DTE, but there was no comparator group of patients on LT4 alone [34]. There are no published studies that have adequately evaluated the long-term efficacy or safety of DTE.

Compounded thyroid hormone preparations from compounding pharmacies are another source available to patients who wish to access combination T4/T3 products. Due to variability and lack of standardization, however, the use of compounded thyroid hormone products cannot be recommended [6–9]. LT3 monotherapy is also not recommended because this approach is clearly not physiologic. Administration of once-daily LT3 is associated with significant excursions of serum total T3 and free T3 levels [35]. Sustained-release LT3 preparations, though not yet available as FDA-approved products in the USA, may provide smoother serum T3 profiles and may be more suitable for future studies of combination T4/T3 therapy.

Current clinical practice guidelines from ATA, AACE, and the European Thyroid Association (ETA) do not recommend combination LT4/LT3 as routine treatment for hypothyroidism because there is no consistent evidence (multiple randomized controlled trials, literature reviews, and meta-analyses) that combination LT4/LT3 treatment is superior to LT4 monotherapy, and there is no long-term safety data. They also recommend against using DTE, citing potential safety concerns regarding the transient supraphysiological T3 levels that occur with DTE and the paucity of long-term safety outcome data [6–9, 36]. However, the guideline authors concede that it is reasonable to consider these regimens in patients who have persistent symptoms consistent with thyroid hormone deficiency despite appropriately dosed LT4 monotherapy or in those who express a strong preference for one of these approaches. When undertaken, both types of combination therapy must be given safely with careful attention to maintaining serum TSH levels within the reference range to avoid the known toxicities of excess thyroid hormone administration [2, 6, 7, 13, 14].

# References

1. Chaker L, Bianco AC, Jonklass J, Peeters RP. Hypothyroidism. Lancet. 2017;390(10101):1550–62.
2. McDermott MT. Hypothyroidism. In: Cooper DS, Sipos J, editors. Medical management of thyroid disease. 3rd ed. New York, NY: Informa Healthcare; 2019. (in press).
3. McDermott MT. Overview of the clinical manifestations of hypothyroidism. In: Braverman LE, Cooper DS, editors. Werner & Ingbar's the thyroid: a fundamental and clinical text. 11th ed. Philadelphia: Lippincott Williams & Wilkins; 2019. (in press).
4. Zulewski HK, Muller B, Exer P, Miserez AR, Staub JJ. Estimation of tissue hypothyroidism by a new clinical score: evaluation of patients with various grades of hypothyroidism and controls. J Clin Endocrinol Metab. 1997;82:771–6.
5. Carle A, Pedersen IB, Knudsen N, et al. Hypothyroid symptoms and the likelihood of overt thyroid failure: a population-based case-control study. Eur J Endocrinol. 2014;171:593–602.
6. Garber JR, Cobin RH, Gharib H, Hennessey JV, Klein I, Mechanick JI, Pessah-Pollack R, For the American Association of Clinical Endocrinologists and American Thyroid Association Task Force on Hypothyroidism in Adults Study Groups, et al. Clinical practice guidelines for hypothyroidism in adults; cosponsored by the American Association of Clinical Endocrinologists and the American Thyroid Association. Endocr Pract. 2012;18(6):988–1028.

7. Jonklaas J, Bianco AC, Bauer AJ, Burman KD, Cappola AR, Celi FS, Cooper DS, For the American Thyroid Association Task Force on Thyroid Hormone Replacement, et al. Guidelines for the treatment of hypothyroidism: prepared by the American Thyroid Association Task Force on thyroid hormone replacement. Thyroid. 2014;24(12):1670–751.
8. Guglielmi R, Frasoldati A, Zini M, Grimaldi F, Gharib H, Garber JR, Papini E. Italian association of clinical endocrinologists statement-replacement therapy for primary hypothyroidism: a brief guide for clinical practice. Endocr Pract. 2016;22(11):1319–26.
9. Santoro N, Braunstein GD, Butts CL, Martin KA, McDermott M, Pinkerton JV. Compounded bioidentical hormones in endocrinology practice: an Endocrine Society scientific statement. J Clin Endocrinol Metab. 2016;101(4):1318–43.
10. Negro R, Valcavi R, Agrimi D, Toulis KA. Levothyroxine liquid solution versus tablet for replacement in hypothyroid patients. Endocr Pract. 2014;20(9):901–6.
11. Bruncato D, Scorsone A, Saura G, Ferrara L, Di Noto A, Aiello V, Fleres M, Provenzano V. Comparison of TSH levels with liquid formulation versus tablet formulations of levothyroxine in the treatment of adult hypothyroidism. Endocr Pract. 2014;20(7):657–62.
12. Vita R, Saraceno G, Trimarchi F, Benvenga S. Switching levothyroxine from the tablet to the oral solution formulation corrects the impaired absorption of levothyroxine induced by proton-pump inhibitors. J Clin Endocrinol Metab. 2014;99(12):4481–6.
13. Biondi B, Wartofsky L. Treatment with thyroid hormone. Endocr Rev. 2014;35(3):433–512.
14. McAninch EA, Bianco AC. The history and future treatment of hypothyroidism. Ann Intern Med. 2016;164(1):50–6.
15. Winther KH, Cramon P, Watt T, Bjorner JB, Ekholm O, Feldt-Rasmussen U, Groenvold M, et al. Disease-specific as well as generic quality of life is widely impacted in autoimmune hypothyroidism and improves during the first six months of levothyroxine therapy. PLoS One. 2016;11(6):e0156925.
16. Lee SY, Braverman LE, Pearce EN. Changes in body weight after treatment of primary hypothyroidism with levothyroxine. Endocr Pract. 2014;20(11):1122–8.
17. Thvilum M, Brandt F, Almind D, Christensen K, Brix TH, Hegedüs L. Increased psychiatric morbidity before and after

the diagnosis of hypothyroidism: a nationwide register study. Thyroid. 2014;24(5):802–8.
18. Quinque EM, Villinger A, Kratzsch J, Karger S. Patient-reported outcomes in adequately treated hypothyroidism – insights from the German versions of ThyQoL, ThySRQ and ThyTSQ. Health Qual Life Outcomes. 2013;11:68.
19. Samuels MH, Kolobova I, Smeraglio A, Peters D, Janowsky JS, Schuff KG. The effects of levothyroxine replacement or suppressive therapy on health status, mood, and cognition. J Clin Endocrinol Metab. 2014;99(3):843–51.
20. Samuels MH, Kolobova I, Smeraglio A, Niederhausen M, Janowsky JS, Schuff KG. Effect of thyroid function variations within the laboratory reference range on health status, mood, and cognition in levothyroxine-treated subjects. Thyroid. 2016;26(9):1173–84.
21. Peterson SJ, Cappola AR, Castro MR, et al. Degrees of satisfaction and coexistent diseases in those responding to a survey exploring perceptions about treatment of hypothyroidism. Thyroid. 2018 Jun;28(6):707–21.
22. Samuels MH, Kolobova I, Smeraglio A, Peters D, Purnell JQ, Schuff KG. Effects of levothyroxine replacement or suppressive therapy on energy expenditure and body composition. Thyroid. 2016;26(3):347–55.
23. Samuels MH, Kolobova I, Antosik M, Niederhausen M, Purnell JQ, Schuff KG. Thyroid function variation in the normal range, energy expenditure, and body composition in L-T4-Treated subjects. J Clin Endocrinol Metab. 2017;102(7):2533–42.
24. Ito M, Miyauchi A, Kang S, Hisakado M, Yoshioka W, Ide A, Kudo T, et al. Effect of the presence of remnant thyroid tissue on the serum thyroid hormone balance in thyroidectomized patients. Eur J Endocrinol. 2015;173(3):333–40.
25. Peterson SJ, McAninch EA, Bianco AC. Is a normal TSH synonymous with "Euthyroidism" in levothyroxine monotherapy? J Clin Endocrinol Metab. 2016;101(12):4964–73.
26. Ott J, Promberger R, Kober F, Neuhold N, Tea M, Huber JC, Hermann M. Hashimoto's thyroiditis affects symptom load and quality of life unrelated to hypothyroidism: a prospective case-control study in women undergoing thyroidectomy for benign goiter. Thyroid. 2011;21(2):161–7.

27. Boelaert K, Newby PR, Simmonds MJ, Holder RL, Carr-Smith JD, Heward JM, Manji N, et al. Prevalence and relative risk of other autoimmune diseases in subjects with autoimmune thyroid disease. Am J Med. 2010;123(2):183.e1–9.
28. Roy A, Laszkowska M, Sundstrom J, Lebwohl B, Green PH, Kämpe O, Ludvigsson JF. Prevalence of celiac disease in patients with autoimmune thyroid disease: a meta-analysis. Thyroid. 2016;26(7):880–90.
29. Bollerslev J, Rejnmark L, Marcocci C, Shoback DM, Sitges-Serra A, van Biesen W, Dekkers OM, European Society of Endocrinology. European Society of Endocrinology Clinical Guideline: treatment of chronic hypoparathyroidism in adults. Eur J Endocrinol. 2015;173(2):G1–20.
30. Panicker V, Saravanan P, Vaidya B, Evans J, Hattersley AT, Frayling TM, Dayan CM. Common variation of in the DIO2 gene predicts baseline psychological well-being and response to combination thyroxine plus triiodothyronine therapy in hypothyroid patients. J Clin Endocrinol Metab. 2009;94(5):1623–9.
31. Appelhof BC, Peeters RP, Wiersinga WM, Visser TJ, Wekking EM, Huyser J, Schene AH, et al. Polymorphisms in type 2 deiodinase are not associated with well-being, neurocognitive functioning, and preference for combined thyroxine/3,5,3′-triiodothyronine therapy. J Clin Endocrinol Metab. 2005;90(11):6296–9.
32. Castagna MG, Dentice M, Cantara S, Ambrosio R, Maino F, Porcelli T, Marzocchi C, et al. DIO2 Thr92Ala reduced deiodinase-2 activity and serum T3 levels in thyroid deficient patients. J Clin Endocrinol Metab. 2017;102(5):1623–30.
33. Hoang TD, Olsen CH, Mai VQ, Clyde PW, Shakir MK. Desiccated thyroid extract compared with levothyroxine in the treatment of hypothyroidism: a randomized, double-blind, crossover study. J Clin Endocrinol Metab. 2013;98(5):1982–90.
34. Shresta RT, Malabanan A, Haugen BR, Levy EG, Hennessey JV. Adverse event reporting in patients treated with thyroid hormone extract. Endocr Pract. 2017;23(5):566–75.
35. Jonklaas J, Burman KD. Daily administration of short-acting liothyronine is associated with significant triiodothyronine excursions and fails to alter thyroid-responsive parameters. Thyroid. 2016;26(6):770–8.
36. Wiersinga WM, Duntas L, Fadeyev V, Nygaard B, Vanderpump MPJ. 2012 European Thyroid Association (ETA) guidelines: the use of L-T4 + L-T3 in the treatment of hypothyroidism. Eur Thyroid J. 2012;1(2):55–71.

# Chapter 24
# Low-Dose Naltrexone Treatment of Hashimoto's Thyroiditis

**Michael T. McDermott**

A 51-year-old man came to the office to establish care with an endocrinologist. He just moved to this community from out of state. He was diagnosed years ago with hypothyroidism and low testosterone; he doesn't recall the tests that were done to establish these diagnoses. He currently takes levothyroxine 225 mcg daily, liothyronine 5 mcg BID and Depo-testosterone 100 mg every week. He feels generally well but has chronic anxiety and trouble sleeping. He has some fatigue but says that his current medication regimen helps considerably. His previous doctor told him that his TSH, which is usually low, is not an accurate measure of his thyroid status since he has severe fatigue when his TSH is normal. He was told that his treatment goal should be to keep his free T4 and free T3 levels within the normal range but that his symptoms are the most reliable indicator of the adequacy of his thyroid hormone therapy. He has done extensive Internet research that has confirmed that, as his previous doctor told him, the

M. T. McDermott (✉)
University of Colorado Hospital, Aurora, CO, USA
e-mail: michael.mcdermott@cuanschutz.edu

© Springer Nature Switzerland AG 2019
M. T. McDermott (ed.), *Management of Patients with Pseudo-Endocrine Disorders*,
https://doi.org/10.1007/978-3-030-22720-3_24

TSH is not a good test for him. A previous MRI of his pituitary gland was normal. He also read information during his research that Hashimoto's thyroiditis may be improved or cured with low-dose extended-release compounded naltrexone therapy. He requests that a prescription for low-dose naltrexone be sent to his local compounding pharmacy that has told him they will compound it for him if he has a prescription from a physician. His most recent labs are as follows: TSH 0.01 mU/L, free T4 1.8 ng/dl, and free T3 2.4 pg/ml.

## Discussion

Hashimoto's thyroiditis (chronic lymphocytic thyroiditis) is the most common etiology of primary hypothyroidism in adults in the United States. Hashimoto's thyroiditis is a genetically based chronic inflammatory condition that leads to gradual but progressive destruction of the thyroid gland, rendering it unable to make sufficient amounts of thyroid hormone to meet the needs of peripheral tissues [1]. Hashimoto' s thyroiditis is the most common of all autoimmune diseases. While a genetic predisposition plays a dominant role in its development, environmental factors may also have an important influence. Nutritional factors, for example, have been linked to a higher risk for developing Hashimoto' s thyroiditis; these include iodine excess, selenium deficiency, and possibly deficiencies of iron and vitamin D [2]. Interestingly, selenium supplementation has been shown to reduce thyroid autoantibody titers in patients with Hashimoto's thyroiditis; however, there is no evidence that selenium reverses or prevents progression of their thyroid dysfunction [3].

The diagnosis of Hashimoto's thyroiditis is made by demonstrating elevated levels of anti-thyroid peroxidase antibodies (anti-TPO) and/or anti-thyroglobulin antibodies (anti-Tg) in the circulation. However, measurement of these anti-thyroid antibodies in hypothyroid subjects is a controversial topic. Routine antibody measurement is not recommended in the current clinical practice guidelines of the American Association of Clinical Endocrinologists (AACE) and the American Thyroid Association (ATA) [4] because adults with hypothyroidism not due to iatrogenic causes (surgery, radioiodine ablation) or medications nearly always have Hashimoto's thyroiditis; therefore, thyroid autoantibody testing offers little additional information and does not usually affect treatment decisions. However, some providers find it beneficial to demonstrate to their patients that their hypothyroidism has an autoimmune etiology; this may also facilitate a discussion about the increased risk of developing other autoimmune disorders for which increased vigilance may be useful. Thyroid sonography is not generally indicated in the evaluation of hypothyroidism unless thyroid nodules are palpable on physical examination or have been identified incidentally by other imaging studies; when performed it often shows a hypoechogenic pattern in the thyroid parenchyma in patients with chronic lymphocytic thyroiditis [1].

The treatment of Hashimoto's thyroiditis is thyroid hormone replacement once hypothyroidism develops as a result of the chronic lymphocytic inflammation. Levothyroxine (LT4) is the recommended replacement medication and should be given in doses sufficient to maintain the serum TSH level within the reference range [4, 5]. The majority of affected patients will have relief or resolution of their symptoms with this therapy. However, as discussed in the previous chapter, some patients may continue to experience symptoms consistent with thyroid hormone deficiency despite adequate LT4 replacement therapy [6–14]. Some providers may then choose a trial of combination LT4 plus liothyronine (LT3) in roughly a 10:1 T4 to T3 ratio or porcine desiccated thyroid extract (DTE), which has approximately a 4:1 T4 to T3 ratio. Neither of these are considered first-line therapy, but the ATA and AACE guideline authors concede that while there is no evidence for superiority of these combined T4/T3 regimens on symptoms or other outcomes and there is no long-term safety data, it is reasonable to consider a trial of combined therapy in patients who continue to suffer symptoms despite adequate LT4 therapy (see more complete discussion of this issue in the previous chapter) [4, 5].

Nonetheless, the ATA survey (discussed in the previous chapter) of 12,000 hypothyroid patients that showed widespread dissatisfaction with their thyroid hormone replacement therapy [13] consisted of 60% who were taking LT4 alone, 25% who were taking combination LT4/LT3, and 10% who were taking DTE or a compounded thyroid hormone preparation. Therefore, even the available combination T4/T3 regimens do not resolve all symptoms in some patients.

# Blogs from a Hashimoto's Disease Website (Unedited)

- I am currently going through this now. I feel like crap, no energy depressed moody dizzy ect. My labs have been in range and my Endo doctor says my symptoms are not related to Hashimoto because my thyroid test are in range. But they cant find any other issues so now they are just treating me like I am crazy and a Hypochonchiac when I tell them what I'm experiencing.
- This is exactly what thyroid patients go through, doctors dismissing our symptoms when labs are in-range. They do not realize they are relying on outdated lab values or that the difference between in-range and optimal can make a dramatic improvement in our quality of life. And yet we continue to be ignored by a majority of endocrinologists and thyroid specialists. Seven out of eight thyroid patients are women. Is it any wonder we are ignored?
- Yes it is BS but what's even worse is being sick for 30 years and them telling you you're fine when you know you aren't. Then you are finally diagnosed and they tell you well this isn't something traditional medicine treats its

more of a holistic health thing. Are you serious!!! I do feel better now on Armour and healthy diet than I ever did on Synthroid so that's a plus.
- Endocrinologists are trained but not educated.

# A Cure for Hashimoto's Thyroiditis Is Not Currently Available

The most commonly cited explanation for persistent symptoms in hypothyroid patients who are treated with LT4 or T4/T3 combinations and have serum TSH levels within the reference range or even within the "optimal range" of 0.45–2.0 mU/L is that the symptoms may not be thyroid-related or endocrine-related at all [15]. However, data from one study suggested that chronic lymphocytic thyroiditis may possibly cause symptoms that are independent of and not related to thyroid hormone levels [16]. Furthermore, multiple other autoimmune conditions are known to occur more commonly in patients with chronic lymphocytic thyroiditis [17, 18], adding to the complexity of symptom management. So, the important question arises: is it possible that Hashimoto's thyroiditis itself could be cured before there is extensive thyroid inflammation and gland destruction?

Autoimmune diseases that destroy some organ systems (joints, kidneys, liver, central nervous system, eyes, skin) are often treated with aggressive immunosuppressive therapies because relatively simple replacement therapies for these organ systems are not available. Due to the frequent side effects and significant toxicities of immunosuppressive agents, they have not been well studied and are not indicated in patients with Hashimoto's thyroiditis. Instead, affected patients are generally monitored until they develop mild hypothyroidism, at which point thyroid hormone replacement therapy is initiated.

Therefore, there is interest in finding therapies that are more benign than currently available immunosuppressive agents and that could potentially be used to reduce or abolish the thyroid inflammation to prevent further thyroid destruction or possibly even allow thyroid regeneration. For example, as mentioned above, selenium supplementation has been shown to reduce thyroid autoantibody titers in patients with this condition; disappointingly, however, there is no evidence that selenium can reverse or prevent progression of thyroid dysfunction [3]. So here is where the murky origins of low-dose naltrexone as a treatment for Hashimoto's thyroiditis begin.

# Background on Low-Dose Naltrexone

Endogenous opioids and opioid antagonists are proposed to play a role in healing and repair of tissues. This has led to the use of low-dose naltrexone (LDN) as a possible treatment for numerous disorders [20]. Dr. Bernard Bihari, "a LDN pioneer and champion" is featured in a 2002 online video describing his work with LDN; an online tribute credits him with improving the lives and relieving symptoms in "tens of thousands (some say hundreds of thousands) of people with multiple sclerosis, rheumatoid arthritis, lupus, HIV/AIDS, and even cancer" [19]. In her book *Honest Medicine*, Julia Schopick proposes LDN as an "effective, time-tested, inexpensive treatment for life-threatening diseases" to include "multiple sclerosis, epilepsy, liver disease, lupus, rheumatoid arthritis, and other disorders" [20].

# Scientific Evidence for Low-Dose Naltrexone

Is there credible science to support these claims? In a 2007 study published in the *American Journal of Gastroenterology*, Dr. Jill Smith did report significant improvements in the Crohn's Disease Activity Index during 12 weeks of treatment with LDN and for 4 weeks after discontinuation of the medication in patients with active Crohn's disease [21]. Other studies followed with mixed results. Subsequently, a 2018

Cochrane Database Systematic Review of this issue concluded that there is "insufficient evidence to allow any firm conclusions regarding the efficacy and safety of LDN for patients with active Crohn's disease" [22].

I have searched all credible sources and have found no published evidence that LDN is beneficial in patients with thyroid or other endocrine disorders, autoimmune or otherwise. As devoted and well-educated clinician scientists and experts in the field, we should always be seeking innovative approaches to evaluation and treatment of our patients who are suffering from endocrine diseases and pseudo-endocrine disorders since our primary goal is to relieve suffering and improve our patients' quality of life. Our evaluation and management recommendations must, in my opinion, be individualized and innovative but should also be evidence-based to ensure that the safety and welfare of our patients is foremost in our plans.

## What Is the Best Way to Manage this Patient's Symptoms and Concerns and to Practice Good Medicine?

It is critically important to educate patients regarding medical information they find on the Internet. This has been well covered in other chapters, so I will briefly say only that patients should be informed that both good information and unreliable and unsubstantiated information can be found on the Internet. One must be careful to determine the source of the information given in order to evaluate its credibility. In this case, some Internet sites make claims of significant beneficial effects of LDN but without solid scientific evidence to substantiate these claims. A review of the existing scientific literature does show some initial reports of benefit in patients with Crohn's disease, but a large Cochrane systemic review of all existing studies did not find evidence for benefit. LDN has not been studied in patients with Hashimoto's thyroiditis.

This information is worth discussing with the patient. Doing so indicates that you acknowledge that he/she is seeking relief of symptoms that are adversely affecting his/her quality of life and respects his/her initiative for investigating measures that might be taken to improve quality of life. At the same time, it emphasizes that you, as the physician, practice evidence-based medicine and do not believe that the use of unproven therapies is good medical practice.

However, because this patient has sought out your opinion and entrusted his healthcare to you, it is incumbent upon the provider to show him respect and compassion. Listening carefully, examining him, offering to order additional testing, if appropriate, and discussing alternative explanations for his symptoms and management options that emphasize healthy lifestyle measures and treatment with evidence-based therapies, if they are available, are always appropriate and can go a long way toward symptom resolution and good quality of life.

# References

1. Chaker L, Bianco AC, Jonklass J, Peeters RP. Hypothyroidism. Lancet. 2017;390(10101):1550–62.
2. Hu S, Rayman MP. Multiple nutritional factors and the risk of Hashimoto's thyroiditis. Thyroid. 2017;27(5):597–610.
3. Wichman J, Winther KH, Bonnema SJ, Hegedus L. Selenium supplementation significantly reduces thyroid autoantibody levels in patients with chronic autoimmune thyroiditis: a systematic review and meta-analysis. Thyroid. 2016;26(12):1681–92.
4. Garber J, et al. Clinical practice guidelines for hypothyroidism in adults: cosponsored by the American Association of Clinical Endocrinologists and the American Thyroid Association. Endocr Pract. 2012;18(6):988–1028. And Thyroid 2012 Dec;22(12):1200–35.
5. Jonklaas J, Bianco AC, Bauer AJ, Burman KD, Cappola AR, Celi FS, Cooper DS, American Thyroid Association Task Force on Thyroid Hormone Replacement, et al. Guidelines for the treatment of hypothyroidism: prepared by the American Thyroid

Association Task Force on thyroid hormone replacement. Thyroid. 2014;24(12):1670–751.
6. Thvilum M, Brandt F, Almind D, Christensen K, Brix TH, Hegedüs L. Increased psychiatric morbidity before and after the diagnosis of hypothyroidism: a nationwide register study. Thyroid. 2014;24(5):802–8.
7. Quinque EM, Villinger A, Kratzsch J, Karger S. Patient-reported outcomes in adequately treated hypothyroidism – insights from the German versions of ThyQoL, ThySRQ and ThyTSQ. Health Qual Life Outcomes. 2013;11:68.
8. Samuels MH, Kolobova I, Smeraglio A, Peters D, Janowsky JS, Schuff KG. The effects of levothyroxine replacement or suppressive therapy on health status, mood, and cognition. J Clin Endocrinol Metab. 2014;99(3):843–51.
9. Samuels MH, Kolobova I, Smeraglio A, Niederhausen M, Janowsky JS, Schuff KG. Effect of thyroid function variations within the laboratory reference range on health status, mood, and cognition in levothyroxine-treated subjects. Thyroid. 2016;26(9):1173–84.
10. Santoro N, Braunstein GD, Butts CL, Martin KA, McDermott M, Pinkerton JV. Compounded bioidentical hormones in endocrinology practice: an Endocrine Society scientific statement. J Clin Endocrinol Metab. 2016;101(4):1318–43.
11. Biondi B, Wartofsky L. Treatment with thyroid hormone. Endocr Rev. 2014;35(3):433–512.
12. Winther KH, Cramon P, Watt T, Bjorner JB, Ekholm O, Feldt-Rasmussen U, Groenvold M, et al. Disease-specific as well as generic quality of life is widely impacted in autoimmune hypothyroidism and improves during the first six months of levothyroxine therapy. PLoS One. 2016;11(6):e0156925.
13. Peterson SJ, Cappola AR, Castro MR, et al. Degrees of satisfaction and coexistent diseases in those responding to a survey exploring perceptions about treatment of hypothyroidism. Thyroid. 2018;28(6):707–21.
14. McAninch EA, Bianco AC. The history and future treatment of hypothyroidism. Ann Intern Med. 2016;164(1):50–6.
15. Guglielmi R, Frasoldati A, Zini M, Grimaldi F, Gharib H, Garber JR, Papini E. Italian Association of Clinical Endocrinologists Statement-Replacement Therapy for Primary Hypothyroidism: a brief guide for clinical practice. Endocr Pract. 2016;22(11):1319–26.

16. Ott J, Promberger R, Kober F, Neuhold N, Tea M, Huber JC, Hermann M. Hashimoto' s thyroiditis affects symptom load and quality of life unrelated to hypothyroidism: a prospective case-control study in women undergoing thyroidectomy for benign goiter. Thyroid. 2011;21(2):161–7.
17. Boelaert K, Newby PR, Simmonds MJ, Holder RL, Carr-Smith JD, Heward JM, Manji N, et al. Prevalence and relative risk of other autoimmune diseases in subjects with autoimmune thyroid disease. Am J Med. 2010;123(2):183.e1–9.
18. Roy A, Laszkowska M, Sundstrom J, Lebwohl B, Green PH, Kämpe O, Ludvigsson JF. Prevalence of celiac disease in patients with autoimmune thyroid disease: a meta-analysis. Thyroid. 2016;26(7):880–90.
19. http://www.lowdosenaltrexone.org.
20. Schopick, Julia E and Berkson Burton M. Honest Medicine. 2011.
21. Smith J. Low dose naltrexone therapy improves active Crohn's disease. Am J Gastroenterol. 2007;102:820–8.
22. Parker CE. Low dose naltrexone for induction of remission in Crohn's disease. Cochrane Database Syst Rev. 2018;4:CD010410. https://doi.org/10.1002/14651858.CD010410.pub3.

# Chapter 25
# Hashimoto Encephalopathy

**Michael T. McDermott**

## Case

A 60-year-old man was admitted to the intensive care unit for a grand mal seizure, confusion, somnolence, tremors, and myoclonus.

- PMH: Hypothyroidism, type 1 diabetes, hypertension, hyperlipidemia.
- Meds: Levothyroxine 88 mcg/day, insulin, ACE inhibitor, statin.
- PE: Ht 5′11″ Wt 193 lb. BP 124/70 P 88 T 99.0.
  - Thyroid: Mildly enlarged, firm.
  - Mental status: Significantly altered.
  - Neurological: Tremors, myoclonus, weakness.
- Lab: TSH 4.4 mU/L, Free T4 0.9 ng/dl, Na 136, K 4.6.
  - TPO antibodies: 1322 (nl < 60), Cortisol 18 ug/dl.
  - LP: High CSF protein MRI: Diffuse white matter changes.

M. T. McDermott (✉)
University of Colorado Hospital, Aurora, CO, USA
e-mail: michael.mcdermott@cuanschutz.edu

© Springer Nature Switzerland AG 2019
M. T. McDermott (ed.), *Management of Patients with Pseudo-Endocrine Disorders*,
https://doi.org/10.1007/978-3-030-22720-3_25

A consult was sent to the Endocrinology Inpatient Consult Service to evaluate and treat this patient for Hashimoto encephalopathy.

**Diagnosis** Steroid-responsive encephalopathy associated with autoimmune thyroid disease (not Hashimoto encephalopathy).

**Recommendation** High-dose glucocorticoid therapy. No change in thyroid hormone dose.

## Discussion

The term "Hashimoto encephalopathy" was first coined in 1966 when a 58-year-old man with treated hypothyroidism due to Hashimoto's thyroiditis presented with a grand mal seizure, impaired mental status, weakness, somnolence, and an unsteady gait [1]. A lumbar puncture showed high protein levels in the cerebrospinal fluid (CSF). Hashimoto's disease was postulated to be the etiology, but the authors wisely cautioned that, "Antibody studies in future cases of unexplained encephalopathy should show whether we have described a syndrome or co-incidence." "Steroid-responsive encephalopathy associated with autoimmune thyroid disease" later emerged as the favored nomenclature for the reasons discussed below.

Steroid-responsive encephalopathy associated with autoimmune thyroid disease (SREAAT) is now characterized as an acute encephalopathy of unknown cause that typically presents with symptoms of impaired mental status, tremors, myoclonus, somnolence, multiple stroke-like episodes, stupor, and seizures [2, 3]. It has further been sub-divided into a vasculitis subtype, characterized by multiple stroke-like episodes, and a diffuse progressive subtype, featuring prominent psychiatric symptoms and dementia. Following the initial case report in 1966 (described above), many affected patients were found to have positive antithyroid antibodies in the serum and the CSF; it was initially believed that these antibodies caused the encephalopathy, possibly by promoting an antibody-mediated cerebritis, and the condition was therefore termed "Hashimoto encephalopathy." However, it was not clear then and remains in doubt now that the antithyroid antibodies play a pathogenic role in this condition. Nor does the disorder appear to be related to thyroid function since reported cases have been hypothyroid, euthyroid, or even hyperthyroid and treatment of hypothyroid patients with thyroid hormone replacement has produced no beneficial effects on the encephalopathy [2, 3].

Importantly, a substantial number of patients experience significant improvement following a course of intravenous or oral glucocorticoid therapy. Treatment typically consists of methylprednisolone 1000 mg intravenously for 5 days or prednisone 60–120 mg orally for 1 week or more. Most patients respond within 1 week and nearly all respond by 4 weeks. Steroid-intolerant or steroid-resistant patients are typically treated with cyclophosphamide, IVIG, or plasma exchange [2, 3].

Because the encephalopathy does not appear to be related to thyroid antibodies or to thyroid dysfunction but does respond well to glucocorticoid therapy and not to any type of thyroid therapy, the term "Hashimoto encephalopathy" fell out of favor, and the condition has become more accurately referred to as steroid-responsive encephalopathy associated with autoimmune thyroid disease (SREAAT) [2, 3].

# References

1. Brain L, Jellinek EH, Ball K. Hashimoto's disease and encephalopathy. Lancet. 1966;2(7462):512–4.
2. Menon V, Subramanian K, Thamizh JS. Psychiatric presentations heralding Hashimoto's encephalopathy: a systematic review and analysis of cases reported in literature. J Neurosci Rural Pract. 2017;8(2):261–7.
3. Zhou JY, Xu B, Lopes J, Blamoun J, Li L. Hashimoto encephalopathy: literature review. Acta Neurol Scand. 2017;135(3):285–90.

# Chapter 26
# Non-thyroidal Illness Syndrome (Euthyroid Sick Syndrome)

Michael T. McDermott

## Case 1

A 52-year-old man was admitted to the hospital 3 weeks ago for a bowel obstruction that required surgery complicated by a bowel perforation and prolonged septic shock. He then developed a pulmonary embolism complicated by a respiratory arrest that required intubation and mechanical ventilation. He subsequently developed a ventilator-associated pneumonia. His diabetes has been difficult to control throughout his hospital stay. He has intermittently required treatment with pressors and steroids. Thyroid tests were ordered during this time and were abnormal, prompting an Endocrinology consult.

- PH: Type 2 diabetes mellitus, hypertension, COPD (smoker).
- PE: BP 110/72 P 92 Ht 5′8″ Wt 225 lb.
  - General exam: Normal   Thyroid: Normal.

M. T. McDermott (✉)
University of Colorado Hospital, Aurora, CO, USA
e-mail: michael.mcdermott@cuanschutz.edu

- Lab: TSH 0.28 mU/L (nl, 0.45–4.5).
  - Free T4: 0.6 ng/dl (nl, 0.8–1.8).
  - Total T3: 23 ng/dl (nl, 80–180).

A consult was sent to the Endocrinology Inpatient Consult Service for urgent evaluation and treatment of the patient for possible central hypothyroidism and to determine if he should be treated with T3 or T4.

**Diagnosis** Non-thyroidal illness syndrome (euthyroid sick syndrome). No evidence of primary or secondary thyroid dysfunction.

**Recommendation** Thyroid replacement is not indicated and could be harmful. Repeat thyroid tests 2–3 months after complete recovery from his hospitalization.

# Case 2

A 66-year-old man was discharged from the hospital 3 days ago after a 10-day hospitalization for community-acquired pneumonia and severe sepsis. He was referred for urgent evaluation of probable hypothyroidism.

- PH: Type 2 diabetes mellitus, hypertension, hyperlipidemia, coronary artery disease.
- PE: BP 142/92 P 80 Ht 5'10" Wt 210 lb.
  - General Exam: Normal   Thyroid: Normal.
- Lab: TSH 12.1 mU/L (nl, 0.45–4.5).
  - Free T4: 0.9 ng/dl (nl, 0.8–1.8).
  - Total T3: 64 ng/dl (nl, 80–180).
  - TPO antibodies: Negative.

A consult was sent to Endocrinology for urgent evaluation and to start treatment for primary hypothyroidism.

**Diagnosis** Recovery from non-thyroidal illness syndrome (euthyroid sick syndrome).

**Recommendation** Thyroid replacement is not indicated at this time. Repeat thyroid tests 2–3 months after complete recovery from his pneumonia.

## Discussion

Non-thyroidal illness syndrome (NTIS) is also commonly called the euthyroid sick syndrome (ESS). It refers to changes in serum levels of triiodothyronine (T3), thyroxine (T4), reverse T3 (RT3), and thyroid stimulating hormone (TSH) and in tissue thyroid hormone levels that occur in patients with various non-thyroidal illnesses and starvation. It is not a primary thyroid disorder but instead results from changes in thyroid hormone secretion, transport, metabolism and action induced by the non-thyroidal illness and may, in fact, be a protective response.

Serious non-thyroidal illnesses cause changes in thyroid hormone levels that can easily be confused with true thyroid disorders, especially central hypothyroidism during the illness and primary hypothyroidism during recovery from the illness. Consequently, thyroid tests should be ordered in seriously ill patients only when there is a reasonably high suspicion for the presence of hyperthyroidism or hypothyroidism. Furthermore, it is generally best to avoid thyroid testing in the first few weeks after recovery from a significant non-thyroidal illness. Considerable experience is often necessary to interpret thyroid tests in these settings.

During a significant non-thyroidal illness, if thyroid testing is deemed necessary, a serum TSH level alone is not adequate to distinguish NTIS from true thyroid disorders. Serum TSH, free T4, and total T3 should be ordered in this situation. RT3 measurement, although rarely indicated in any other situation, can sometimes be helpful in distinguishing NTIS from central hypothyroidism.

Even in mild-to-moderate non-thyroidal illnesses in the inpatient or ambulatory settings, serum total T3 can drop to low normal or frankly low levels because of decreased T4 to T3 conversion, due to reduced hepatic deiodinase type 1 (D1) activity. The magnitude of the serum T3 reduction correlates well with the severity of the non-thyroidal illness. Serum free T4 and TSH levels usually remain within the reference range in the mildest form of this condition. In more severe non-thyroidal illnesses, serum total T3 drops to very low levels, generally in proportion to the underlying illness severity. Serum TSH levels also decrease below the reference range at this stage because of cytokine-mediated suppression of TRH and TSH secretion. TSH secretion can also be inhibited by numerous medications, most notably glucocorticoids and dopamine. Reduced TSH secretion further decreases serum T3 levels and most often also decreases serum free T4 levels. However, free T4 values can be highly variable (normal, decreased, or increased) depending on the underlying illness, concomitant medications, and the assay technique. The most common pattern, therefore, is low TSH, low free T4, and very low total T3 (Fig. 26.1), which can often be difficult to distinguish from central hypothyroidism. However, serum RT3 tends to be high in NTIS and low in central hypothyroidism.

When patients begin to recover from severe non-thyroidal illnesses, serum TSH levels increase and may become transiently elevated above the reference range. Serum total T3 levels begin to increase but may remain low, while free T4 levels often decrease due to recovery of hepatic production of thyroid hormone-binding proteins. Thyroid hormone tests during recovery from non-thyroidal illnesses can therefore show an elevated serum TSH level (transiently) along with low levels of free T4 and total T3 (Fig. 26.1), making this condition difficult to distinguish from mild primary hypothyroidism. Considering the transient nature of thyroid hormone changes during recovery from NTIS/ESS and the lack of urgency for immediate treatment of mild primary hypothyroidism, it is best to simply repeat thyroid testing 2–3 months after full recovery from the non-thyroidal illness.

NTIS (ESS) is believed to be caused by increased circulating cytokines and other inflammation mediators resulting from the underlying non-thyroidal illness. These mediators inhibit the thyroid axis at multiple levels, including the hypothalamus (decreased TRH secretion), pituitary gland

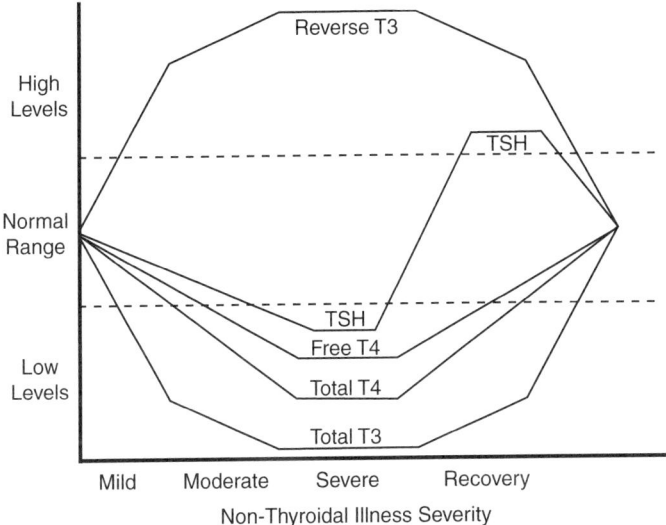

FIGURE 26.1 Changes in thyroid hormone levels in patients with non-thyroidal illnesses of varying severity and during recovery

(decreased TSH secretion), thyroid gland (decreased $T_4$ and $T_3$ responses to TSH), transport proteins (decreased thyroid hormone binding), and peripheral tissues (decreased T4 to T3 conversion by tissue deiodinases).

Deiodinases are selenocysteine enzymes that activate and deactivate thyroid hormones by removing iodine molecules. Deiodinase enzymes have three major subtypes: deiodinase 1 (D1), deiodinase 2 (D2), and deiodinase 3 (D3) (Table 26.1 and Fig. 26.2). D1 converts T4 to T3 in the liver and kidneys, producing the majority of circulating T3, and converts RT3 to diiodothyronine (T2); D1 has a higher affinity for RT3 than for T4. D2 converts T4 to T3 in the brain and pituitary gland, increasing intracellular T3 in these tissues; D2 has a higher affinity for T4 than for RT3. D3 converts T4 to RT3 and T3 to T2. D1 activity is significantly reduced and D3 activity is enhanced in NTIS. These changes are responsible for the low serum T3 and high serum RT3 levels that are characteristic of this condition.

TABLE 26.1 Deiodinase enzymes: Selenocysteine enzymes that deiodinate thyroid hormones

|  | Deiodinase 1 (D1) | Deiodinase 2 (D2) | Deiodinase 3 (D3) |
|---|---|---|---|
| Substrate | RT3 >> T4 | T4 >> RT3 | T4 + T3 |
| Tissue | Liver | Brain | Placenta |
|  | Kidney | Pituitary | Brain |
|  |  | Fat |  |
| Function | Clear RT3 | ↑ cellular T3 | Protect fetus |
|  | ↑ serum T3 | ↑ serum T3 | ↓ cellular T3 |
|  |  |  | Clear T4 + T3 |

*RT3* reverse triiodothyronine, *T4* thyroxine, *T3* triiodothyronine

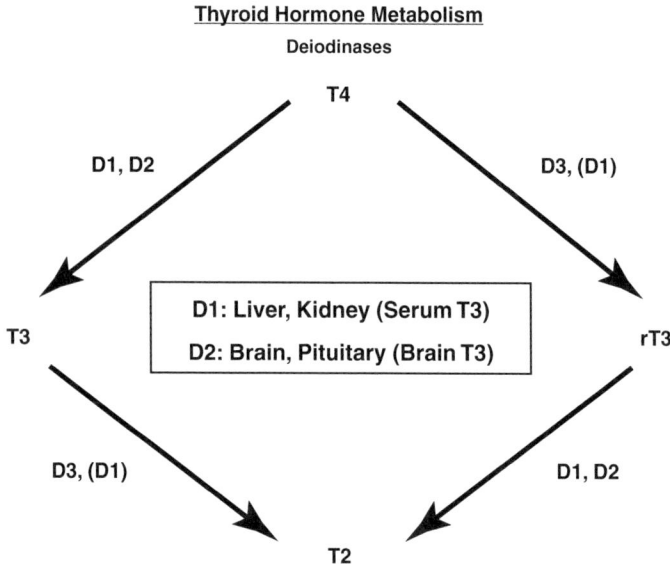

FIGURE 26.2 Thyroid hormone metabolism by deiodinases. T4 thyroxine, T3 triiodothyronine, rT3 reverse triiodothyronine, T2 diiodothyronine. D1 deiodinase 1, D2 deiodinase 2, D3 deiodinase 3

Most experts consider NTIS/ESS to be an adaptive mechanism developed to reduce peripheral tissue energy expenditure during the non-thyroidal illness. Conversely, some argue that the alterations in circulating thyroid hormone levels may be harmful and may accentuate the effects of the non-thyroidal illness. The majority favor the former view, but the issue is likely to remain controversial for years to come.

Management of NTIS is also controversial. Interventional studies have not reported consistent or convincing evidence of benefit from treating NTIS patients with either liothyronine (LT3) or levothyroxine (LT4), and there is some evidence that thyroid hormone treatment may actually be harmful. LT3 therapy was shown to improve ventricular performance and neuroendocrine profiles in chronic heart failure patients in one randomized controlled trial. Experts agree that large, prospective studies in a variety of settings are needed. Therefore, thyroid hormone therapy cannot, at present, be recommended for patients with NTIS (euthyroid sick syndrome), except possibly those with chronic heart failure.

## General References

1. Adler SM, Wartofsky L. The nonthyroidal illness syndrome. Endocrinol Metab Clin NA. 2007;36:657–72.
2. Boonen E, Van den Berghe G. Endocrine responses to critical illness: novel insights and therapeutic implications. J Clin Endocrinol Metab. 2014;99:1569–82.
3. Debaveye Y, Ellger B, Mebis L, Darras VM, Van den Berghe G. Regulation of tissue iodothyronine deiodinase activity in a model of prolonged critical illness. Thyroid. 2008;18:551–60.
4. den Brinker M, Joosten KFM, Visser T, et al. Euthyroid sick syndrome in meningococcal sepsis: the impact of peripheral thyroid hormone metabolism and binding proteins. J Clin Endocrinol Metab. 2005;90:5613–20.
5. Fliers E, Bianco AC, Langouche L, Boelen A. Thyroid function in critically ill patients. Lancet Diabetes Endocrinol. 2015;3:816–25.

6. Huang SA, Bianco AC. Reawakened interest in type III iodothyronine deiodinase in critical illness and injury. Nature Clin Pract Endocrinol Metab. 2008;4:148–54.
7. Iervasi G, Pingitore A, Landi P, et al. Low serum free triiodothyronine values predict mortality in patients with cardiac disease. Circulation. 2003;107:708–11.
8. Kaptein EM, Sanchez A, Beale E, Chan LS. Clinical review: thyroid hormone therapy for postoperative nonthyroidal illnesses: a systematic review and synthesis. J Clin Endocrinol Metab. 2010;95:4526–34.
9. Kimura T, Kanda T, Kotajima N, et al. Involvement of circulating interleukin-6 and its receptor in the development of euthyroid sick syndrome in patients with acute myocardial infarction. Eur J Endocrinol. 2000;143:179–84.
10. Langouche L, Vander Perre S, Marques M, et al. Impact of early nutrition restriction during critical illness on the nonthyroidal illness syndrome and its' relation with outcome: a randomized, controlled study. J Clin Endocrinol Metab. 2013;98:1006–13.
11. Liu J, Wu X, Lu F, et al. Low T3 syndrome is a strong predictor of poor outcomes in patients with community-acquired pneumonia. Sci Rep. 2016;6:22271.
12. Nagaya T, Fujieda M, Otsuka G, et al. A potential role of activated NF-kappa B in the pathogenesis of euthyroid sick syndrome. J Clin Invest. 2000;106:393–402.
13. Pasqualetti G, Calsolaro V, Bernardini S, et al. Degree of peripheral thyroxin deiodination, frailty, and long-term survival in hospitalized older patients. J Clin Endocrinol Metab. 2018;103:1867–76.
14. Peeters RP, Wouters PJ, Kaptein E, et al. Reduced activation and increased inactivation of thyroid hormone in tissues of critically ill patients. J Clin Endocrinol Metab. 2003;88:3202–11.
15. Peeters RP, Wouters PJ, van Toor H, et al. Serum 3, 3′, 5′-triiodothyronine and 3, 5, 3′- triiodothyronine/rT3 are prognostic markers in critically ill patients and are associated with tissue deiodinase activities. J Clin Endocrinol Metab. 2005;90:4559–65.
16. Peeters RP, Kester MHA, Wouters PJ, et al. Increased thyroxine sulfate levels in critically ill patients as a result of a decreased hepatic type I deiodinase activity. J Clin Endocrinol Metab. 2005;90:6460–5.
17. Peeters RP, van der Geyten S, Wouters PJ, et al. Tissue thyroid hormone levels in critical illness. J Clin Endocrinol Metab. 2005;90:6498–507.

18. Pingitore A, Landi P, Taddei MC, et al. Triiodothyronine levels for risk stratification of patients with chronic heart failure. Am J Med. 2005;118:132–6.
19. Pingitore A, Galli E, Barison A, et al. Acute effects of triiodothyronine (T3) replacement therapy in patients with chronic heart failure and Low-T3 syndrome: a randomized, placebo-controlled study. J Clin Endocrinol Metab. 2008;93:1351–8.
20. Plikat K, Langgartner J, Buettner R, et al. Increasing thyroid dysfunction is correlated with degree of illness and mortality in intensive care unit patients. Metabolism. 2007;56:239–44.
21. Rothberger GD, Gadhvi S, Michelakis N, et al. Usefulness of serum triiodothyronine (T3) to predict outcomes in patients hospitalized with acute heart failure. Am J Cardiol. 2017;119:599–603.
22. Schmidt RL, LoPresti JS, McDermott MT, Zick SM, Straseski JA. Is reverse triiodothyronine ordered appropriately? Data from reference lab shows wide practice variation in orders for reverse triiodothyronine. Thyroid. 2018;28(7):842–8.
23. Spratt DI, Frohnauer M, Cyr-Alves H, et al. Triiodothyronine replacement does not alter the hemodynamic, metabolic, and hormonal responses to coronary artery surgery. Am J Physiol Endocrinol Metab. 2007;293:E310–5.
24. Van den Berghe G. Non-thyroidal illnesses in the ICU: a syndrome with different faces. Thyroid. 2014;24:1456–65.
25. Vanhorebeek I, Langouche L, Van den Berghe G. Endocrine aspects of acute and prolonged critical illness. Nat Clin Pract Endocrinol Metab. 2006;2:20–31.
26. Zhang K, Meng X, Wang W, et al. Prognostic value of free triiodothyronine level in patients with hypertrophic obstructive cardiomyopathy. J Clin Endocrinol. 2018;103:1198–205.

# Index

**A**
Acetaminophen, 104
Acid-labile subunit (ALS)
    functions, 236
Addison's disease, 144
Adrenal abnormalities, 38
Adrenal fatigue, 24, 44–46
    ACTH stimulation test, 129, 130
    adrenal supplements, 135
    clinical history, 3
    clinical outcomes, 136
    cortisol, 130
    definition, 131
    diagnosis, 135
    Hormone Foundation website, 133
    HPA, 131
    internet, 135
    Mayo Clinic website, 133
    primary adrenal insufficiency, 128
    screening test, 129
    secondary adrenal insufficiency, 128
    stages, 130, 131
    symptoms, 129, 134
    treatment, 132
Adrenal Fatigue and Thyroid Care, 32

Adrenal insufficiency (AI), 32, 128
    ACTH stimulation test, 144, 147, 149–152
    acute illness and sepsis, 147–149
    albuterol-ipratropium nebulizers, 140
    chronic hyponatremia, 146
    COPD, 140
    critical illness, 147
    diagnostic criteria, 152–154
    dyspnea and abdominal pain., 139
    flexible sigmoidoscopy and colonoscopy, 140
    gabapentin, amitriptyline and quetiapine, 140
    hepatic encephalopathy, 140, 141
    hypotension, 140
    liver disease and hypoalbuminemia, 140
    neuropathy and mood disorder, 140
    physical exam, 140
    soft and non-tender abdomen, 141
Adrenocorticotropic hormone (ACTH), 129, 141, 143, 144, 149–152, 160

© Springer Nature Switzerland AG 2019
M. T. McDermott (ed.), *Management of Patients with Pseudo-Endocrine Disorders*,
https://doi.org/10.1007/978-3-030-22720-3

Alcohol-induced cortisol hypersecretion, 162, 163
Allopurinol, 228
American Association of Clinical Endocrinologists (AACE), 25, 312, 319
American College of Physicians (ACP), 25
American Medical Association (AMA), 25
American Thyroid Association (ATA), 24, 25, 40, 282, 305, 319
Amitriptyline, 228
Androgen replacement therapy, 42
Antidepressants, 79
Anti-thyroid peroxidase antibodies (anti-TPO), 318
Ascorbic acid, 103
Autoimmune diseases, 321
Autoimmune thyroid disease, 328
Autonomous cortisol secretion, 230, 231

# B
Biotin
  advantages, 61
  Beckman Coulter assays, 57
  biotinylated anti-T4 antibody, 56, 57
  clearance, 53
  competitive immunoassays, 56
  daily requirement, 51
  Graves' disease, 52
  hormone immunoassays, 57, 60
  immunometric assays, 55, 56
  laboratory test, 61
  multiple sclerosis, 53
  pathological hormonal condition, 57–59
  pharmacokinetic study, 53
  pseudo-thyroid abnormalities (*see* Pseudo-thyroid abnormalities)
  RocheElecsys assays, 57
  serum biotin concentration, 54
  *vs.* streptavidin, 54
Bio-T programs, 26, 27
Borderline hypertension, 216
Brexpiprazole, 228
Brief Fatigue Inventory (BFI), 262

# C
Chronic fatigue, 8
  acceptance, 124
  case presentation, 109–111
  causes of, 112, 113
  diagnosis, 117
  emotional health, 123, 124
  evaluation, 114, 117
  mental health, 122, 123
  movement, 121, 122
  nutrition, 120, 121
  SEEN, 118
  sleep, 119
  time and patience, 111
  treatment, 118
Chronic obstructive pulmonary disease (COPD), 140
Continuous positive airway pressure (CPAP), 184
Coolens' equation, 151
Corticotropin releasing hormone (CRH), 141, 162
Cortisol, 130
Cortisol binding globulin (CBG), 144
Critical illness related corticosteroid insufficiency (CIRCI), 147
Crohn's disease, 323

Cushing's syndrome, 79
Cyclic Cushing's disease, 189

# D
Debunking internet myths
  adrenal fatigue, 44–46
  improve patient-physician relationship, 38
  increased patient anxiety and overutilization, 38
  non-specific symptoms, 38
  self-diagnose conditions, 38
  testosterone
    androgen replacement therapy, 42
    assessing readability, credibility and quality of patient information, 42
    diagnosis and treatment, 43, 44
    low testosterone, 42, 44
    medications, 39
  thyroid
    biochemical marker, 41
    diagnosing and treating hypothyroidism, 40, 41
    fatigue, 39
    Hashimoto's hypothyroidism, 40
    hypothyroidism, 39
    "inflammatory" foods, 40
    naturopath, 39
    physiology, 40
Dehydroepiandrosterone sulfate (DHEA-S), 160
Desiccated thyroid extract (DTE), 304, 319
Desmopressin (DDAVP), 163
Dexamethasone-CRH (Dex-CRH) test, 169, 188
Dexamethasone suppression test (DST), 160, 161, 165, 228
Diabetes medications, 78
Dulaglutide, 228
Dyslipidemia, 185

# E
Eisenmenger syndrome, 100
Empagliflozin, 228
Endocrine disorders
  adrenal insufficiency, 32
  hypercortisolism, 32
  hyperthyroidism, 32
  hypothyroidism, 32
  social media sites, 32
  testosterone deficiency, 32
  top-listed search engine sites, 32
  trustworthy information, 32
Equilibrium dialysis, 151
European Thyroid Association (ETA), 312
Euthyroid sick syndrome (ESS), 333
  see also Non-thyroidal illness syndrome (NTIS)

# F
First- and second-generation antipsychotics, 78–79
Follicle stimulating hormone (FSH), 218
Free cortisol index (FCI), 151
Furosemide, 140

# G
General Health Questionnaire-12 (GHQ-12), 262
Glucocorticoids, 78
  resistance, 148
Gonadotropin releasing hormone (GnRH), 217
Google Trends, 33

Graves' disease
    pseudo-overt
        hyperthyroidism, 62, 63
    pseudo-subclinical
        hyperthyroidism, 63–66
Growth hormone deficiency
    (GHD), 4, 5, 79, 237
Guillain-Barre syndrome, 140

**H**

Harris–Benedict equation, 84
Hashimoto encephalopathy
    anti-thyroid antibodies, 328
    confusion, 327
    grand mal seizure, 327, 328
    impaired mental status, 328
    oral glucocorticoid therapy, 329
    somnolence, 327
    steroid-responsive
        encephalopathy, 328
    thyroid antibodies, 329
    thyroid dysfunction, 329
    tremors and myoclonus, 327
Hashimoto's hypothyroidism, 40
Hashimoto's thyroiditis, 306
    ATA and AACE guideline, 319
    ATA survey, 320
    autoimmune disorders, 318, 319
    chronic inflammatory
        condition, 318
    chronic lymphocytic
        thyroiditis, 321
    DTE, 319
    iodine excess, 318
    iron and vitamin D, 318
    LDN, 322, 323
    LT4 replacement therapy, 319
    manage patient's symptoms, 323, 324
    optimal range, 321
    selenium deficiency, 318
    simple replacement therapie, 321
    thyroid hormone
        replacement, 319
    thyroid regeneration, 322
    thyroid sonography, 319
    website blogs, 320
"Hepato-adrenal" syndrome, 150
High performance liquid
    chromatography
    (HPLC), 166
Holistic hypercalcemia
    epidemiology, 207
    laboratory evaluation, 204, 205
    multiple sclerosis, 204
    PTH-independent
        hypercalcemia, 204, 206
    vitamin D deficiency, 207–210
Hormone Foundation
    (Endocrine Society), 24, 133
Hospital anxiety and depression
    scale (HADS), 263
Hypercortisolism, 32
Hypertension, 231
Hyperthyroidism, 32
Hyperviscosity syndromes, 103
Hypoglycemia, *see* Idiopathic
    postprandial syndrome
Hypogonadism, 79, 217, 223
Hypothalamic-pituitary-adrenal
    (HPA) axis, 130, 161, 181
Hypothyroidism, 32, 38, 301, 302

**I**

Idiopathic postprandial
    syndrome
    alpha-glucosidase inhibitor, 96
    causes of, 93, 94
    clinical history, 91
    medications, 93

MMTT, 95
neurogenic symptoms, 92
neuroglycopenic symptoms, 92
pseudohypoglycemia, 95
reactive hypoglycemia, 94
Whipple's triad, 93
IGF-1-binding proteins (IGF-BP), 236
Inferior petrosal sinus sampling (IPSS), 160, 169, 170
Insulin-like growth factor-1 (IGF-1)
 ALS deficiency, 236
 autocrine functions, 236
 clinical causes, 239
 diagnosis of, 237, 238
 GHD, 237
 hypothyroidism, 240
 Laron syndrome, 240, 241
 long-term survival rates, 239
 low IGF-1 levels, 242, 243
 MAMC, 239
 molecular causes, 238
 nutritional disturbances, 241, 242
 pituitary gland stimulates, 235
 primary IGF-1 deficiency, 237
 secondary IGF-1 deficiency, 237
 storage pools, 236
 treatment guidelines for, 244
International Physical Activity Questionnaire (IPAQ-7), 262
Internet, endocrinology practice
 access medical information, 31
 adrenal fatigue, 33
 celebrity testimonials and popular news stories, 32
 Hormone Health Network, 32
 media coverage, 33
 health information, 31, 32
 online health information, 34
 pseudo-endocrine disorders, 32
 reputable online medical information resources, 34
 treatment options, 31
 WebMD patient reviews, 33–34

**K**
Klinefelter syndrome, 219

**L**
Laron syndrome, 240–242
Late night salivary cortisol (LNSC) test, 166, 167
Leucocytes, 103
Levothyroxine, 228
Lifestyle behaviors
 acceptance, 124
 emotional health, 123, 124
 mental health, 122, 123
 movement, 121, 122
 nutrition, 120, 121
 sleep, 119
Liothyronine (LT3), 337
Liquid chromatography tandem mass spectrometry (LC-MS/MS), 166
Low-dose dexamethasone test (LDDST), 188
Low dose naltrexone (LDN), 322
Low metabolism
 calorie restriction and diet composition, 84, 85
 energy balance/energy homeostasis, 81
 evaluation, 78, 79
 fat-free mass, 79
 FDA-approved anti-obesity medications, 85
 GABA receptor activation, 86

Low metabolism (cont.)
  genetics and epigenetics, 80
  GLP-1 receptor agonist, 86
  levothyroxine, 78
  low-carb and low-fat foods, 78
  management, 82, 83
  metabolism boosters, 86
  methylphenidate, 85
  mobile application, 77
  PAEE, 79
  REE, 79, 80
  serotonin, 86
  social-ecological model, 81, 82
  supplements/herbs, 78
  sympathomimetics, 85
  TDEE, 79
  24-hour energy expenditure, 79
Low testosterone, 42, 44
  axillary gels, 224
  borderline hypertension, 216
  diurnal and circadian variation, 220
  equilibrium dialysis, 221
  erectile dysfunction and decreased libido, 216
  hypogonadism, 223
  injections of pellets, 224
  intramuscular injections, 224
  LH and FSH, 218
  low serum testosterone levels, 225
  male hypogonadism, 217
  obesity, sleep apnea and depression, 223
  online calculators, 221
  persistent fatigue, 215
  primary hypogonadism, 217, 219
  secondary hypogonadism, 217, 219, 222
  secondary sex characteristics, 219
  serum FSH and LH, 222
  serum total testosterone level, 222
  SHBG levels, 220
  supraphysiologic testosterone, 225
  symptoms of hypogonadism, 220
  testosterone assays, 217
  testosterone pellet injections, 224
  testosterone replacement therapy, 217, 224
  trans-buccal patches, 224
  transdermal gels, 224
  transdermal patches, 224
Low T3 syndrome, *see* Wilson's syndrome
LT4 replacement therapy, 319
Lubiprostone, 228
Luteinizing hormone (LH), 218

# M
Male hypogonadism, 216
Mayo Clinic, 24
Medical intensive care unit (MICU), 141
Messenger RNA (mRNA), 131
Metabolism boosters, 86
Metformin, 228
Midarm muscle circumference (MAMC), 239
Midnight salivary cortisol (MSC), 230
Midnight serum cortisol test, 168, 169
Mifepristone, 228–230, 232, 233
Mindfulness-based stress reduction(MBSR), 123
Mixed meal tolerance test (MMTT), 95
Monocarboxylate transporter 8 (MCT8), 276
Mood stabilizers, 79
Multidimensional fatigue inventory (MFI), 261
Multiple sclerosis (MS), 204
Myasthenia gravis, 99

## N

Neuropsychiatric disorders, 187
Non-alcoholic steato-hepatitits (NASH), 243
Non-thyroidal hypothyroidism
 alternative physical etiologies, 266
 anti-thyroid antibodies, 258
 BFI, 262
 biochemical hypothyroidism, 252
 chronic disease, 263
 dry skin, 252
 FT4 and TT3, 261
 GHQ-12 and TSQ-12, 263
 hypothyroid symptoms, 264
 IPAQ-7, 262
 LT4 therapy, 255, 260, 261, 263, 264
 NHANES III population, 257
 OHypo *vs.* euthyroid controls, 252
 psychological morbidity, 255
 QOL assessments, 259
 SCHypo, 252, 256, 259
 TFTs, 253
 thyroid condition, 265
 thyroid function testing, 253, 254
 thyroid hormone intervention, 265
 tiredness and feeling depressed, 251
 TSH, 255–258
 TSQ score, 254
Non-thyroidal illness syndrome (NTIS)
 central hypothyroidism, 332, 333
 coronary artery disease, 332
 deiodinase enzymes, 335, 336
 ESS, 333
 hyperlipidemia, 332
 hypertension, 332
 intubation and mechanical ventilation, 331
 LT3 therapy, 337
 NTIS/ESS, 334, 337
 serum free T4 and TSH levels, 333, 334
 thyroid hormone levels, 335
 thyroid hormone metabolism, 336
 thyroid replacement, 333
 thyroid testing, 331, 333
 type 2 diabetes mellitus, 332

## O

Obesity, 6, 7
Obstructive sleep apnea (OSA), 79, 184
1 mg Dexamethasone suppression test (1 mg DST), 167, 168, 230
Oral contraceptive pill (OCP), 159
Oral glucose tolerance test (OGTT), 95
Oral levothyroxine (LT4), 304
Osteoarthritis, 79
Overt hypothyroidism (OHypo), 251

## P

Parathyroid hormone (PTH), 55
Parkinson's disease, 27
Persistent hypothyroid symptoms, 6
Physical activity-related energy expenditure (PAEE), 79
Plasma metanephrine, 228
Politico, 33
Polycystic ovarian syndrome, 79
Polyglandular autoimmune syndrome type 1 and 2, 144

Primary hypogonadism, 217, 219
Primary IGF-1 deficiency, 237
Progestins, 79
Pseudo-central hyperthyroidism/
 thyroid hormone
 resistance, 67, 68
Pseudo-Cushing's syndrome,
 68–70
 ACTH, 160
 adenohypophysis and
  neurohypophysis, 160
 alcohol-induced cortisol
  hypersecretion, 162,
  163
 alcohol intake, 185–187
 assessments, 190
 causes of physiologic
  hypercortisolism, 161,
  162
 challenging diagnosis, 181
 clinical features, 182, 183
 cyclic Cushing's disease, 189
 definition, 180
 Dex-CRH test, 169
 DHEA-S, 160
 endogenous hypercortisolism,
  161
 endorsed insomnia, 159
 estrogen-containing OCP, 161,
  170
 evidence of hypercortisolism,
  159
 hypercortisolism evaluation,
  179
 IPSS, 169, 170, 172
 LNSC test, 166, 167, 171, 172
 midnight serum cortisol test,
  168, 169
 neuropsychiatric illnesses, 163
 non-specific features, 183
 obese patients, 185
 obesity, 184
 OCP therapy, 159, 171
 1 mg DST, 167, 168
 pathological/neoplastic
  causes, 182
 physiologic *vs*. pathological
  causes, 189
 pregnancy, 164
 salivary cortisol values, 170
 screening tests, 187, 188
 starvation equivalent
  disorders, 165
 24-hour UFC, 170, 171
 type 2 diabetes mellitus, 164
 UFC, 160, 166
 vital signs, 161
Pseudo-endocrine disorder
 definition, 1, 2
 patients management, 15–17, 19
Pseudo-exogenous thyroid
 excess/ thyrotoxicosis,
 66, 67
Pseudohypoglycemia
 classification, 101
 diabetes, 102
 Eisenmenger syndrome, 100
 evaluation, 104, 105
 glucose monitoring analytic
  errors, 102
 insulin therapy, 100
 myasthenia gravis, 99
 PHG-1, 102
 PHG-2, 102
 Raynaud's phenomenon, 99
Pseudohypoglycemia type 1
 (PHG-1), 102
Pseudohypoglycemia type 2
 (PHG-2), 102
Pseudo-non-parathyroid
 hypercalcemia, 72
Pseudo-overt hyperthyroidism,
 62, 63
Pseudopheochromocytoma
 abdominal striae and
  hirsutism, 228
 anti-hypertensive
  medications, 199

autonomous cortisol
  secretion, 230, 231
comfort foods, 229
coronary artery disease, 227
depression/anxiety/PTSD, 227
dexamethasone suppression
  test, 228
diabetes, morbid obesity, 227
differential diagnosis, 197, 198
DST, 231
exogenous steroids, 229
gout, 227
hypercortisolism and
  comorbidities, 232
interfering substances, 196
irritable bowel syndrome, 227
mifepristone, 228, 230, 232, 233
multiple comorbidities, 229
multiple medications, 228
1 mg DST, 231
panic disorder, 198
patient history, 193, 194
potassium and renal function, 228
recurrent upper respiratory
  infections, 227
single best test, 233
stress eater, 229
trichotillomania, 227
type 2 diabetes mellitus, 232
untreated sleep apnea, 227
Pseudo-subclinical
  hyperthyroidism, 63–66
Pseudo-testosterone excess, 71
Pseudo-thyroid abnormalities
  Graves' disease
    pseudo-overt
      hyperthyroidism, 62, 63
    pseudo-subclinical
      hyperthyroidism, 63–66
  negative pregnancy testing, 70
  pseudo-central
    hyperthyroidism/
      thyroid hormone
        resistance, 67, 68
  Pseudo-Cushing's syndrome, 68–70
  pseudo-exogenous thyroid
    excess/ thyrotoxicosis, 66, 67
  pseudo-non-parathyroid
    hypercalcemia, 72
  pseudo-testosterone excess, 71

# R
Radioimmunoassay (RIA), 185
Raynaud's phenomenon, 100
Recommended daily allowance
  (RDA), 207
Relative adrenal insufficiency
  (RAI), 147
Resting energy expenditure
  (REE), 79, 80
Retinoid X receptor
  (RXR), 277
Reverse T3 syndrome
  cellular thyroid binding
    receptor, 294
  citing insulin resistance, 296
  clinical history, 3–5
  de-iodinase enzymes, 293
  diet, 297
  elevated rT3 causes
    hypothyroidism, 293
  gut imbalances, 296
  inflammation, food/chemical
    sensitivities, 296
  nonthyroidal illness, 294, 295
  rT3 production, 296, 297
  selenium, zinc and thyroid
    support formulations, 295
  thyroid hormone levels, 295
  thyroxine, 293
Rivaroxaban (Xarelto), 161

Rogue practitioners and practices
  adrenal fatigue, 24
  animal whole organ, 23
  endocrinologists letters, 26–28
  local state medical board, 25
  phony diagnosis, 25
  promote hormonal treatments, 23
  testosterone, 23, 24
  thyroid-related health sites, 26
  thyroid treatment programs, 24
  Wilson's syndrome, 24, 25
Rosuvastatin, 228

**S**
Secondary hypogonadism, 217, 219, 222
Secondary IGF-1 deficiency, 237
Selective serotonin reuptake inhibitors (SSRIs), 194
Serum free cortisol (SFC), 151
Sex hormone binding globulin (SHBG), 71, 220
Social media sites, 32
Social-ecological model, 81, 82
Spironolactone, 140
Starvation equivalent disorders, 165
Steroidogenic acute regulatory protein (StAR), 143
Steroid responsive encephalopathy associated with autoimmune thyroid disease (SREAAT), 328, 329
Streptavidin, 54
Subclinical hypothyroidism (SCHypo), 251, 252
Support, educate, empower, and nurture (SEEN), 118, 119
Synthetic liothyronine (LT3), 304

**T**
Testosterone deficiency, 32, 38, 39
Testosterone level, 5–7
Testosterone replacement therapy, 42, 217
Testosterone therapy, 24
Thiamine, 140
Thyroglobulin, 55
Thyroid function tests (TFTs), 253, 275
Thyroid hormone deficiency, 39, 41
Thyroid hormone replacement
  chronic lymphocytic thyroiditis, 306
  classification and etiology, 303–304
  clinical data, 309
  coexisting disease, 308
  congenital hypothyroidism, 303
  D2 polymorphism, 310
  D2 Thr92Ala polymorphism, 310
  deiodinase 2 polymorphisms, 308
  despite levothyroxine therapy, 301
  DTE, 306, 311, 312
  Hashimoto' thyroiditis, 306
  hypothalamic-pituitary disorders, 303
  hypothyroidism, 302, 307
  infiltrative disease, 303
  levothyroxine sodium, 305
  lifestyle measures suboptimal, 308
  LT3 monotherapy, 312
  LT4 replacement, 306
  LT4/LT3/DTE therapy, 305, 309–311
  management advice, 309
  oral levothyroxine, 304, 305
  patients' quality of life, 307
  peripheral hypothyroidism, 304

satisfactory outcomes, 307
synthetic liothyronine, 304
T4/T3 therapy, 311
Thr92Ala polymorphism, 310
thyroid function, 307
thyroxine, 304, 305
Thyroid hormone response elements (TRE), 277
Thyroid Hormone Therapy, 259
Thyroid Related Quality of Life Patient Reported Outcome (ThyPRO), 259
Thyroid sonography, 319
Thyroid stimulating hormone (TSH), 55, 255, 333
Thyroid Symptom Questionnaire-12 (TSQ-12), 262
Thyroxine (T4), 293, 304
Total daily energy expenditure (TDEE), 79
Type 2 diabetes mellitus, 164, 185

**U**

Urinary free cortisol (UFC), 159, 166
US National Health and Nutrition Examination Survey (NHANES), 282

**V**

Valproic acid, 228
Vanity Fair, 33
Vitamin D deficiency, 209, 210
Vitamin D supplementation, 123

**W**

Washington Postt, 33
Whipple's triad, 92, 93, 101
Wilson's Low T3 syndrome, 4, 5
Wilson's syndrome, 24, 25
dry skin, 274
evaluation and management, 284–286
fatigue and insomnia, 273
hair loss, 274
herbal supplements, 275
hypothyroidism, 274
intermittent nausea, 274
occasional dizziness, 274
physical examination/laboratory tests, 274
thyroid hormone intracellular regulation of, 275–276
mechanism of, 276–278
T3 in hypothyroidism, 278, 282–284

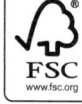

MIX
Papier aus verantwortungsvollen Quellen
Paper from responsible sources
FSC® C105338

If you have any concerns about our products,
you can contact us on
**ProductSafety@springernature.com**

In case Publisher is established outside the EU,
the EU authorized representative is:
**Springer Nature Customer Service Center GmbH
Europaplatz 3, 69115 Heidelberg, Germany**

Printed by Libri Plureos GmbH
in Hamburg, Germany